SBTU/ZAYB

Evaluating Stress

A Book of Resources, Volume 2

Edited by
Carlos P. Zalaquett
and
Richard J. Wood

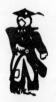

The Scarecrow Press, Inc.
Lanham, Md., & London
1998

SCARECROW PRESS, INC.

Published in the United States of America
by Scarecrow Press, Inc.
4720 Boston Way
Lanham, Maryland 20706

4 Pleydell Gardens
Kent CT20 2DN, England

British Library Cataloguing in Publication Information Available

Library of Congress Cataloging-in-Publication Data

Evaluating stress : a book of resources / Edited by Carlos P. Zalaquett
    and Richard Wood.
        p.   cm.
        Includes bibliographical references and index.
        1. Stress (Psychology)—Measurement.   I. Zalaquett, Carlos P.,
    1952–   .   II. Wood, Richard J. (Richard John)
    RC455.4.S87E83   1998   96-42961
    155.9′042′0287—dc20   CIP
    ISBN 0-8108-3231-3 (v. 1 : alk. paper)
    ISBN 0-8108-3522-3 (v. 2 : alk. paper)

∞ ™ The paper used in this publication meets the minimum
requirements of American National Standard for Information
Sciences—Permanence of Paper for Printed Library Materials,
ANSI Z39.48–1984. Manufactured in the United States of America.

Contents

iii

Introduction

It is a pleasure for us to present the second volume of *Evaluating Stress: A Book of Resources*. Compiling and editing this second resource book of stress evaluation instruments has helped us appreciate even more the dynamic and creative character of the field of stress evaluation. Working with the contributors of 38 stress evaluation instruments represented by the two volumes has given us the opportunity to fully appreciate the multiplicity and depth of knowledge that the research in this area is generating. We hope that our two volumes about stress evaluation instruments convey this breadth and depth of the field to everyone who consults the books.

The developers of stress instruments included in the two volumes masterfully illustrate that the area of stress evaluation has grown and diversified well beyond its early beginnings with W. E. Cannon and Hans Selye. There are good reasons for this. The population of the United States and other countries has become more, not less, diverse and complex as the economy has moved from an essentially agrarian to industrial base, then to an information and digital economy. Individuals today may choose from many hundreds of careers and, within each, usually many kinds or levels of positions. Clerical, paraprofessional, technical, professional, management, and executive positions represent different kinds of stress and stress interventions. The expansion of stress assessment instruments have followed behind, and in some cases mirrored, such societal changes. Researchers, practitioners, and others have responded by producing ad-hoc instruments to cover these new populations or situations, thereby enriching and widening the scope of stress evaluation efforts. The current challenge is to assess, in general, the impact of these rapid societal changes and to measure, in particular, the consequences of societal changes on individuals' stress levels.

The rapid development and assessment of these instruments created a need for a unified source of information about such tools. Literature searches revealed a myriad of citations about a vast array of instruments but no single source for finding detailed information about the history, characteristics, applicability, case illustration, and benefits or limitations of the instruments referenced in our book. This is usually the case in new fields of knowledge, particularly when research and development, as well as clinical practices, occur rapidly. In such cases, many studies and research reports are reported in proceedings of conferences, regional publications, and dissertations. Among the sources used for this search were the PsycLit and ERIC on-line systems and the following comprehensive handbooks: *Tests: A Comprehensive Reference for Assessments in Psychology, Education, and Business* (Sweetland & Keyser, 1991), *Test Critiques* (Keyser & Sweetland, 1994), *Tests in Print IV: An Index to Tests, Test Reviews, and the Literature on Specific Tests* (Murphy, Conoley, & Impara, 1994), and *The Eleventh Mental Measurements Yearbook* (Kramer & Conoley, 1992). Until stress tests have been proven valid and reliable, they are not included in *Mental Measurements Yearbook* volumes or other reference sources like it.

The need for a resource or reference book to assist practitioners and researchers alike led us to contact the developers of the instruments now included in the two volumes of *Evaluating Stress: A Book of Resources*. Our objective was to include newly revised editions of known instruments and new instruments originated within a known line of research or theory. We are grateful to all of the developers of these instruments and the authors of the chapters for their responsiveness and cooperation with us in meeting our objective.

In essence, this book is the natural continuation of our *Evaluating Stress: A Book of Resources* (Scarecrow Press,

1997). We say "natural" because this second volume adds new elements to help us in our efforts to measure stress. The two volumes put at your fingers a vast array of instruments for the assessment of stress, providing a convenient reference tool to facilitate a search for finding summaries of a diverse number of stress instruments. All of the chapters provide a list of references for background information or additional research.

Underlying our objective in compiling and editing the two volumes is the contention that the selection of one or more stress tests is an essential first step for counselors, psychologists, psychiatrists, and other professionals who are helping their clients cope with stress. The choice of the right instrument to evaluate stress objectively is basic to developing effective stress reduction strategies or interventions. Counselors, psychologists, medical doctors, psychiatrists, and others know that finding the right stress evaluation instrument often is key to determining the parameters of the interventions that they need to apply. The evaluation of stress, in any case, is a necessary element in assessing the efficacy of their interventions. In these respects, the instruments included in *Evaluating Stress: A Book of Resources* shows that considerable progress has been made in understanding the evaluation of stress in humans. The instruments included in our two volumes show that stress is correlated with hardiness, wellness, happiness, and successfully coping with challenging life events.

The chapters in volume 1 include general as well as specific measures of stress, measures of daily or weekly stress, and measures that produce stress profiles, "thermometers," or maps. Still others assess the stress effects of a variety of activities such as parenting, teaching, nursing, and computer use. Likewise, a variety of instruments measure coping responses, anxiety, the stress of being ill or having low self-esteem, and burnout. Volume 1 collects key information about the stress evaluation instruments of nationally and internationally regarded people like Aaron T. Beck, Cary Cooper, Christina Maslach, Elaine Wethington, Esther Orioli, Glen Greenberg, James Battle, Leonard Derogatis, Phillip Brantley, Richard

Abidin, Richard Hudiburg, Robert Steer, Rudolf Moos, Salvatore Maddi, and Stephen Williams. Specifically, the stress evaluation instruments (alphabetically listed by the instrument title, along with chapter authors) in volume 1 are as follows:

- Anxiety Scales for Children and Adults by James Battle
- Beck Anxiety Inventory by Robert A. Steer and Aaron T. Beck
- Computer Hassles Scale: A Measure of Computer Stress by Richard A. Hudiburg
- Coping Responses Inventory: A Measure of Approach and Avoidance Coping Skills by Rudolf H. Moss
- Culture-Free Self-Esteem Inventories for Children and Adults by James Battle
- Daily Stress Inventory by Phillip J. Brantley, Sheryl L. Catz, and Edwin Boudreaux
- The Derogatis Stress Profile (DSP)® by Leonard R. Derogatis and Megan P. Fleming
- Illness Effects Questionnaire by Glen D. Greenberg and Rolf A. Peterson
- The Index of Teaching Stress: Student-Teacher Transactions by Richard R. Abidin and Ross W. Greene
- Life Stressors and Social Resources Inventory: A Measure of Adults' and Youths' Life Contexts by Rudolf H. Moos and Bernice S. Moos
- Maslach Burnout Inventory (3rd ed.) by Christina Maslach, Susan E. Jackson, and Michael P. Leiter
- North American Depression Inventories for Children and Adults by James Battle
- Nurse Stress Index by Stephen Williams and Cary L. Cooper
- Occupational Stress Indicator by Stephen Williams and Cary L. Cooper
- Parenting Stress Index: A Measure of the Parent-Child System by Richard R. Abidin.
- Personal Views Survey II: A Measure of Dispositional Hardiness by Salvatore R. Maddi

- StressMap® by Esther M. Orioli and Karen F. Trocki
- Stress Resiliency Profile: A Measure of Interpretive Styles That Contribute to Stress by Kenneth W. Thomas and Walter G. Tymon, Jr.
- Stress Schedule by Loren Sauer, Edmond C. Hallberg, and Rochelle Noday-Aschieris
- Structured Life Events Inventory by Elaine Wethington
- Weekly Stress Inventory by Phillip J. Brantley, Glenn N. Jones, Edwin Boudreaux, and Sheryl Catz.

Volume 1 is successful in bringing together information about the stress evaluation instruments listed here. The literature about the instruments in volume 2 includes instruments that are more recently developed or more specialized as to their targeted population. Together, these two volumes capture and illustrate the diversity and richness of instruments that attempt to measure the stress of individuals in society today.

As with volume 1, each contributor was asked to provide essential information about their instruments such as the following:

The name of the instrument and developer
Contact information
A brief history of the instrument
Its underlying assumptions, premises, and objectives
A summary of the research
Conditions for its use
Benefits and limitations in the use of this instrument
Major references for research
Key references for finding the measure, psychometrics, and instructions for use.

In addition, the contributors were asked to provide a case example to illustrate the type of information provided by their instrument.

Evaluating Stress: A Book of Resources, Volume Two, brings together 17 different instruments for the evaluation of stress or stress-related factors. Each instrument (see Contents page) is presented by its original author(s), which includes the developer of the instrument in most cases. As with the first volume, a book outline is provided to help the reader easily find the location of each instrument, with the page numbers of its description, research, benefits, administration, scoring, application, case examples, and references in the main text. Used with the book outline of volume one, the chart shows the great number of instruments available and makes the task of finding the appropriate instrument(s) for differing goals far easier than looking through the index or contents pages of the two volumes. The outline shows how the books complement each other and why the reader will want to acquire both volumes.

With respect to this second volume, the outline shows that the instruments do reflect the cultural diversity and societal changes discussed previously. For example, the Sandhu/Asrabadi instrument, titled An Acculturative Stress Scale for International Students, and the Watts-Jones instrument, titled African-American Women's Stress Scale, measure stress in two particular populations: international students and African-American women, respectively. These instruments happen to be the first two chapters or instruments of volume two. They also point to the need of all individuals to develop personal resources to handle stressors.

Self-reliance or personal security, for example, is one resource that can help individuals meet daily demands and stressors successfully. The Self-Reliance Inventory: An Approach to Interdependence and Secure Social Attachments was developed by Whittington, Joplin, Nelson, Quick, and Quick as a self-report assessment of an individual's interpersonal attachment orientation. The instrument contains items that relate to the concepts of interdependence, counterdependence, and overdependence.

The Inventory of Positive Psychological Attitudes: Measuring Attitudes That Buffer and Facilitate Primary Prevention Using Constructs Responsive to Diverse Cultural World Views by Jared Kass certainly speaks to some aspects of cultural diversity, as well as positive affectivity and its relationship to health. Kass also emphasizes the need for connectedness to family and community and the clinical use of assessment instruments.

In a rapidly changing world, people are vulnerable to many stressors but need to be resilient to them. The Personal Style Inventory: A Measure of Stress Resiliency by Charles Sheridan and Sally Radmacher addresses and identifies stress resistance resources and dimensions. For example, the authors identify significant dimensions described by other researchers in constructing the Personal Style Inventory. When people cannot cope with stress effectively, however, their personal well-being is impaired; Leonard Derogatis's instrument, the Derogatis Affects Balance Scale: A Measure of Affective Balance and Disregulation, addresses such emotional consequences of stress. Similarly, Zimet's The Multidemensional Scale of Perceived Social Support addresses the adequacy of emotional social support on individuals in any population.

The Global Inventory of Stress, while the first inventory of the Comprehensive Scale of Stress Assessment, is a standalone instrument to measure an individual's status on the major dimensions of stress. Sheridan and Radmacher say that this generic property of the Global Inventory of Stress circumvents the common problem of other instruments—ommision of unique or unusual stressors. It also includes an appraisal of the effectiveness of the subjects' stress-coping resources. The importance of coping to the health of individuals is also recognized by Kenneth Matheny and William Curlette. Their Coping Resources Inventory for Stress: A Comprehensive Measure of Resources for Stress-Coping effectively measures this variable. The development of the Ways of Religious Coping Scale grew out of the realization that stress research investigating religion and degree of religiosity was lacking and needed to remediate a few problems of previous measures of religious coping. It assesses the degree to which subjects engage in religious behaviors as a coping strategy.

Students and adolescents represent other populations covered by the developers of several instruments: (1) The Daily Life Stressors Scale by Christopher Kearney and Bonnie Horne, (2) the School Refusal Assessment Scale by Christopher Kearney and Cheryl Tillotson, (3) the Stress Response Scale: A Measure of Children's Behavioral Adjustment by Louis Chandler, (4) the Stress Response Scale for Adolescents by Gerald R. Adams, and (5) the Student-Life Stress Inventory by Bernadette Gadzella. The Daily Life Stressors Scale by Christopher Kearney and Bonnie Horne identifies the severity of general daily stressors in youngsters aged 6 to 17 years, as the stress related to both objective external events and subjective internal discomfort. A strength of their instrument is that children answer this 30-item measure. Chandler's Stress Response Scale, on the other hand, relies on a parent's or teacher's responses. Developed for use in clinics, schools, and community agencies, it assesses a child's emotional adjustment using a 40-item behavior rating scale. The School Refusal Assessment Scale considers the linkage between children who refuse to go to school and common internalizing problems such as general anxiety, fear, depression, suicide, withdrawal, and fatigue. Adams's Stress Response Scale for Adolescents is a brief measure designed to be a self-perceived stress response measure for children as young as 10 years of age and up to 20 years. As a simple screening device of the subject's current stress response, it can also detect changes in the respondent's state of stress. Gadzella's instrument is also a self-reporting questionnaire that asks subjects whether they perceive their stress to be mild, moderate, or severe. The Student-Life Stress Inventory was designed by Gadzella to get college-age students actively engaged in evaluating their stressors and reactions to them.

The life of a child begins, of course, as an infant, and one instrument in this volume addresses the stressful, sometimes traumatic experience of childbirth for the infant's parents when the newborn requires hospitalization: Michael Hynan's The Perinatal Posttraumatic Stress Disorder (PTSD) Questionniare (PPQ). Parents of newborn infants requiring hospitalization in a neonatal intensive care unit, Hynan says, have provided him with the qualitative descriptions of the stressors parents face in their experiences. Chandler's Stress Response Scale, on the other hand, does rely on a parent's or teacher's responses to a 40-item behavior rating scale. Developed for use in clinics, schools, and community agencies, it assesses children's emotional adjustment.

Many hundreds more career choices are available today compared with just three or four decades ago; the Hilson Career Satisfaction/Stress Index included in this volume will likely be the first of many to come in the 21st century. Readers may want to consult the The Nurse Stress Index by Stephen Williams and Cary L. Cooper, as well as the The Occupational Stress Indicator by Stephen Williams and Cary L. Cooper; they are related chapters in volume one of our book.

In summary, this second volume, like the first, is intended for practitioners at all levels of practice and education in the social sciences. The two volumes present a broader number of instruments used in the field and capture the breadth, depth, and complexity of stress instruments. The instruments evaluating stress and the case examples provided in most of the chapters show the diverse possibilities for evaluating stress in individuals, groups, and organizations. In addition, the chapter authors present cases or guidelines of how these stress instruments might be used best. The two volumes should be an invaluable resource for neophytes, advanced practitioners, and researchers in the field. Persons devoted to stress management programs should find studying and applying the instruments described here enriching and gratifying. All those interested in evaluating stress should find that the two volumes are indeed valuable resources.

References

Keyser, D. J., & Sweetland, R. C. (Eds.). (1994). *Test critiques*. Austin, TX: Pro-Ed.

Kramer, J. J., and Conoley, J. C. (Eds.). (1992). *The eleventh mental measurements yearbook*. Lincoln: Buros Institute of Mental Measurements, University of Nebraska.

Murphy, L. L., Conoley, J. C., & Impara, J. C. (Eds.). (1994). *Tests in print IV: An index to tests, test reviews, and the literature on specific tests*. Lincoln: Buros Institute of Mental Measurements, University of Nebraska.

Sweetland, R. C., & Keyser, D. J. (Eds.). (1991). *Tests: A comprehensive reference for assessments in psychology, education, and business*. Austin, TX: Pro-Ed.

Outline of Book

Continued on next page

Outline of Book (*Continued*)

Acronyms

For the convenience of readers, acronyms used throughout the book are listed here.

ASSI	Acculturative Stress Scale for International Students
APA	American Psychological Association
CRIS	Coping Resources Inventory for Stress
DABS	Derogatis Affects Balance Scale
DLSS	Daily Life Stressors Scale
DSM-III-R	Diagnostic and Statistical Manual of Mental Disorders (3rd ed., rev.)
Ed.D.	Doctor of education (degree)
GIS	Global Inventory of Stress
HCSSI	Hilson Career Satisfaction/Stress Index
HIV	Human immunodeficiency virus
IPPA	Inventory of Positive Psychological Attitudes
IQ	Intelligence quotient
M.D.	Medical doctor
MMPI	Minnesota Multiphasic Personality Inventory
MSPSS	Multidimensional Scale of Perceived Social Support
Ph.D.	Doctor of philosophy (degree)
PTSD	Perinatal posttraumatic stress disorder
SLSI	Student-Life Stress Inventory
SRAS	School Refusal Assessment Scale
SRI	Self-Reliance Inventory
SRS	The Stress Response Scale
SRSA	The Stress Response Scale for Adolescents
STAI	State and Trait Anxiety Inventory
WAIS	Wechsler Adult Intelligence Scale
WORCS	Ways of Religious Coping Scale

An Acculturative Stress Scale for International Students

A Practical Approach to Stress Measurement

Daya S. Sandhu, University of Louisville
Badiolah R. Asrabadi, Nicholls State University

■ Instrument Name

An Acculturative Stress Scale for International Students (ASSIS)

■ Developers

Daya Singh Sandhu, Ed.D., NCC, NCSC, NCCC, DAC; Professor and Chair, Department of Educational and Counseling Psychology, University of Louisville, Louisville, KY 40292

Badiolah R. Asrabadi, Ph.D., Professor, Department of Mathematics, Nicholls State University, Thibodaux, LA 70310

■ Contact Information

Dr. Daya Singh Sandhu, Chair, Department of Educational & Counseling Psychology, 320 Education Building, University of Louisville, Louisville, KY 40292
Telephone: (502) 852-6646; fax: (502) 852-0629;
e-mail: dssand0i@ulkyvm.louisville.edu
To conduct research using this scale, please also contact:
Editor, The Psychological Reports, Box 9229, Missoula, MN 59807

Description and History of the Instrument

The pursuit of learning beyond indigenous boundaries is quite old (Bois, 1956; Fasheh, 1984). The United States of America has become the *Mecca* for foreign students in recent times because many of them believe it is the world's center of technology and sophisticated knowledge. Both students and scholars perceive U.S. higher education as the best system in the world (Johnson, 1993). As a result, the United States ranks first among all countries of the world that host foreign students.

The most recent data available indicate that 453,787 foreign students were enrolled in U.S. colleges and universities in 1997, almost half of the world's total number of foreign students (Altbach, 1997). Previously, Zikopoulos (1993) reported 438,618 foreign students enrolled in the United States in fall 1992–1993, a steady increase of 23.14% over 5 years. Economic, cultural, and political factors indicate that the number of international students in the United States will continue to increase significantly into the next century (Hayes & Lin, 1994; Huang, 1993; Pedersen, 1991). The presence of these students provide an opportunity for college administrators and faculty to promote understanding of other cultures. They can encourage these "cultural ambassadors" not only to achieve their personal goals and enjoyment of a foreign land but also enhance international understanding and collaboration to tackle global problems such as hunger, AIDS, and drug abuse.

The reality of being a "foreigner," however, makes living in a strange land difficult when a person has to make a number of personal, social, and environmental changes upon arrival. Many foreign students experience culture shock, cultural distance, differences in communication styles, isolation, language problems, and loneliness (Aubrey, 1991; Cross, 1995; Leong & Chou, 1996; Redmond & Bunyi, 1993; Sandhu, 1993). Naturally, issues relating to adjustment and acculturative stress of international students seem to dominate the related literature (Altbach, Kelly, & Lulat, 1985). Berry, Kim, Minde, and Mok (1987) defined this *acculturative stress* as a special form of stress that manifests in physical, social, and psychological problems when people move across different cultures.

Because international students living in the United States are many miles away from home, they are likely to find it frightening to establish sense of belonging. When cultural contexts change, so do values, priorities, and behavior (Sandhu, 1997). The demands of the host culture might be totally at odds with their experiences in the native country (Ozbay, 1994). For this reason, persons moving from one culture to another experience unique stressors that natives never even imagine (Cross, 1995; Smart & Smart, 1995). A large majority of foreign students coming from the underdeveloped countries to the United States face such dilemmas when they are expected to make several adjustments. Immediately after the international students arrive in the United States, their cultural transformation begins. As a consequence of these acculturating processes, "threats to cultural identity, powerlessness, feelings of marginality, a sense of inferiority, loneliness, hostility, and perceived alienation and discrimination become major mental health concerns" (Sandhu, Portes, & McPhee, 1996, p. 16).

The seriousness of emotional pain associated with migration is so real and sometimes so traumatic that it has been given many special names. Ward (1967) calls it "a foreign student syndrome," affecting an individual suffering from an extremely high level of anxiety-related problems but having no recognizable physical signs and symptoms. Zwingman (1978) calls the migration experience of foreign students a phenomenon of "uprooting disorder" with identifiable psychological symptoms of alienation, nostalgia, depression, and a sense of helplessness. Based on their clinical findings, Alexander, Klein, Workneh, & Miller (1981, p. 228) assert that the vast majority of non-Western third world students "feel vulnerable during much of their time in the United States. In addition to suffering culture shock when dealing with external matters such as differences in food, climate, language, manners and communication, these students also suffer from status change and status loss."

After reviewing 96,804 diagnoses of international students, Ebbin and Blackenship (1986) report insomnia, anxiety, depression, and sexual dysfunctions as the most frequent health problems of international students. Aubrey (1991) notes additional stress-related somaticized problems such as colds, dizziness, epigastric pain, fatigue, headaches, neurasthenia (a generalized feeling of body weakness), and skin disorders that afflict the foreign students. It is estimated that 15% to 25% of all international students are at risk of experiencing psychological and psychiatric problems due to acculturative stress, and they are likely to be impaired in some ways (Church, 1982; Leong & Chou, 1996).

Unfortunately, we found that the research conducted on the psychological problems of international students is isolated, sporadic, inconsistent, varied, and desultory. Most of the psychological problems of international students, for instance, have been conceptualized with very little supporting empirical data. As a result, few instruments have been designed to assess the psychological needs of foreign students in a comprehensive manner. Crano and Crano (1993) asserted that rigorous studies on adjustment especially those focusing on international students are plagued due to the failure of valid and reliable measures. This chapter summarizes our attempt to construct and test an instrument for the acculturative stress of international students that might fill this gap as a composite measure of adjustment problems of international students.

Instrument Development

An initial pool of 125 statements in Likert-type format was constructed by using two strategies. First, 13 international students, 8 men and 5 women, were interviewed at an urban university in the southern United States to take into consideration their personal experiences and perspectives. These students included two from China, one from Egypt, one from Ethiopia, two from Germany, two from India, one from Iran, one from Japan, two from Venezuela, and one from Nicaragua. Second, recurrent themes of adjustment difficulties with high face validity were identified from the prevalent counseling literature related to international students. Specifically, works of Alexander et al. (1981), Allen and Cole (1987), Altbach and Wang (1989), Anderson and Myer (1985), Berry (1984), Dillard and Chisolm (1983), Furnham (1988), Furnham and Bochner (1986), Heikinheimo and Shute (1986), Johnson (1971), Klineburg and Hull (1979), Manese, Sedlacek and Leong (1988), Pedersen (1991), Spaulding and Flack (1976), Walton (1971), and Zikopoulos (1993) were closely examined for this purpose. The initial 125-item *Acculturative Stress Scale for International Students* was pilot tested with 17 undergraduate and 9 graduate international students. The first draft was also reviewed by three university professors at two different universities. These professors taught graduate courses in multicultural counseling and were familiar with issues relating to international students.

A number of items were eliminated or revised to avoid confusion, repetition, and ambiguity regarding the intent of meaning. In its refined and polished version, this scale resulted in 78 items, with 6 to 9 items under different themes. After the statistical procedures were done as explained here, this scale yielded 36 items in its final version.

Psychometric Characteristics

The procedure used to analyze the data included Cronbach's coefficient alpha, Guttman split-half coefficient, two measures of reliability, correlation, factor analysis (with principal component extraction and varimax rotation), and Kaiser-Meyer-Olkin (KMO), a measure of sampling adequacy. SPSS

7.0 for Windows 95 was used to perform all necessary computations. Barlett's test of sphericity was used to test the hypothesis that the population correlation matrix is an identity matrix. The value of the test statistic for sphericity was 3,424.78, with an associated significance level of $p < .00000$. Although this test was based on the assumption that the data were sampled from a multivariate population, the value of the test statistic was large enough to overcome the lack of normality. Therefore, the hypothesis that the population correlation matrix was an identity was rejected. The Cronbach's coefficient alpha is calculated to be 0.9464 for 36 items. The calculated value of the Guttman split-half statistic is 0.9690 with 0.9399 as the correlation between halves. All of these statistics support a very high measure of reliability. The anti-image correlation (the negative of the partial correlation coefficient) supported the feasibility of using factor analysis. The overall KMO measure of sampling adequacy was found to be quite large (0.86853) and meritorious, as defined by Kaiser (1974). These statistics are summarized in Table 1.

In addition to the large value of the overall measure of sampling adequacy, almost all of the individual measures of sampling adequacy were more than 0.74, suggesting a strong support for the application of factor analysis for the data. The

Table 1: Summary Statistics for Sphericity, Reliability, and Sampling Adequacy

Statistics	Value	Measure of	Significance
Bartlett's test	3,424.78	Sphericity	High
Cronbach's coefficient alpha	0.9464	Reliability	Very high
Guttman split-half	0.9690	Reliability	Very high
Kaiser-Meyer-Olkin	0.86853	Sample adequacy	Very good, meritorious

individual measures of sampling adequacy are listed in Table 1.

The method of principal components extracted 7 factors (using factors with eigenvalues of more than one) accounting for 69.7% of the total population variance. These factors with their eigenvalues, percentages of variance, cumulative percentages, and the coefficient alphas for items in each factor are presented in Table 2.

These results are clearly recognizable: six principal factors capture about two-thirds of the total population variance. These principal factors and their respective items with their factor loadings, communalities (proportion of the variance of an item explained by the factor), and the individual measures of sampling adequacy are shown in Table 3.

Discussion of Results

Since Factor 1, Perceived Deprivation, captured the highest percentage of total variation (37.6%), one can conclude that

Table 2: Summary of Extracted Principal Factors

Factor	Eigenvalue	Percentage Variance	Cumulative Variance	Alpha
1. Perceived Discrimination	13.54	37.6	37.6	0.90
2. Homesickness	3.08	8.6	46.2	0.89
3 Perceived Hate/ Rejection	2.66	7.4	53.6	0.90
4. Fear	1.91	5.3	58.9	0.88
5. Stress Due to Change	1.58	4.4	63.2	0.79
6. Guilt	1.21	3.4	66.6	0.44
7. Nonspecific	1.11	3.1	79.7	0.84

Table 3: Principal Factors and Representative Items with Their Loadings, Communalities, and Individual Measures of Sampling (IMS) for Variables Contributing to Each Factor

Factor Name and Item Content	Loading KMO	Communality	IMS
1. Perceived Discrimination			
Many opportunities are denied to me	0.71	0.618	0.924
I am treated differently in social situations	0.52	0.718	0.940
Others are biased toward me	0.78	0.730	0.882
I feel that I receive unequal treatment	0.73	0.669	0.874
I am denied what I deserve	0.56	0.630	0.851
I feel that my people are discriminated against	0.70	0.610	0.854
I am treated differently because of my race	0.65	0.638	0.888
I am treated differently because of my color	0.67	0.665	0.907
2. Homesickness			
I feel sad leaving my relatives behind	0.88	0.813	0.847
Homesickness bothers me	0.87	0.821	0.895
I feel sad living in unfamiliar surroundings	0.78	0.727	0.921
I miss the people and country of my origin	0.74	0.701	0.892
3. Perceived Hate/Rejection			
People show hatred toward me nonverbally	0.64	0.851	0.908
People show hatred toward me verbally	0.73	0.699	0.896
People show hatred toward me through actions	0.68	0.807	0.916

Continued on next page

Table 3 (*Continued*)

Others are sarcastic toward my cultural values	0.55	0.697	0.909
Others don't appreciate my cultural values	0.56	0.766	0.868
4. Fear			
I fear for my personal safety because of my different cultural background	0.86	0.828	0.823
I generally keep a low profile due to fear	0.86	0.859	0.752
I feel insecure here	0.82	0.796	0.798
I frequently relocate for fear of others	0.59	0.610	0.789
5. Stress Due to Change/ Culture Shock			
I feel uncomfortable to adjust to new foods	0.80	0.714	0.851
Multiple pressures are placed upon me after migration	0.79	0.672	0.741
I feet uncomfortable to adjust to new cultural values	0.73	0.631	0.677
6. Guilt			
I feel guilty to leave family and friends behind	0.77	0.757	0.842
I feel guilty because I am living a different lifestyle here	0.67	0.555	0.897

perceived deprivation/alienation is of the most concern with the item "Others are biased toward me" as the highest contributor. This item has a loading of 0.78 and communality of 0.73. The second-highest contributor of Factor 1 is the item "I feel that I receive unequal treatment," with loading of 0.73 and communality of 0.699. These findings are consistent with some previous studies. Bois's (1956) observations made about perceived discrimination over four decades ago seem to still hold true: "Probably relatively few foreign students have had personal experiences with the cruder varieties of racial discrimination. More suffer from difficulties of strangeness . . . sensitive students may interpret social distance as racial discrimination" (p. 47).

The process of alienation is doublefold. First, the natural response of foreign students during the acculturative process is to seek other conationals for their primary support and not to make any special efforts to reach out to Americans. On the other side, American students, being complacent with their situation, do not feel the need to go out of the way to socialize with foreign students. Unfortunately, both foreign and native students dwell on what Pedersen (1991) calls "superficial pleasantries." The end result is a sense of alienation that is far more severe among foreign students than others (Schram & Lauver, 1988). Three major elements of alienation—feelings of powerlessness, meaninglessness, and social estrangement, as defined by Burbach (1972)—are very characteristic of foreign students' perceived sense of alienation.

The second major factor was found to be loneliness, which contributed 8.6% to the total variance. This sense of loneliness is caused by homesickness, missing significant others in the native country, and a sense of being lost in the unfamiliar surroundings. Most of all, this perceived sense of loss is caused by the lack of emotional and social support as indicated by the items "I feel sad leaving my relatives behind" and "Homesickness bothers me." Coping with loss of family, friends, and country could be a very painful and an extremely stressful experience (Aubrey, 1991). Siegel (1991) seems to have captured the very essence of the loneliness problem of foreign students by reporting, in the words of a student from India: "An international student is a sapling or a tree, depending on his age, but his roots are still there in his home country" (p. 75). Hull (1987) presents another picturesque description of loneliness as experienced by a foreign student, Kabul:

"I am not doing anything but sitting in my room drinking coffee and smoking cigarettes. None of this has any meaning. Sometimes I think I should just kill myself. My roommate thinks it is because I have no parents, no country, and no religion. The psychiatrist keeps giving me pills but they aren't working. Why do I feel like this? What should I do? My grades are O.K." (p. 307).

The third factor, which contributed 7.4% to the total variance and is named Perceived Hate Rejection in this study seems to be unique in the existing counseling psychology literature on international students. The item "People show hatred toward me verbally," with loading of 0.73, is the highest contributor. The participants reported strong negative feelings toward host nationals in response to culturally biased verbal and nonverbal communications and actual derogatory behaviors.

The fourth factor, Fear, contributing 5.3% to the total variance, was also found unusual in the literature on foreign students. This fear seems to be related to the perceived sense of insecurity in unfamiliar surroundings, perceived sense of racial discrimination, sense of inferiority, and off-and-on hostile relations between the foreign student's native country and the United States. The items "I fear for my personal safety because of my different cultural background" and "I generally keep a low profile due to fear," with a loading of 0.86, are the highest contributors to this factor.

The fifth factor, Stress Due to Change, is the most researched topic in the literature of foreign students (Alexander et al., 1981; Bochner, 1986; Mena, Padilla, & Maldonado, 1987; Padilla, Alvarez & Lindhom, 1986; Thomas and Althen, 1989). Most of the stress is caused by multiple pressures placed on international students because of migration to a strange land. We agree that "foreign students are a high risk group, under considerable stress; this stress is more likely to be experienced in the form of physical complaints than psychological complaints" (Alexander et al., 1981, p. 235). It may be noted, however, that in our study, variance due to this factor contributed only 4.4% with the items "I feel uncomfortable to adjust to new foods" and "Multiple pressures are placed upon me after migration" with factor loadings of 0.80 and 0.79, respectively, being the two highest contributors.

The last factor, Guilt, contributed 3.4% to the total variance and, like the factors of Perceived Hate/Rejection and Fear in this study, was also found to be unique. Adjusting to the host culture meant betrayal to the native culture for many foreign students. Adopting the host culture's values was perceived as being insincere to their own culture by these participants. International students seem to be in a double bind, caught between the old values of their cherished native culture and the new values of the host culture, which they are pressured to adopt.

Studies in Progress

Even though published in 1994, this scale is relatively new. Several studies ($n = 29$) using the Acculturative Stress Scale for International Students are currently in progress. It is interesting to note how swiftly ASSIS attracted the attention of students and scholars worldwide. In addition to several studies in the United States, a number of studies are being conducted in Australia, Canada, China, Croatia, Cyprus, Germany, India, Israel, Korea, Mexico, and the United Kingdom. The major focus of these studies is to empirically examine the acculturative stress of international students by using the ASSIS.

Studies Completed

The results of some studies have already become available. These results are persuasive and are consistent with our preliminary findings. Ansari (1996) studied the validity of the ASSIS by examining the difference in acculturative stress between American and international students. The participants consisted of 51 American college students and 53 international college students. The data on seven subscales were submitted to multivariate analysis of variance (MANOVA). The MANOVA indicated the groups were significantly different on the linear combination of the seven subscales, F (7, 96) = 5.59, p = .0001 (Wilks's lambda − .71), with the international students scoring higher than the American students. This indicated that international students experienced significantly higher acculturative stress than American students. Since the MANOVA indicated a significant difference between the two groups on the linear combination of the seven subscales, Univariate analysis of variance (ANOVA) was utilized to test the significant *difference* between the groups on each subscale. ANOVA indicated that the groups were significantly different on Perceived Discrimination, F (1,102) = 11.68, p = .0009, Perceived Hate/Rejection, F (1,102) = 6.75, p = .0108, and the Nonspecific factor, F (1,102) = 12.14, p = .0007, with the international students scoring higher than the American students on each of these subscales. This indicated that compared with American students, international students experienced more stress regarding Perceived Discrimination, Perceived Hate/Rejection and the items on the Nonspecific subscale. The Nonspecific subscale included items as follows:

I feel nervous to communicate in English
I feel intimidated to participate in social activities
I feel angry that my people are considered inferior here
It hurts when people don't understand cultural values

Additional items included some as follows:

I feel low because of my cultural background
I feel that my status in this society is low due to my cultural background
I don't feel a sense of belonging (community) here
I feel sad to consider my people's problems
I feel some people don't associate with me because of my ethnicity

*I worry about my future for not being able to decide
whether to stay here or to go back.*

Since all these items were hard to classify under one specific
factor, these nonspecific items were grouped as *Miscellaneous.*

Ansari (1996) reported the internal consistency of the total
ASSIS scores as .87. In addition, the reliabilities for all the
subscales were relatively high, ranging from .74 to .87 except
for Guilt (.58) and Culture Shock (.55), which are considered
moderate.

Using ASSIS, Buseh, McElmurry, and Fox (1997) conducted a study to address the health and psychosocial factors
that influence the acculturation process of male Liberian immigrants. Interestingly, these authors hypothesized the same
psychoacculturative processes between the international students and the immigrants from Liberia to the United States.
As several investigators (Berry & Kim, 1988; Westermyer,
1989) have suggested, the new lifestyle often induces changes
in behavior that can compromise health.

A cross-sectional descriptive study of male Liberian immigrants in a large midwestern U.S. city was designed to describe
the acculturative stress experienced by this group and the impact of stress on the emotional health status. A convenience
sample of (*n* = 50) Liberian males (median age 36) completed
a self-administered survey that included the Center for Epidemiologic Studies Depression Scale (CES-D) developed by
Radloff (1977) and our 1994 Acculturative Stress Scale for International Students along with sociodemographic variables.
Using the ASSIS, the following factors were measured: Perceived Discrimination, Homesickness, Perceived Hate/Rejec-
tion, Fear of living in a new environment, and Fear for safety
due to cultural background. Other factors measured by the
scale were: Culture Shock, Stress due to culture change, and
feelings of Guilt for leaving relatives and friends behind in the
homeland. Sociodemographic information (e.g., age at migration, length of stay in the U.S., income employment status,
etc.) was obtained from the participants.

The CES-D scores indicated that 16% of the subjects had scores from the cutoff point of 1.16 or greater on the scale, indicating "caseness" or depressive symptomatology. However, the mean depressive score (8.8) was lower relative to other ethnic populations. The acculturative stress significantly correlated with emotional health ($r = .51, p < .05$), age ($r = .31, p < .05$), and employment ($r = .54, p < .05$). With multiple-regression analysis, the most powerful correlates of acculturative stress were emotional health ($R^2 = .258$) and age, ($R^2 = .461, p < .05$) when independent variables were entered in the regression equation. The CES-D scale had an alpha coefficient of .85, while the Acculturative Stress Scale for International Students (1994) demonstrated a high internal consistency with a Cronbach's alpha of .93 in this study.

Principal component factor analysis was performed on both scales. Among the six factors extracted from the principal component analysis of the ASSIS, Factor I (Perceived Discrimination) accounted for the highest percentage of total variation (29.8%). Perceived Discrimination was therefore the major factor of concern among the Liberian male immigrants in the current study. Other factors extracted from the factor analysis with eigenvalues are as follows: Culture Shock/Stress due to culture change (8.5%), Perceived Hate/Rejection (7.4%), feelings of Guilt (6.8%), perceived Fear (5.5%); and Homesickness (4.4%). The findings suggested that the factors of discrimination and cultural isolation are major concerns to male Liberian immigrants. The authors of this study pointed out that the Factor 1, Perceived Discrimination, mirrors the ASSIS results.

Using ASSIS, Michailidis (1996) conducted a study to research the factors that contribute to gender differences in acculturative stress. This study also investigated differences existing in acculturative stress among students from first, second, and third world countries. A total of 118 full-time international undergraduate and graduate students enrolled at a university in the northeastern United States participated, 83 males and 35 females. The highest percentage of undergraduate students were juniors (30.2%) and the highest percentage of the graduate students were doctoral students (33.9%). The age range was 19 to 48 with a mode of 30 and median of 27. Engineering majors were the highest percentage (33.1%). Most of the students (63.3%) had been in the United States for 3 years or less. First world students in the total sample had the highest percentage rate (38%), followed by the third and second world students (32% and 30%, respectively).

Possible gender differences were examined as they related to acculturative stress. ANOVA and the students' Gender and Origin were used as the independent variables with the sub-scale scores of Perceived Discrimination, Safety, and Adjustment used one at a time as the dependent variables. ANOVA was used to determine whether the factors exhibited a statistically significant difference across Gender and Origin and to examine any potential interaction between these factors. The results indicated that only the Perceived Discrimination factor was significant with gender, with highly significant difference at the .01 alpha level (df $= 2, 116; p < .01$).

The statistical analysis also indicated that the students' gender influenced the amount of acculturative stress they experienced; male students experienced more discrimination than female students. A post hoc Tukey (HSD) test was performed on Perceived Discrimination and males to determine where the significance mostly existed. The Tukey results indicated that the group with the highest significant difference on Perceived Discrimination was the male students from the third world countries, with an unweighted mean of 19.5, which was the greatest value of the three Origin factors (first world $=$ 14.2, second world $= 11.6$).

Michailidis (1996) concluded that the Perceived Discrimination factor was of greatest concern for international students, a finding consistent with earlier research (Sandhu & Asrabadi, 1994). This study also reported gender differences in acculturative stress among international students: international male students suffer higher levels of acculturative stress than females. As a result, they should be considered at higher risk for academic and social failures. Another important implication of this study is that the interventions to assist international students in adjusting to U.S. campuses should focus more on the group at risk: male students from the third world countries.

Since foreign students in the United States from third world countries are torn between two cultures, this recommendation supports the assertions of Martinez, Huang, Johnson, and Edwards (1989) that foreign students who do not identify with American mainstream culture are at a greater risk of acculturative stress-related problems. In another study, Gholamrezaei (1996) reported that a higher level of acculturative stress is associated with a lower level of acculturation. Heikinheimo and Shute (1986) reported that students from third world countries in Canadian universities generally had to make more substantial adjustments than their counterparts from Europe and Caribbean countries.

Case Examples

Four different case examples of foreign university students are presented in this section to demonstrate the afflictions of acculturative stress that such students endure, as well as the use of the Acculturative Stress Scale. The four students were randomly interviewed and were asked to write a paragraph or two to express their acculturative stress-related experiences.

Case Example 1

Angelia Farc, a 28-year-old female Romanian, came to the United States as an international student in 1990, right after the revolution that swept across Eastern Europe. After receiving her Master of Divinity degree in pastoral care and counseling, she enrolled in the doctoral program in counseling psychology. Angelia described her experiences as an international student as follows:

I knew I was supposed to be happy. After all I had just arrived in the promised land. Everyone I knew back home would have given their most prized possessions to be in my place. But, instead of feeling happy I felt disconnected from myself like I had been ripped apart from me. My greatest loss did not seem to be that of my culture, my parents, my status or my safety. I had lost myself. It was almost as if somewhere over the Atlantic my soul had slipped away and dropped from the airplane. I couldn't get in touch with myself because I was nowhere to be found. I didn't cry. The chance of a lifetime had been given to me and I had no right to cry. I did not complain. I did not speak the words to explain what I felt, even if say, by some miracle I would have felt anything at all. The only thing I knew to do was deny completely everything I had been before, deny my longing for my homeland (why should I miss it after all, it was a rotten communist place), deny my passion for its litera-ture and art (it was infantile and lacking modernity), deny my need for old friends and family (my mother mistreated me and my friends had always been jealous). I kept telling myself I was an American now, and I forced myself to better start behaving like one. When some mentioned "culture shock" I laughed at them and said "You've got to be kidding! What shock? I have everything I could possibly want, I'm fine!" I just went through the motions for months and months until bits of pieces of my old identity and my new identity met and I started feeling again. Boy, I started feeling. It hurt so much I could barely stand it.

We found Angelia's statement an extremely powerful ex-pression of deep hurt, homesickness, guilt, and culture shock. If the ASSIS were administered to Angelia, her scores on sev-eral statements such as, "Homesickness bothers me," "I feel sad living in unfamiliar surroundings," "I don't feel a sense of belonging (community) here," etc., would be much higher than her counterpart, American students. Without disclosing background information, we asked a licensed psychologist to review Angelia's statement and prepare a psychological inter-pretation. We wanted to make an objective assessment of Angelia's acculturative stress. A summary of this interpreta-tion follows:

Most theories of identity acknowledge the strong influence of role expectations upon the psychological functioning of the individual. In fact, many theorists believe that the bulk of individual's personal identity is defined in terms of the multiple roles that all of us enact. Angelia experienced the total eradication of roles as she had known them. Her sense of self was assailed and she was no longer able to define herself as an individual in relation to others, e.g., fulfilling specific and well-defined roles. Instead, there were expectations of emotions unattached to specific role expectation. In order not to risk the loss of her self, she attempted to split off the hurt and bury it deep in her subconscious. So not to experience devastating multiple losses, she denied the importance of her relationships and roles as parts of her self. This allowed her to function physically, but it also retarded her ability to grieve her losses and experience the emotional growth necessary to recognize, feel, and accept them, and ultimately integrate change with her sense of self.

All of us use denials or detachment to facilitate functioning. In order to perform efficiently and effectively, surgeons distance themselves from the physical pain that patients feel as a result of their actions; parents try not to empathize too closely with the disappointments of their children in order to model a healthy view of loss. Problems occur when, under stress from the imposed anticipations of self or others, the individuals deny their emotions, dismiss their losses, and deconstruct their sense of self without allowing adequate time for integration of change. Such is often the case with international students who are expected to adjust quickly to their new surroundings, "fit in," appreciate, and enjoy their new experiences without mourning their loss of relationships, rituals, and roles. Sadly, few individuals understand the cycle of denial of loss, psuedo-adaptation, recognition of loss, experience of mourning, and reintegration of self, leading to an appropriate adaptation that most international students experience. Messages from host families, new acquaintances, faculty, and other students is often one of "getting over and on with it" rather than "respecting the ability to negotiate such tremendous and overwhelming change."

Case Example 2

Twenty-two-year-old Fikre Kassie aspires to complete his degree in chemical engineering before returning to Ethiopia. Fikre admires the American educational system and is very much surprised by how easily one can gain admission to a university in America. He is also delighted by the availability of books and career opportunities. But he feels extremely lonely and homesick and is not sure when he will be able to see his family and friends again. In addition, he feels guilty for not being able to attend an Ethiopian church here. Fikre wrote the following as one of his acculturative stress-related experiences:

> I was in a university-run campus gym exercising while waiting for a "stair master." I was next in the line to use the machine. This was a common practice amongst the gym users to wait in line. However, a young Caucasian male came by and announced that he should be allowed to use the first available machine since "foreigners should be kicked out and sent back to where they came from." I ignored his statement and proceeded to exercise. He came within six inches of my face and said, "why don't you go back to wherever the hell you came from." I was scared and did not know how to respond. Luckily, the manager showed up and this man left.

Fikre's episode is indicative of many statements of the Acculturative Stress Scale for international students. Some of these statements include, "Others are biased toward me," "People show hatred toward me through actions," and "I fear for my personal safety because of my different cultural background."

Case Example 3:

The Gulf War and the most recent conflict over Iraq's refusal to cooperate with United Nations arms inspectors again brought forth anti-Iraqi feelings and open hostility to many

Arab Americans. Here is an episode of a student from Bangladesh who became a target of anger and abuse presumably due to the mistaken identity. Akbar Sayed, a 27-year-old male computer engineering major was verbally assaulted at a university dining area and reported:

> A male Caucasian student told me: "I wish the government would just throw the likes of you out of *our* country. And you, Saddam, a man like you, should never have been allowed in our Christian country." I told him that I was born and raised in Bangladesh. He continued to tell me that all non-Christians should just be kicked out— and people like me did not deserve to live here. Not only had this man insulted me for my appearance, but also for my religion.

In the context of this episode, several statements of the ASSIS represent Sayed's feelings: "I am treated differently in social situations," "I feel that I receive unequal treatment," "I feel insecure here," etc.

Case Example 4

Emotional wounds are generally hard to heal, but it seems that acculturative stress experiences are even more difficult to forget and forgive. Such a painful acculturative experience was shared by Prafula P. Sheth, a 51-year-old female doctoral student in college student personnel. She was borne and raised in Sudan, Africa. Her ancestral heritage is rooted in the Gujrati culture of India. Prafula's acculturative stress-related experiences after 28 years are evoked in the following passage:

> What follows is the first encounter with my assigned roommate: a Caucasian, 18 years old, walked in our room, took one look at me and announced to her parents (who were helping her move in), "I ain't living with a 'ni . . .' This was my *first* encounter with race/color discrimination. The housing administration refused to let her move. Because of her attitude, I spent my first semester with a roommate who openly treated

me as though I had some sort of terrible, communicable disease that she would catch if she only passed within a foot of me. I survived that incident. However, even after 28 years, I can relive that moment and the semester with clarity and with pain.

Several statements on the ASSIS capture Prafula's painful and hard-to-forget feelings: "I am treated differently because of my race," "People show hatred toward me verbally," "I am treated differently because of my color," etc.

Administration and Scoring

Several steps, described in the following sections, should be taken to ensure the effective use of the ASSIS.

Purpose

Before administering the ASSIS, we recommend that the rationale or purpose for administering this scale is explained to subjects. The administration of the scale should be presented as an important task. It is also important that the international students completing this scale are instructed to respond to all the statements as honestly as possible for the data to be meaningful. In addition to oral directions, we recommend that written instructions be provided. It is crucial that these students receive feedback about their performance on the ASSIS.

Administration

Generally speaking, the administration of the ASSIS should be easy and straightforward. The completion of a personal data sheet and the ASSIS generally takes 20 to 25 minutes. An eighth-grade reading level should be adequate to respond to the statements. Because English is a foreign language for most international students, however, some students may take longer than others to complete this scale. These students may also seek clarification about certain statements if they do not understand the meaning of certain words. As a caveat, administrators should ensure that subjects are able to read and comprehend what is being asked. Greene (1991) noted that the inconsistent responding is mostly attributed to poor reading ability.

Scoring

The scoring of the ASSIS may easily be accomplished by hand. The score range of the ASSIS is 36 to 180. Higher scores are indicative of higher levels of acculturative stress. The total acculturative stress scores in raw form are obtained by summing all the scores of the 36 statements of the ASSIS. The separate subscales scores can be obtained by summing up the responses on the respective statements as stated below:

1. Perceived Discrimination   3, 9, 11, 14, 17, 23, 26, 29
2. Homesickness   1, 6, 21, 35
3. Perceived Hate   4, 15, 20, 24, 33
4. Fear   7, 18, 27, 31
5. Stress due to change   2, 13, 22 (Culture shock)
6. Guilt   10, 34
7. Nonspecific Miscellaneous   5, 8, 12, 16, 19, 25, 28, 30, 32, 36

The scores on subscales may be important in finding the specific sources of acculturative stress afflicting individual international students. This information might be very useful to counselors and psychologists in developing strategies to help international students focus on relieving a particular area of acculturative stress.

Interpretation

The global scores on the ASSIS range from 36 to 180. The mean score of this scale is 66.32 and the standard deviation is

21.16. So, within two standard deviations, mean scores from 108.64 or 109 are normal. Since not all international students experience the same level of acculturative stress, a score higher than 109 should be interpreted as a warning sign for some sort of counseling and psychological intervention. Therefore, we recommend that the ASSIS should be used only as a screening scale. A substantial number of additional studies need to be completed before ASSIS can be recommended for clinical purposes.

Implications for Counseling and Psychotherapy

As a silent and powerless group, international students can be described as another minority population. To work effectively with this special group, it is imperative that counselors, psychologists, and other mental health professionals are familiar with cross-cultural competencies as advocated by Sue, Arredondo, and McDavis (1992). To alleviate acculturative stress of international students, the ASSIS can be employed as a valuable tool to implement the following recommendations for foreign student directors, advisors, counselors, and other mental health professionals.

Proactive approaches

Generally speaking, international students do not actively seek out counseling and psychological help. They may not be aware of the availability of psychological services or are reluctant to discuss personal problems with strangers due to various stigmas. For this reason, counseling services should be preplanned, well structured, and offered on the regular basis as an integral part of the educational programs for foreign students. The ASSIS can be used as a preliminary screening tool to assess the acculturative stress level of foreign students and improvise necessary strategies for providing counseling and psychological help. In case of severe acculturative stress, appropriate referrals should be made to seek outside help.

Continuous and comprehensive approaches

It is important that counseling services for international students are provided on a continuous basis. We agree with Pedersen (1991) that "orientation is a continuous process requiring contact with students before they arrive, during their stay, and after they have returned home, as the student experiences a continuous process of adjustment" (p. 44). The ASSIS can be used as a continuous assessment instrument to gain insight into the unique acculturative concerns and problems of foreign students at the various stages of their sojourning experiences.

Counseling and Psychotherapy Groups

Due to cultural inhibitions, foreign students are generally reluctant to discuss their personal problems. It is a major challenge to make them share their concerns in individual counseling sessions where they feel embarrassed and guilty to discuss personal matters with authority figures (Wehrly, 1988). However, Aubrey (1991) suggested that group therapy is the treatment of choice for a majority of international students. It is through group therapy that these students can be helped to acknowledge and mourn their loss of family, friends, home, status, and language. The counseling groups could also become a great process through which foreign students' anxieties, fears, and inhibitions can be explored and resolved.

The ASSIS can be very useful in identifying the special concerns of foreign students due to their acculturative stress-related problems. Based on ASSIS research, various counseling and psychotherapy groups can be formed to alleviate the psychological pain associated with acculturative stress. Some of these counseling groups might include problem-solving for prejudice and discrimination reduction, therapy to ease the pain of hate, fear, and guilt, and support for loneliness and homesickness.

These groups can serve as a surrogate family and provide psychological bonding and social support for many foreign students. As the effects of acculturative stress are mitigated by social support (Mallinckrodt & Leong, 1992), we hope that participation of international students in various groups will alleviate their acculturative distress.

Limitations

There are several factors that contribute to the acculturative stress of the international students. Sandhu (1995) broadly classified these factors into two major categories: interpersonal and intrapersonal. The ASSIS is developed mainly to assess the acculturative stress of international students relating to intrapersonal factors aimed at psychological difficulties such as perceived discrimination, loneliness, homesickness, fear, hate, and guilt.

The ASSIS precluded many factors identified in literature that generate acculturative stress. For instance, Coleman (1997) identified academic pressures, academic difficulties, and problems with language as the major source of psychological difficulties of the foreign students. Charles & Stewart (1991) added academic overload, differences in educational systems, and financial problems to this list. Cheng, Leong, & Geist (1993) suggested immigration difficulties, culture fatigue, and the need to become independent as some additional causes of acculturative stress. The ASSIS has a limitation in that it does not assess factors that mainly relate to the environment of the foreign students.

Although the ASSIS has a promising beginning, much research remains to be done to evaluate the utility of this instrument in the assessment of clinical problems of foreign students. Since identification of psychiatric symptomatology requires much more careful evaluation, we do not recommend ASSIS for the diagnosis of psychiatric disorders of foreign students.

Conclusion

Recently, many other countries such as Australia, Canada, England, France, Germany, and Japan have mobilized their efforts and resources to attract foreign students. Desruisseaux (1996, 1997) noted that many countries, especially Australia, have recently become very aggressive in recruiting foreign students and are now finding new ways to deliver education in Asia and Pacific in partnership with the local institutions. On the other hand, perceptions about the quality of American education is beginning to change. Maslen (1997a) reported the findings of a study that examined Asian students' perceptions of educational quality in Australia, Canada, Great Britain, and the United States. The students in this study ranked British universities as the best in standards. They also perceived Australia and Great Britain as the safest places to study. Even after more than 15 years, Dunnett's (1981, p. xi) criticism about treatment of foreign students in America is still very legitimate.

"Not only have U.S. institutions of higher education been indifferent to the adjustment problems of foreign students, they have also given little attention to problems such as the relevancy of American educational programs for the developing world. Today, many developing countries are themselves questioning the suitability of western technology, education, and culture for their countries."

In the face of such present and future challenges, American institutions of higher education cannot afford to be complacent and not proactively recruit foreign students. Universities are already being advised that they need new strategies to compete for foreign students (Maslen, 1997b). And when these students are here, it is important that their sojourning experience is made pleasant, safe, and rewarding. We cannot remain apathetic to the acculturative stress-related psychological problems of international students, nor let them suffer silently, if we hope to keep America as the center and cynosure of this special group of students. In this effort, the ASSIS could serve as one of the most important tools to identify and ameliorate the psychological problems of foreign students.

Chapter References

Alexander, A. A., Klein, M. H., Workneh, F., & Miller, M. H. (1981). Psychotherapy and the foreign student. In P. B. Pedersen, J. G. Draguns, W. J. Lonner, & J. E. Trimble (Eds.), *Counseling across cultures,* 2nd ed. (pp. 227–243). Honolulu: University Press of Hawaii.

Allen, F. C. L., & Cole, J. B. (1987). Foreign student syndrome: Fact or fable? *Journal of American Health, 35,* 182–186.

Altbach, P. G. (1997). Opinion/essays: Come study in America. *Christian Science Monitor, 89*(52), p. 18.

Altbach, P. G., Kelly, D. H., & Lulat, Y. M. (1985). *Research on foreign students and international study: An overview and bibliography.* New York: Praeger.

Altbach, P. G., & Wang, J. (1989). *Foreign students and international study: Bibliography and analysis, 1984–1988.* Lanham, MD: University Press of America.

Anderson, T. R., & Myer, T. E. (1985). Presenting problems, counselor contacts, and "no shows": international and American college students. *Journal of College Student Personnel, 26,* 500–503.

Ansari, F. P. (1996). Assessing the validity of the acculturative stress scale for international students (ASSIS). Unpublished master's thesis, Middle Tennessee State University, Murfreesboro, TN.

Aubrey, R. (1991). International students on campus: A challenge for counselors, medical providers, and clinicians. *Smith College Studies in Social Work, 62*(1), 20–33.

Berry, J. W. (1984). Psychological adaptation of foreign students. In R. Samuda & A. Wolfgang (Eds.), *Intercultural counseling and assessment* (pp. 235–248). Toronto: Hogrefe.

Berry, J. W., & Kim, U. (1988). Acculturation and mental health. In P. R. Dasen, J. W. Berry, & N. Sartorius (Eds.), *Health and cross-cultural psychology: Toward application* (pp. 207–235). Newbury Park, CA: Sage.

Berry, J. W., Kim, U., Minde, T., & Mok, D. (1987). Comparative studies of acculturative stress. *International Migration Review, 21,* 491–511.

Bochner, S. (1986). Coping with unfamiliar cultures: Adjustment or cultural learning. *Australian Journal of Psychology, 38*(3), 347–358.

Bois, C. D. (1956). *Foreign students and higher education in the United States.* Washington, DC: American Council on Education.

Burbach, H. J. (1972). The development of a contextual measure of alienation. *Pacific Sociological Review, 15,* 225–234.

Buseh, A. G., McElmurry, B. J., & Fox, P. G. (1997). *A description of the acculturative stress process and the emotional health status of Liberian male immigrants in a large Midwestern U.S. city.* Unpublished manuscript.

Charles, H., & Stewart, M. A. (1991). Academic advising of international students. *Journal of Multicultural Counseling and Development, 19,* 173–181.

Cheng, D., Leong, F. T. L., & Geist, R. (1993). Cultural differences in psychological distress between Asian and Caucasian American college students. *Journal of Multicultural Counseling and Development, 21*(3), 182–190.

Church, A. T. (1982). Sojourner adjustment. *Psychological Bulletin, 91,* 540–572.

Coleman, S. (1997). International students in the classroom: a resource and an opportunity. *International Education, 26,* 52–61.

Crano, S. L., & Crano, W. D. (1993). A measure of adjustment strain in international students. *Journal of Cross-Cultural Psychology, 24*(3), 267–283.

Cross, S. E. (1995). Self-construals, coping, and stress in cross-cultural adaptation. *Journal of Cross-Cultural Psychology, 26*(6), 673–697.

Desruisseaux, P. (1996, December 6). A record number of foreign students enrolled at U.S. colleges last year. *The Chronicle of Higher Education, 43,* pp. A64–A69.

Desruisseaux, P. (1997, November 28). Canada's 2-year colleges seek a bigger role in educating overseas students. *The Chronicle of Higher Education, 44,* p. A49.

Dillard, J. M., & Chisolm, G. B. (1983). Counseling the international student in a Multicultural context. *Journal of College Student Personnel, 24,* 101–105.

Dunnett, S. C. (Ed.) (1981). *Needs of foreign students from develop-*

ing nations at U.S. college and universities. Washington, DC: National Association for Foreign Student Affairs.

Ebbin, A. J., & Blackenship, E. S. (1986). A longitudinal health care study: International versus domestic students. *Journal of American College Health, 34*(4), 177–182.

Fasheh, M. (1984). Foreign students in the United States: An enriching experience or a wasteful one? *Contemporary Educational Psychology, 9,* 313–320.

Furnham, A. (1988). The adjustment of sojourners. In Y. Y. Kim & W. Gundykunst (Eds.), *Cross-cultural adaptation: Current approaches* (pp. 42–61). Newbury Park, CA: Sage.

Furnham, A., & Bochner, S. (1986). *Culture shock: Psychological reactions to unfamiliar environments.*

Gholamrezaei, A. (1996). Acculturation and self-esteem as predictors of acculturative stress among international students at the University of Wollongong (Australia). *Dissertation Abstracts International, 57,* 6648A. (University Microfilms No. AAG0597573)

Greene, R. L. (1991). *The MMPI-2/MMPI: An interpretative manual.* Boston: Allyn and Bacon.

Hayes, R. L., & Lin, H. (1994). Coming to America: developing social support systems for international students. *Journal of Multicultural Counseling and Development, 22*(1), 7–16.

Heikinheimo, P. S., & Shute, J. C. M. (1986). The adaptation of foreign students: student views and institutional implications. *Journal of College Student Personnel, 27,* 399–406.

Huang, J. (1993). The relationship of cognitive styles, cognitive profiles, and thinking styles among selected Chinese and North-American adult students in higher education. *Dissertation Abstracts International, 54,* 3294A. (University Microfilms No. AAG9405075)

Hull, F. W. (1987). Counseling and therapy with the non-immigrant in the educational environment. In P. Pedersen (ed.). *Handbook of cross-cultural counseling and therapy* (pp. 307–313). New York: Praeger.

Johnson, D. (1971). Problems of foreign students. *International Educational and Cultural Exchange, 7,* 61–68.

Johnson, K. A. (1993). Correlates of the organizational structure of international students services in higher education. *Dissertation Abstracts International, 54,* 3280A. (University Microfilms No. AAG9402536)

Kaiser., H. F. (1974). An index of factorial simplicity. *Psychometrika, 39*(1), 31–36.

Klineburg, O., & Hull, W. F. (1979). *At a foreign university: An international study of adaptation and coping.* New York: Praeger.

Leong. F. T. L., & Chou, E. L. (1996). Counseling international students. In P. B. Pedersen, J. G. Draguns, W. J. Lonner, & J. E. Trimble (Eds.), *Counseling across cultures* (4th ed.) (pp. 210–242). Thousand Oaks, CA: Sage.

Mallinckrodt, B., & Leong, F. T. L. (1992). International graduate students, stress, and social support. *Journal of College Student Development, 33,* 71–78.

Manese, J. E., Sedlacek, W. E., & Leong, F. T. L. (1988). Needs and perceptions of female and male international undergraduate students. *Journal of Multicultural Counseling and Development, 16*(1), 24–29.

Martinez, A. M., Huang, K. H. C., Johnson, S. D., Jr., & Edwards, S. (1989). Ethnic and international students. In. P. A. Grayson, & K. Cauley (Eds.). *College Psychotherapy* (pp. 298–315). New York: Guilford.

Maslen, G. (1997a, October 24). Asians praise British quality. *The Times Higher Education Supplement, no. 1303,* p. 18.

Maslen, G. (1997b, November 28). Universities told they need new strategies to compete for students from Asia. *The Chronicle of Higher Education, 44,* pp. A48–A49.

Mena, F., Padilla, A., & Maldonado, M. (1987). Acculturative stress and specific coping strategies among immigrant and later generation college students. *Hispanic Journal of Behavioral Sciences, 9,* 207–225.

Michailidis, M. P. (1996). A study of factors that contribute to stress within international students (Acculturation). *Dissertation Abstracts International, 57,* 2333A. (University Microfilms No. AAG 9635183)

Ozbay, Y. (1994). An investigation of the relationship between adaptational coping process and self-perceived negative feelings on international students. *Dissertation Abstracts International, 54,* 2958 A. (University Microfilms No. AAG 9404099)

Padilla, A. M., Alvarez, M., & Lindholm, K. J. (1986). Generational status and personality factors as predictors of stress in students. *Hispanic Journal of Behavioral Sciences, 8*(3), 275–288.

Pedersen, P. B. (1985). *Handbook of cross-cultural counseling and therapy.* Westport, CT: Greenwood.

Pedersen, P. B. (1991). Counseling international students. *Counseling Psychologist, 19*(1), 10–58.

Radloff, L. S. (1977). The Center for Epidemiologic Studies Depression Scale (CES-D) for research in the general population. *Applied Psychological Measurements, 1*(3), 385–401.

Redmond, M. V., & Bunyi, J. M. (1993). The relationship of intercultural communication competence with stress and the handling of stress as reported by international students. *International Journal of Intercultural Relations, 17,* 235–254.

Sandhu, D. S. (1993). Making the foreign familiar. *American Counselor, 2*(2), 22–25.

Sandhu, D. S. (1995). An examination of the psychological needs of the international students: Implications for counselling and psychotherapy. *International Journal for the Advancement of Counselling, 17,* 229–239.

Sandhu, D. S. (1997). Psychocultural profiles of Asian and Pacific Islander Americans: Implications for counseling and psychotherapy. *Journal of Multicultural Counseling and Development, 25*(1), 7–22.

Sandhu, D. S., & Asrabadi, B. R. (1994). Development of an acculturative stress scale for international students: Preliminary findings. *Psychological Reports, 75,* 435–448.

Sandhu, D. S., Portes, P. R., & McPhee, S. (1996). Assessing cultural adaptation: Psychometric properties of the Cultural Adaptation Pain Scale. *Journal of Multicultural Counseling and Development, 24,* 15–25.

Schram, J. L., & Lauver, P. J. (1988). Alienation in international students. *Journal of College Student Development, 29*(2), 146–150.

Siegel, C. (1991). Counseling international students: A clinician's comments. *The Counseling Psychologist, 19*(1), 72–75.

Smart, J. F., & Smart, D. W. (1995). Acculturative stress: the experience of the Hispanic immigrant. *The Counseling Psychologist, 23*(1), 25–42.

Spaulding, S., & Flack, M. (1976). *The world's students in the United States: A review and evaluation of research on foreign students.* New York: Praeger.

Sue, D. W., Arredondo, P., & McDavis, R. J. (1992). Multicultural counseling competencies and standards: A call to the profession. *Journal of Counseling and Development, 70,* 477–483.

Thomas, K., & Althen, G. (1989). Counseling foreign students. In

P. B. Pedersen, J. G. Draguns, W. J. Lonner, & J. E. Trimble (Eds.), *Counseling across cultures* (3rd ed.) (pp. 205–241). Honolulu: University of Hawaii Press.

Walton, B. J. (1971). Research on foreign graduate students. *International Educational and Cultural Exchange, 6,* 17–29.

Ward, L., (1967). Some observations on the underlying dynamics of conflict in a foreign student. *Journal of the College Health Association, 10,* 430–440.

Wehrly, B. (1988). Cultural diversity from an international perspective. *Journal of Multicultural Counseling and Development, 16*(1), 7–15.

Westermyer, J. (1989). *Mental health for refugees and other migrants: Social and preventive approaches.* Thomas: Springfield, IL.

Zikopoulos, M. (Ed.). (1993). *Open doors: 1992–1993: report on international educational exchange.* New York: Institute of International Education.

Zwingman, C. A. A. (1978). *Uprooting and related phenomena: a descriptive bibliotherapy* (Doc. MNH/78.23). Geneva: World Health Organization.

African-American Women's Stress Scale (AWSS)

Darielle Watts-Jones, Rockland Children's Psychiatric Center

■ Instrument Names

African-American Women's Stress Scale
AWSS

■ Developer

Darielle Watts-Jones, Ph.D., Rockland Children's Psychiatric Center, Orangeburg, NY

■ Contact Information

Dr. Darielle Watts-Jones, Rockland Children's Psychiatric Center, Orangeburg, NY 10962
Telephone: (914) 961-7220 or (914) 235-8528

Description and History of the Instrument

I developed the AWSS when I was a doctoral candidate in clinical psychology at Duke University (Watts-Jones, 1983). The impetus for its development emerged from my interest in looking at the relationship among stress, social support, and depression among African-American women. A review of the stress literature at that time revealed a predominance of stress scales based on the conceptualization of stress as a function of change (life events) and/or an acute situation (Dohrenwend, Krasnoff, Askenasy, & Dohrenwend, 1978; Holmes & Rahe,

1967). In those few instances in which stressors were either elicited from or rated by African-Americans, the life events model of stress was utilized (Dohrenwend et al., 1978; Rosenberg & Dohrenwend, 1975).

In my view, much of the stress in the lives of African-American women is associated with ongoing situations (lack of change) and/or chronic stressors. Many African-American women of low or marginal income face the stress accompanying inadequate or inferior resources on a daily basis. The demands of parenting and running a household become even more stressful in this context. For example, living in a drug-ridden community introduces an ongoing concern about the safety of one's children, especially when they are outside.

The value of including this conceptualization is reflected in much of the subsequent stress literature (Brown, Bhrolchain & Harris, 1975; Ilfeld, 1977; Myers, 1982). For example, in his study of the relationship between stress and depression, Ilfeld (1977) identifies social stressors as different from life events in that the former are usually tied to a social role, consist of an ongoing circumstance as opposed to a discrete event, and are commonly regarded as problematic or undesirable. His findings indicate that five stressor realms—marital, parental, financial, job, and neighborhood—accounted for 25% of the variance in depression. Brown et al. (1975) found that including major long-term difficulties as stressors strengthened the association between stress and the incidence of affective disturbance beyond that based on life events alone.

The AWSS represents an attempt to develop an ecologically valid stress scale for African-American women. Both the content and the ratings of the stressors were drawn from this population. A major assumption of this instrument is that African-American women provide the best source of identifying the meaningful and relevant stressors in their lives and determining how stressful they are in their experience.

The scale reflects a model of stress as a function of the interaction between an environmental demand (stressor), acute or ongoing, and the subjective elements brought to bear by the individual in perceiving and responding to the stressor. It is an interactive model of stress in that it recognizes that the degree of stress experienced by an individual depends on the interplay of the stimulus demand and the degree to which it is perceived to tax one's resources in meeting the demand. Resources can be spiritual, material, cognitive, physical, or emotional. Thus, a stimulus demand that one perceives can easily be met by one's resources would generate little or no stress, in comparison with one that appears to challenge or override one's resources. This model is consistent with Lazarus's assertion that there are multiple appraisals involved in this process: an initial appraisal involving an assessment of the potential threat of a stressor, followed by an appraisal of one's ability to handle the challenge or threat presented by the stressor (Lazarus, 1966, as cited in Monat & Lazarus, 1991).

The stressors included in the scale were among the most frequent stressors identified by two independent, self-selected samples of African-American women between the ages of 25 and 50. The first sample ($n = 12$) consisted of four women from each socioeconomic class level—middle, working, and lower (Watts-Jones, 1981). The socioeconomic status (SES) of the second sample ($n = 35$) was 25% middle class, 50% working class, and 25% lower class. The SES of this sample resembles that of African-American families in 1986, although the lower class was underrepresented by 5%, and the working class was overrepresented by 16% (U.S. Bureau of the Census, 1986, as cited in Billingsley, 1992).

In both samples, women were asked to identify situations and/or events they considered or would consider stressful, in the sense of "hard to deal with," ranging from a "little hard" to "extremely hard to deal with." Of the entire pool of stressors generated by both samples, a list of 100 stressors was compiled, using the following criteria as guidelines:

■ Similar content: stressors expressing the same or similar situation were treated as one stressor category (e.g., "exam time" and "trying to pass a test" were condensed into "preparing for an exam").

- Frequency of occurrence: all stressors cited by 48% (highest) to 10% (lowest) of the sample were included in the list, accounting for approximately half of the stressors retained. The remaining half varied in frequency from 8% to 2% in the original pool.
- Specificity: retention of stressors was biased toward stressors being as specific as possible. Thus, for example, "not getting a promotion for nonracial reasons" was considered distinct from "not getting a promotion due to race."

These stressors were then rated by 35 of these women as to degree of stressfulness, by placing a mark on a line with opposite ends reflecting least and most stressful. Four of the ratings were eliminated because of an apparent response bias. Thus, the weightings of the stressors in the AWSS are based on a sample of 31 women. The median score across subjects for each stressor was utilized instead of the mean, as the former is less sensitive to extreme scores, and nearly half of the distributions of stressor scores were negatively skewed.

Reliability and Validity

Test-retest reliability of the AWSS was examined in the original research, using a sample of African-American women (n = 64), independent of the sample used to establish stressors and their weightings (Watts-Jones, 1983). The socioeconomic status of this sample was 50% middle class, 38% working class, and 12% lower class; it is not representative of the population of African-American women, being substantially biased toward the higher SES levels. Women ranged in age from 23 to 50 years.

In this study, the AWSS was administered at three 6-week intervals, and respondents were asked to indicate stressors experienced during the preceding 6 weeks. Reliability at 6 weeks was .76, and at 12 weeks was .73.

Internal consistency of the AWSS was found to be .87 among a predominantly African-American sample of mothers (n = 123), in a study of stress, coping, and homelessness (Banyard &, Graham-Bermann, 1997). Two groups of mothers who had at least one child below the age of 12 participated. One group (n = 64) consisted of women living in temporary emgergency shelters. The other group (n = 59) were receiving public assistance and living in their own residences. The two groups were not significantly different in number of children, education level or marital status; however, the homeless group had significantly more African-American women among them than the housed group. Using factor analysis on the 27 items most frequently endorsed by the homeless women (n = 65), Banyard (1995) identified three significant factors that she labeled resource problems, caretaking stress, and relational stress. It is noteworthy that nearly two-thirds of the most frequently endorsed stressors were ongoing situations.

Nearly half of the stressors comprising the AWSS reflect ongoing or chronic situations. Six subgroups were identified (Watts-Jones 1990):

- Inadequate resources (e.g., "unable to afford your own place" [living in another's home], "unsure you can pay rent, utilities and buy food," "unable to afford necessities for your children")
- Work related (e.g., "working at a boring job," "being unemployed")
- Relationship conflict/dissatisfaction (e.g., "your man is possessive/jealous," "trying to find male companionship")
- Role functioning (e.g., "getting children ready in the mornings," "being the only parent")
- Race and ethnicity (e.g. "working with prejudiced co-workers," "not getting a promotion due to race")
- Personal health (e.g., "being overweight," "not enough time for yourself").

The predictive validity of the AWSS has been established in regard to depressive symptomatology. To date, I am unaware of any studies using the AWSS to predict any other outcome measures. In the originating study, the AWSS was able to account for 18% of the variance in depressive symptoms over a 4.5-month period and 23% of the variance over a 6-week period. It is important to note that these figures were obtained using a limited measure of stress. That is, although women identified the total number of stressors experienced over each of three 6-week time intervals, the stress score used was restricted to the 10 stressors identified by respondents as the most stressful.

This approach was taken for reasons of time feasibility, given that support data was being collected for each of these stressors. However, post hoc analyses indicated that this restricted measure was grossly inadequate in representing the level of stress experienced by these women. When the total number of stressors (each stressor weighted by 1) was used as the stress measure, 40% of the variance in depression over a 4.5-month interval and a maximum 49% of the variance in depression over a 6-week interval were accounted for (Watts-Jones, 1990). Additional post hoc analyses using the total number of stressors (each weighted by its median score) revealed 36% of the variance in depression over a 4.5-month period, and a maximum 40% over a 6-week interval were accounted for. Thus, the simpler scheme of weighting stressors by 1 appears to be as or more efficient in predicting depression than using the median as the weighting factor. However, this finding requires further evaluation to determine whether it can be replicated.

Using correlational analysis, Banyard et al. (1997) found that stress (determined by summing the number of AWSS stressors endorsed, each weighted by 1) accounted for 16% of the variance in depressed mood among homeless women. Using hierarchical regression analysis, stress and three measures of coping (active-behavioral, active-cognitive, and avoidance) were entered as step 2, with depressed mood as the outcome measure. Once ethnicity was entered as step 1, the step 2 measures accounted for an additional 28% of the variance in depressed mood. Beta scores were significant for two of the measures—total stress (beta = .36, p < .001) and avoidance coping (beta .32, p < .01). Stress was not a significant predictor of depression among the housed sample of women. When stress and coping measures were introduced at step 2, a nonsignificant 13% of the variance in depression was accounted for. The only significant beta score was for avoidance coping (.32, p < .05).

Benefits and Limitations

The AWSS is a self-report inventory that is easily administered by an interviewer or self-administered in a relatively short time. The items are drawn from a socioeconomic cross-section of African-American women and therefore is not biased toward a particular socioeconomic lifestyle. The scoring procedure for the AWSS is straightforward, especially if the number of stressors is simply totaled. As noted, there is some support for this being as effective as using the median scores as weightings. However, more research evaluating these two weighting schemes is necessary before abandoning the median scores for the more simpler weighting scheme.

Limitations include the self-selected and relatively small samples of African-American women used to derive the AWSS and to examine its ability to predict depressive symptoms. More studies are needed to determine whether this scale can predict depression among African-American women of varying regional and urban-rural backgrounds. Additional research is also needed to examine whether the AWSS can predict other kinds of symptomatology associated with stress.

Chapter References

Banyard, V. and Graham-Bermann, S. (1997). *Survival on the streets: A comparative study of stress and coping in the lives of housed and homeless mothers.* Unpublished manuscript. University of New Hampshire, Durham.

Banyard, V. (1995). Survival on the streets: Coping strategies of mothers who are homeless. *Dissertation Abstracts International,* 55(8), 3578B.

Billingsley, A. (1992). *Climbing Jacob's ladder.* New York: Touchstone.

Brown, G., Bhrolchain, M., & Harris, T. (1975). Social class and psychiatric disturbance among women in an urban population. *Sociology, 9,* 225–254.

Dohrenwend, B., Krasnoff, L., Askenasy, A., & Dohrenwend, B. (1978). Exemplification of a method for scaling life events: The Peri Life Events Scale. *Journal of Health and Social Behavior, 19,* 205–229.

Holmes, T., & Rahe, R. (1967). The Social Readjustment Ratiner Scale. *Journal of Psychosomatic Research, 11,* 213–218.

Ilfeld, F. (1977). Current social stressors and symptoms of depression. *American Journal of Psychiatry, 134,* 161–166.

Monat, A. & Lazarus, R. (1991). *Stress and Coping: An Anthology.* New York: Columbia University Press.

Myers, H. (1982). Stress, ethnicity and social class: A model for research with black populations. In E. Jones and S. Korchin (Eds.), *Minority mental health,* (pp. 118–148). New York: Praeger.

Rosenberg, E. & Dohrenwend, B. (1975). Effects of experience and ethnicity on ratings of life events as stressors. *Journal of Health and Social Behavior, 16,* 127–129.

Watts-Jones, D. (1981). The effect of socioeconomic class on African-American womens' stress perceptions and social support networks. Unpublished master's thesis, Duke University, Durham, NC.

Watts-Jones, D. (1983). The quality of social support among African-American women and its effect as a mediator of the relationship between stress and depression. *Dissertation Abstracts International, 45–11,* 3636B.

Watts-Jones, D. (1990). Toward a stress scale for African-American women. *Psychology of Women Quarterly, 14,* 271–275.

The Coping Resources Inventory for Stress

A Comprehensive Measure of Resources for Stress-Coping

Kenneth B. Matheny and William L. Curlette,
Georgia State University

■ Instrument Names

The Coping Resources Inventory for Stress
The Coping Resources Inventory for Stress: A
  Comprehensive Measure of Resources for Stress-Coping
CRIS

■ Developers

Kenneth B. Matheny, Ph.D.; William L. Curlette, Ph.D.;
  David W. Aycock, Ph.D.; James L. Pugh, Ph.D.; Harry F.
  Taylor, Ed.D.*

■ Contact Information

The CRIS is distributed by Health Prisms, Inc., 130 Pleasant
  Pointe Way, Fayetteville, GA 30214.
Telephone: (770) 460–0808

Description and History of the Instrument

Transactional stress models, such as that offered by Lazarus
(1966, 1981), maintain that objective measures of potentially

---

*The Coping Resources Inventory for Stress (CRIS) is copyrighted by
its developers named here.

43

stressful events (e.g., unemployment, indebtedness, family members leaving home, changes in address, high noise levels) are weak predictors of stress symptoms because they discount personal reactions to these events. Indeed, correlations of life events with stress symptoms such as illness often are quite modest—usually in the range of .2 to .3 (Rabkin & Struening, 1976). Consequently, modern stress theories accord a pivotal role to person variables (e.g., perceptual filters and cognitions) that determine whether life demands will be viewed as stressors, challenges, or perfunctory tasks eliciting no emotional involvement. Lazarus (1981) focused upon the role of appraisal, the primary appraisal of demands and the secondary appraisal of the resources one has for dealing with these demands. Features of the demand (e.g., its intensity and the perceived consequences of failure to deal successfully with it) and resources (e.g., their appropriateness and sufficiency) are taken into consideration in appraising the seriousness of the situation.

Early efforts to measure stress largely were limited to self-reported measures of major environmental demands (Coddington, 1972; Dohrenwend & Dohrenwend, 1974; Holmes & Rahe, 1967; Sarason, Johnson, & Siegel, 1978). Kanner, Coyne, Schaefer, and Lazarus (1981) complemented these measures of macroevents with perceptual measures of microevents—hassles and uplifts. All of these measures, however, attended only to one-half of the stress equation—namely, the measurement of perceived demands. Hobfoll (1988), however, contends that the focus of stress models should be directed mainly to the resource side of the equation. According to his conservation of resources model, people constantly strive to retain, protect, and build coping resources, and they react stressfully to the loss, or potential for loss, of these resources. He argues that the measurement of perceived coping resources will prove more useful in predicting stress symptoms than will the measurement of demands.

Most stress-coping instruments have been designed to measure coping *responses* rather than coping *resources* (Carver,

Scheier, & Weintraub, 1989; Folkman & Lazarus, 1980; Stone & Neale, 1984). Coping responses are behaviors occurring *after* stressors have been engaged, whereas coping resources are factors in place *before* stressors occur (Pearlin & Schooler, 1978). One may draw upon these resource factors to adapt to stressors (Wheaton, 1983). Antonovsky (1979) referred to these resources as general resistance factors.

Some instruments such as the Derogatis Stress Profile (Derogatis, 1980) and the Health and Daily Living Form (Moos, Cronkite, Billings, & Finney, 1985) measure multidimensional aspects of adaptation including stressors, symptoms, and coping. However, because of the ambitious scope of the domains covered and the limitations on testing time, such instruments often fail to offer a comprehensive measurement of coping resources. The Coping Resources Inventory for Stress CRIS (Matheny, Curlette, Aycock, Pugh, & Taylor, 1987) was designed to measure coping resources only, and, because it is a rather lengthy test, it is able to offer a comprehensive array of perceived coping resources.

Data on 700-plus items obtained from over 3,500 subjects were analyzed through disparate group studies, factor analyses, item analysis, item bias studies, and reliability coefficients in order to select the 280 items now appearing on the current version of the inventory. CRIS scales reflect the results of extensive literature reviews (Matheny, Aycock, Pugh, Curlette, & Cannella, 1986), two meta-analyses of the effectiveness of coping resources (Cannella, 1987; Matheny et al., 1986), and several factor analyses of its items (Curlette, Aycock, Matheny, Pugh, & Taylor, 1990). These scales have relatively high internal consistency reliabilities (.84 to .97; median = .88; n = 814) and test-retest reliabilities (.76 to .95 over a 4 week period; $\overline{X}$ = .86; median = .87; n = 34 college students). The 15 scales have moderate to low intercorrelations (range .05 to .62; $\overline{X}$ = .35, median = .33) (Curlette et al., 1990). These features allow it to be used as an inventory offering stable measures of subconstructs all of which contribute to one superordinate construct: coping resources. The relatively high Kuder-Richardson formula 20 (K-R20) reliabilities and large number of items for the scales (20 or more) lead to smaller errors of measurement and more variability in the observed scores. Therefore, differences between scales for the same individual can be used more appropriately for clinical interventions. Evidence of the modifiability of each of the CRIS scales (Aycock & Matheny, 1985) adds further to its clinical usefulness.

The CRIS offers 37 scores: an overall Coping Resources Effectiveness CRE score, 12 Primary Scales, three Composite Scales, 16 Wellness Inhibiting items, and five validity keys. The Primary Scales do not share items with each other and hence offer independent assessments of each resource. The Composite Scales themselves do not have overlapping items but do share some items with six of the Primary Scales.

Scale Descriptors

The following list briefly describes each resource scale along with an example of the items appearing on the scale:

- *Self-Disclosure* is a measure of the tendency to disclose freely one's feelings, troubles, thoughts, and opinions. Item: "I freely share my thoughts and feelings with others."
- *Self-Directedness* measures the degree to which persons respect their own judgment for decision making and therefore demonstrate assertiveness in interpersonal relationships. Item: "I'm very good at standing up for my rights."
- *Confidence* measures the ability to cope successfully—that is, to gain mastery over one's environment and to control one's emotions in the interest of reaching personal goals. Item: "I cope with difficult situations better than most people do."
- *Acceptance* measures the degree to which persons accept their shortcomings and imperfections and maintain a

positive and tolerant attitude toward others and the world at large. Item: "I do not expect too much of myself."

■ *Social Support* measures the availability and use of a network of caring others (usually family members and friends) that acts as a buffer against stressful life events. Item: "I have a satisfying loving relationship with someone."

■ *Financial Freedom* measures the extent to which persons are free of stressful financial restraints to their lifestyles. Item: "I have financial problems because I manage money poorly."

■ *Physical Health* measures the person's overall health condition, including the absence of chronic disease and disabilities. Item: "My health does not restrict my daily activities."

■ *Physical Fitness* measures one's personal health practices, especially physical exercise. Item: "I engage in an exercise program for stretching."

■ *Stress Monitoring* measures one's awareness of tension buildup, situations, and events that are likely to prove stressful, and one's optimal stimulation range. Item: "I'm good at recognizing early signs of tension build-up in my body."

■ *Tension Control* measures one's ability to lower arousal through relaxation procedures and thought control. Item: "I often reduce my stress through physical activity."

■ *Structuring* measures the ability to organize and manage resources such as time and energy. Item: "I am satisfied with my time management skills."

■ *Problem Solving* measures the ability to resolve personal problems. Item: "I often take action on a problem before I fully understand it."

The three Composite Scales are Cognitive Restructuring, Functional Beliefs, and Social Ease:

- *Cognitive Restructuring* measures the ability to change one's thinking in the interest of reducing stress. Item: "When facing frightening tasks, I have learned to rehearse past successes to help calm myself."
- *Functional Beliefs* measures beliefs that are helpful in preventing stressful situations and in lowering stressful arousal. Item: "I have a hard time accepting the fact that many things are different than I would like them to be."
- *Social Ease* measures the degree of comfort one experiences in the presence of others. Item: "I generally feel at ease when I meet people."

Administration, Scoring, and Norms

The CRIS may be administered by either test booklet or personal computer. A seventh-grade reading ability is required; consequently, it is an appropriate instrument for high school students and adults. Typically it takes 45 minutes to an hour to complete with test booklet and roughly 30 to 45 minutes with the personal computer (PC) version. The PC-CRIS is the personal computer program for administering and scoring the CRIS. The PC-CRIS Test Administration Program administers all 280 items as well as the demographic items on the screen of a personal computer. In addition to providing computer administration for the test, this program offers a method of data entry for item responses when the CRIS is administered in a paper-and-pencil format. If the user prefers to scan the data in from the CRIS answer sheet, the PC-CRIS software contains the variable format file for interfacing with National Computer Systems scanners. The PC-CRIS Scoring Program produces Score Reports, Interpretive Reports, Group Summary Reports with means and standard deviations, and a data file of individual scores appropriate for use in statistical analysis programs. For persons using the test booklet, answer sheets may be faxed in for scoring. The computer-generated interpretive report discusses strengths and weaknesses across each of the 15 scales and offers remedial strategies and reading assignments for each weakness noted. The report is written in essay form for the lay public. Consequently, the report typically is given to the client for reading as a homework assignment. The normative sample (n = 1,199) is weighted by race, gender, and age so as to be somewhat representative of the United States population.

Psychometric Characteristics

Instrument Development

During instrument development, all primary standards presented in the Standards for Educational and Psychological Testing were addressed (American Educational Research Association, 1985). This included efforts to eliminate racial, ethnic, and sexual bias from the CRIS through panels using item review procedures and statistical analyses. Overall, the instrument development process took 8 years and involved seven versions of the test prior to the final version. The types of studies conducted during those 8 years included content validity studies and tables of specifications, item format studies (true/false vs. Likert), investigations involving common stems for items, group difference studies, factor analyses, item analyses, fake good versus fake bad studies, correlations of CRIS items with items and scales of other tests, and interscale correlations.

Factor Analyses

Factor analysis studies were conducted on two different data sets to ensure that CRIS scales have construct validity in terms of representing underlying dimensions in the data. The factor analysis procedure used was iterated principle factor analysis with communality estimates obtained from squared multiple correlations and an oblique rotation (direct quartimin) where the default value for gamma was used to rotate factors with eigenvalues greater than one. Factor analyses were conducted using the responses of 1,352 people to 240 items on the fourth version of the CRIS (Pugh, 1984). These factor analyses supported 12 primary factors, while a Second-order factor analysis upheld the notion of one overall coping effectiveness score. Then a new item pool of 438 items was constructed by writing enough items for each of the hypothesized factors to have approximately 40 items assigned a priori to each hypothesized factor. Using a new data set of 2,450 people, factor analyses were run along with item to scale correlations to create the final (eighth) version of the CRIS. A detailed description of these studies is provided in the *Coping Resources Inventory for Stress Manual* (Curlette, et al., 1990).

A concern during instrument development was increasing unnecessarily the number of items on the CRIS. Two of the weakest factors were Social Ease and Functional Beliefs. It was decided to keep these factors but overlap items with the Primary Scales in order to use fewer items on the CRIS. One additional scale, Cognitive Restructuring, was created, primarily based on the examining the correlations of items. These three scales—Social Ease, Functional Beliefs, and Cognitive Restructuring—are referred to as Composite Scales. The domains covered by these scales match the content of many stress management training efforts and, consequently, often prove useful in measuring the effectiveness of such training.

Interscale Correlations

The intercorrelations for the scales derived from the factor analyses are reported in the CRIS manual (Curlette et al., 1990) based on a sample ($n = 814$) different from the samples used in the factor analyses. The intercorrelations of the Primary Scales typically fall in the moderate range, as would be expected for variables from the same general domain. Correlations of the Primary Scales with the CRE ranged from .81

for Confidence to .43 for Physical Fitness. All the correlations of the Social Desirability scale and the Infrequency scale were negative, with every Primary Scale providing additional support for the Validity scales.

Reliability

Internal Consistency. Studies were conducted throughout the instrument development process to ensure that all the Primary and Composite Scales would have internal consistency reliabilities of at least .80 in the final version. The K-R20 reliabilities for the 12 Primary and the 3 Composite Scales ranged from .92 to .84 using a cross validation sample not used in instrument development (n = 814). The overall coping resource score, named the Coping Resource Effectiveness (CRE) score, had 260 items and a K-R20 reliability of .97.

Test-Retest Reliability. Test-retest reliabilities for the coping resource scales indicate a high level of stability. The CRIS was administered twice to a sample of 34 undergraduates with 4 weeks between administrations. The test-retest reliabilities for the Primary and Composite scales ranged from .95 to .76. The CRE had a test-retest reliability of .95.

Critical Items. Items were retained in the test as Wellness Inhibiting Items to alert test takers about practices or conditions that interfere with their optimal health. These items refer to conditions and practices such as being seriously overweight, smoking, and crash dieting. The test takers' responses to these items are printed out separately on the Score Report, and a remediation paragraph for each of these items not responded to in the keyed direction is provided in the Interpretive Report.

Validity Studies

Foremost among a test's characteristics is its validity. Although we use the terms *content* and *criterion-referenced* to describe validity, we subscribe to Messick's (1995) view that ultimately these types of validity support construct validity. Establishing validity is a matter of accumulating evidence for the meaningfulness, usefulness, and appropriateness of test scores for making inferences.

Since the instrument development process for the CRIS was completed in 1988, multiple studies have been conducted to establish the validity of the instrument. We review studies demonstrating the usefulness of the CRIS in contributing to theory development, in establishing the coping resource profiles of drug abusers, in pretest/posttest group difference studies, and in medical research. Some of the validity studies provide descriptions of treatments used in the research studies that exemplify ways the CRIS can be applied in practical situations. Furthermore, correlations between scales on the CRIS and many other psychological instruments are presented.

Theory Development

Roseman's Model. A study by McCarthy, Lambert, and Brack (1996) provides some construct validity evidence for grouping CRIS Primary Scales into two groups (preventive and combative coping resources) as well as showing relationships between CRIS scores and emotional appraisals. Using a path analysis model, McCarthy et al. (1996) investigated the relationships between two sets of CRIS coping resources termed preventive (self-directedness, confidence, acceptance, financial freedom, and physical health) and combative (self-disclosure, social support, physical fitness, tension control, and problem solving) along with three measures derived from Roseman, Spindel, and Jose's (1990) cognitive appraisals on the end of a romantic relationship assessed at two different times. The 231 participants were graduate students. The results suggest that preventive coping resources influence the appraised desirability of the event, ending the romantic relationship, and the initial emotional reactions. Combative coping resources were more related to subsequent emotional responses.

Laygo's (1996) comparison of Roseman's model with Ellsworth's and Smith's model (1988) involved the CRIS. He supported Roseman's model and found that the Functional Beliefs scale on the CRIS was related to the degree to which one experiences negative emotions in a stressful situation.

Adlerian Theory. In one study (Kern, Gfroerer, Summers, Curlette, & Matheny, 1996), stress coping as measured by the CRIS was related to personality variables based on the constructs of Adlerian psychology. These personality variables were assessed with the Basic Adlerian Scales for Interpersonal Success—Adult Form (BASIS-A; Wheeler, Kern, & Curlette, 1993). A unique feature of the 65-item BASIS-A inventory is that it asks an individual to recollect childhood experiences rather than describe present functioning. Correlations between BASIS-A and CRIS scales support Adlerian theory, which emphasizes that perceptions of early childhood experiences are indicative of a person's approach to life. For example, the Belonging–Social Interest scale on the BASIS-A inventory is statistically significant ($p < .05$) with 11 of the 12 Primary CRIS scales. The largest correlation is between the BASIS-A Being Cautious scale (which measures hurt in the family of origin) and Social Support on the CRIS ($r = -.59$, $p < .001$). This implies that people who see the environment for their family of origin as unpredictable, unfair, or dangerous will tend to lack Social Support as a coping resource.

These results have implications for counseling by providing evidence that a person's perceptions of early childhood experiences are related to coping resources. Other researchers have found relationships between personality variables and coping resources (Fleishman, 1984; Houtman, 1990) but not from the Adlerian perspective.

Jungian Theory. In a study of 101 school teachers, Davis-Johnson (1991) found that teachers designated as Extroverts on the Myers-Briggs Type Indicator ($\overline{X} = 75.8$) were significantly different ($p < .001$) than Introverts ($\overline{X} = 57.9$) on the CRIS Self-Disclosure scale. On the CRIS Structuring scale, Perceptive types ($\overline{X} = 55.5$) were significantly different

($p > .001$) than Judging types ($\overline{X} = 79.1$). In addition, she found the CRE and seven CRIS scales to correlate negatively ($p < .008–.001$) with burnout as measured by the Pines-Aronson Burnout Scale. She also found that Extroversion and Intuition are related to greater overall coping resources ($p < .001$). Davis-Johnson concluded that Jungian theory may provide a key to understanding people's affinity for certain coping resources. That relationships exist between coping resources and psychological type is independently supported by Hammer (1988).

Clinical Applications

Drug Dependency and Counseling

The CRIS was administered to 45 inpatients for drug or alcohol abuse in the addiction unit of a major hospital. Research results reported by Longine, Cannella, Gilead, and Mulaik (1995) show that the mean CRIS Coping Resource Effectiveness score of the inpatients was 1.45 standard deviations below the mean for the norm group on the CRIS. The means for the inpatient group on all 15 CRIS scales were below the norm group, with effect sizes expressed in standard deviation units ranging from $-.81$ to -1.57. Granade (1990) compared the mean scores of alcoholics on the CRIS scales with the CRIS norms and found significant differences on each scale. The differences between the groups were approximately one standard deviation on most scales. Thus, two separate studies have shown drug abusers to exhibit low coping resources.

In a study of 414 college students (Sineath, Curlette, & Brack, 1995), scores on four of five CRIS scales (Social Support, Structuring, Cognitive Restructuring, and Social Ease) were significantly different for dysfunctional adult children of alcoholics (ACAs), functional ACAs, dysfunctional non-ACAs, and functional non-ACAs. Correlational analyses revealed low to moderate correlations between each of the CRIS scales and the other two tests used in this study: the Children of Alcoholics Screening Test (CAST) and the Family Adaptability and Cohesion Evaluation Scales (FACES II).

At a leading rehabilitation center for drug-addicted professionals, the CRIS is being used (a) as an intake assessment to assist in patient recovery and (b) to document program effectiveness by pretest and posttest assessment. Pretest and posttest differences roughly average 30 percentile points for most CRIS scales. Over 200 people have gone through this program to date.

The CRIS was administered to 263 participants in a smoking cessation treatment program (Matheny & Weatherman, 1997). Follow-up t-tests to a multivariate analysis indicated that relapsers were found to have significantly lower scores than abstainers on the CRIS scales Confidence ($\overline{X} = 66.2$ and $62.6, p < .05$), Physical Fitness ($\overline{X} = 45.8$ and $36.7, p < .001$), and Physical Health ($\overline{X} = 73.4$ and $65.4, p < .001$). The CRIS Physical Fitness scale was predictive of participants who were abstainers versus relapsers 6 months later.

Pretest and Posttest Studies with Interventions

Sensitivity to Instruction. In an instrument development study on the fourth version of the CRIS (Aycock & Matheny, 1985), the modifiability of stress-coping resources was examined in a group of 72 graduate students enrolled in a 10-week psychoeducational training course. Pretest and posttest scores were obtained on the CRIS. Hotelling's T^2 was significant ($p < .001$), and each of the follow-up univariate t-tests indicated gains ($p < .001$) for each of the eight resources being measured. This study provides some evidence that coping resources are modifiable within a relatively short period of time through structured psychoeducational training and that the CRIS is sensitive enough to detect these changes.

The CRIS Interpretive Report as a Treatment. The effectiveness of the CRIS Interpretive Report in improving stress-coping resources in associate degree nursing students was investigated by Rollant & Curlette (1994). The study used two alternative treatment groups and a control group. Treatment group 1 ($n = 46$) participants (a) contracted to work on relaxation, time management, body scanning, problem solving, and confidence; (b) had structured tension control experiences (relaxation exercises and massage instruction); and (c) received a CRIS Interpretive Report. Treatment group 2 ($n = 61$) merely received the CRIS Interpretive Report and were given an opportunity to ask questions about the CRIS. The control group ($n = 54$) took the CRIS pretest and posttest but received no feedback before posttesting.

Although the treatment was designed to improve stress monitoring and tension control, results indicated that members of treatment group 1 (the CRIS Interpretive Report + contracting for change + structured relaxation experiences) attained significantly higher ($p < .05$) posttest scores than control group members on the CRIS scales Self-Disclosure, Self-Directedness, Acceptance, Social Support, Stress Monitoring, and Tension Control. This result seems to demonstrate that effecting changes in some resources may have an effect on others if these resources are correlated. Because the CRIS scales are moderately correlated with each other, improvement in regard to one resource may have a rippling effect upon others. Also, these interpretations provide more support for the construct validity of the CRIS. Members of treatment group 2 (CRIS Interpretive Report only) attained significantly higher ($p < .05$) posttest scores than the control group members on the CRIS scales Self-Disclosure and Tension Control. Thus, it appears that the CRIS Interpretive Report alone may be an effective stress-coping treatment.

Drug Education and Relapse Prevention Interventions. In Junker's (1993) study, 122 federal inmates were randomly assigned to drug education, relapse prevention, or control groups. The CRIS along with the Alcohol Expectancy Questionnaire, Cocaine Effects Expectancy Questionnaire, and the Drug-Taking Confidence Questionnaire were administered as pretests and posttests. The male inmates had knowledge of their pretest CRIS scores prior to a series of group training sessions. Inmates assigned to the drug education condition received 20 hours of didactic instruction corresponding to biological and physiological explanations for addiction. The relapse prevention skills training condition consisted of small group interaction and followed a social learning theory model (Donovan & Chaney, 1985; Marlatt & Gordon, 1985) of addiction. Data analyses were run for three of the CRIS scales hypothesized to be influenced by the treatment. Because of incomplete data or invalid responses, the scores of only 94 of the 122 inmates were included in the data analyses. Effect sizes were calculated by subtracting a control group mean from the treatment group mean and dividing by a standard deviation. The effect sizes representing the differences between the relapse prevention and control groups on the CRIS scales Acceptance, Confidence, and Self-Directedness were .52, .55, and .66, respectively. The effect size representing the difference between the drug education and the control group on Self-Directedness was .70, and for Acceptance and Confidence the effect sizes were .20 and .35, respectively.

Psychoeducational Intervention. In a model dissertation at the University of Florida, Stewart (1991) provided a psychoeducational counseling intervention for adults who were responsible for the care of a parent at least 60 years old. The intervention consisted of four 2-hour, weekly sessions in which the research discussed the aging process, communication skills, stress and time management, and developmental issues related to mid- and late life. In a delayed treatment control group design with pretests and posttests, significant differences using version 5 of the CRIS were found on the CRE and the Self-Disclosure scale.

Cooperative Education Intervention. A study by Bono (1995) examined the feasibility of looking at CRIS scores as outcome variables for a 12-week cooperative education experience for undergraduate college students in a Fortune 500 company. Using a nonequivalent pretest/posttest control group design, no significant differences were found on the CRIS scales in comparison with a control group of undergraduate students not in cooperative education. There was no specific instruction on stress coping; the intervention consisted only of the usual work experience in a national technical support center for computers. However, using multiple regression, two CRIS scales (Confidence, $p = .020$, and Physical Health, $p = .020$) were statistically significant predictors of the supervisors ratings of the overall job performance of these students.

Correlations of the CRIS with other Instruments

Strong support was found for the convergent and divergent validity of the CRIS scales (Matheny, Aycock, Curlette, & Junker, 1993). Administered concurrently with the Interpersonal Behavior Survey, the Social Support Questionnaire, the State-Trait Anxiety Inventory, the Depression Adjective Checklist, the Beck Depression Inventory, the Social Reticence Scale, and the Shipley Institute of Living Scale, the CRIS scales provided significant convergent correlations in 29 of 32 instances. Also as hypothesized, none of the 37 divergent correlations were significant. Table 1 summarizes the correlations of six CRIS scales with the Beck Depression Inventory and the State-Trait Anxiety Inventory. Table 2 summarizes the correlations of the overall score on the CRIS, the Coping Resource Effectiveness score, with other tests taken from several studies. All correlations reported in Table 2 are statistically significant with $p < .05$ except those reported in parentheses. In regard to the magnitude of the correlations, it should be noted that the correlations are not with tests purporting to measure "coping resources" but with tests addressing other aspects of stress coping models. The sample sizes on which the correlations are based are furnished in the table in order to indicate the stability of the correlation.

Wedl (1986) found the CRE score on version 5 of the CRIS to correlate with the *Life Satisfaction Index* for a sample of

Table 1: Correlations of CRIS Scales with the Beck Depression Inventory (BDI) and the State-Trait Anxiety Inventory (STAI)

CRIS Scale	Other Psychological Instrument	Pearson Correlation*
Self-Disclosure	BDI	-.30
Problem Solving	BDI	-.34
Social Ease	BDI	-.42
Confidence	BDI	-.46
Social Support	BDI	-.35
Acceptance	BDI	-.45
Self-Disclosure	STAI	-.37
Problem Solving	STAI	-.44
Social Ease	STAI	-.43
Confidence	STAI	-.64
Social Support	STAI	-.45
Acceptance	STAI	-.46

* *Note*: $n = 68$.

older persons ($n = 55$, $p < .05$). Four of the primary CRIS scales also correlated significantly with the *Life Satisfaction Index*: Social Support, Confidence, Acceptance, and Problem Solving (p values ranging from .05 to .01). This finding suggests that the greater one's coping resources, the greater is one's satisfaction with life.

Medical Studies

HIV Infection. Hughes (1993) studied 89 HIV-infected individuals according to the Centers for Disease Control

Table 2: Correlations of the CRIS Overall Score Coping Resource Effectiveness (CRE) with Other Tests

CRIS Scale	Other Psychological Instrument	Pearson Correlation	Reference & Sample Size
CRE	Tennessee Self-Concept Scale	.53	Bird (1992), $n = 48$
CRE	Self-Profile Chart	.28	Bird (1992), $n = 48$
CRE	Hs Scale of the MMPI	-.50	Seitz (1989), $n = 166$
CRE	Pines-Aronson Burnout Scale	-.61	Davis-Johnson (1991), $n = 101$
CRE	Seriousness of Illness Rating Scale	-.35	Rapp (1988), $n = 102$
CRE	Seriousness of Illness Rating Scale	-.38	Ellett (1991), $n = 91$
CRE	Beck Depression Inventory	-.63	Ellett (1991), $n = 92$
CRE	Taylor Manifest Anxiety	-.63	Ellett (1991), $n = 92$
CRE	Uplifts Frequency	.44	Ellett (1991), $n = 91$
CRE	Uplifts Severity	(-.13)	Ellett (1991), $n = 91$
CRE	Hassles Frequency	(-.15)	Ellett (1991), $n = 90$
CRE	Hassles Severity	-.27	Ellett (1991), $n = 91$
CRE	Dean Scale of Alienation	-.43	Ellett (1992), $n = 92$
CRE	BASIS A Belonging-Social Interest	.38	Kern et al. (1996), n = 173
CRE	BASIS-A Softness	.53	Kern et al. (1996), n = 173
CRE	Positive Symptom Distress	-.38	Peeler (1991), $n = 213$
CRE	Positive Symptom Total	(-.08)	Peeler (1991), $n = 213$
CRE	General Severity Index	-.23	Peeler (1991), $n = 213$

groupings II, III, and IVC2. Using multiple regression with the Global Severity Index of the SCL-90 R as the dependent variable, a statistically significant ($F = 34.9$, $p < .0001$) predictive equation was derived that included significant contributions by Confidence, Physical Health, and Acceptance.

This model had a multiple R of .74 and according to an adjusted R^2 accounted for 54% of the variance in the Global Severity Index scores.

Another multiple regression was run using a measure of the body's cellular immune response, CD4 T-lymphocytes, as the dependent variable. Of all the CRIS Primary scales, only Financial Freedom predicted ($p = .03$) the CD4 count by accounting for 5% of the variability.

A comparison of the HIV sample to a user norm group of 1,187 subjects resulted in 12 of the 15 CRIS scales showing significant mean differences ($p < .001$, except for Tension Control where $p = .012$). No mean differences were found on Self-Directedness ($p = .296$), Acceptance ($p = .083$), and Functional Beliefs ($p = .082$).

Eating Disorders. Buchanan (1993) compared 17 restricting anorexics, 24 bulimic anorexics, 50 bulimics, and 51 binge eaters on the CRIS, the Eating Disorder Inventory, Dissociative Experiences Scale, Symptoms Checklist-90 R, and the Zung Self-Rating Depression Scale. Significant differences between at least two of the eating disorder groups were observed on the CRIS scales of Functional Beliefs, Social Ease, Social Support, Self-Directedness, Confidence, and Physical Health.

Psychotropic Medications. Peeler (1991) compared the coping resources (CRIS) of 213 medical patients who were prescribed psychotropic medications by their primary care physicians to those patients who were not given psychotropic medications. In addition to the CRIS, the Symptom Checklist, Revised (SCL-R 90), and a medication checklist were administered to the 213 outpatients. A multivariate analysis of variance run on the CRIS compared the 12 Primary Scales and CRE for the two groups of medical patients. Not only was the overall Wilks's lambda significant ($p < .001$), but every one of the 12 Primary Scales and the CRE had statistically significant mean differences ($p < .001$). The effect sizes were moderate to large.

Cardiac Reactivity. Buzzell (1991) found significant correlations between certain CRIS scales and heart rate reactivity and systolic blood pressure for 80 university student volunteers (40 African Americans and 40 Caucasians) with a family history of hypertension when confronted with stressors. More particularly, scores for African Americans on Tension Control were inversely correlated with both heart rate reactivity (i.e., the degree of change in heart rate) ($r = -.37$, $p < .05$) and systolic blood pressure ($r = -.40, p < .05$) when confronting stressful arithmetical computations. Scores for African Americans on Tension Control were also correlated significantly with systolic blood pressure ($r = -.40, p < .05$) when stressed by the Stroop color-naming task. Scores for African Americans on Cognitive Restructuring were correlated significantly with both heart rate reactivity ($r = -.33$, $p < .05$) when stressed by the Stroop color-naming task and with blood pressure ($r = -.47, p < .01$) when confronting stressful arithmetical computation. Scores for African Americans and whites on the Confidence scale were significantly correlated with heart rate reactivity when confronting stressful arithmetic computation ($r = -.44, p < .01$ and $r = -.31$, $p < .01$, respectively).

Nutrition. In an investigation of the effects of nutrition on stress coping, Brock (1991) studied 90 adults from health centers and counseling centers who responded to inventories regarding nutrient intake (Right Byte Nutrition Evaluator), stressors (Schedule of Recent Experiences), and stress coping resources (CRIS). Using a blocks-by-treatment analysis of variance design with anxiety (State-Trait Anxiety Inventory) as the outcome measure, a three way interaction was statistically significant ($p = .004$), and the three levels of coping (high, medium, and low categorization of the CRIS CRE) were significant ($p < .000001$). In general, greater coping resources as measured by the CRIS was found related to reduced anxiety in a variety of treatment conditions.

Occupational Choice

Walker (1991) found significant differences on the CRIS Problem Solving and CRE scores between African American women in occupations traditionally dominated by women and those traditionally dominated by men ($\overline{X}$ = 70.9 and 78.6, p < .05; $\overline{X}$ = 68.74 and 75.57, p < .01, respectively). Moreover, she found significant differences in favor of white women over African-American women on five of the CRIS scales.

Acculturation

Miranda, Hill, and Timberlake (1993) studied the acculturation of Spanish-speaking immigrants who were living in a large metropolitan area of the southeastern United States. The CRE correlated .78 with the Hispanic Acculturation Scale. Five CRIS scales—Self-Directedness, Social Ease, Confidence, Acceptance, and Structuring—all entered a regression equation predicting acculturation. Three of the five (Confidence, Self-Directedness, and Social Ease) alone accounted for 48.54% of the variance in acculturation scores. These results suggest that the higher the coping resources, the higher the level of acculturation.

Validity Scales

In general, self-report instruments for which the more desirable response on a item is fairly self-evident are more susceptible to faking. An advantage of the CRIS is that it provides five measures of test taking validity: Social Desirability; Infrequency (tending to fake for lower scores); Random Response (X-ZERO) starting at the beginning of the test; Random Response (X-100), which measures random responding that starts after the first 100 items; and the Number of Omitted Items on a scale. Elevated Social Desirability scores were found in two studies with convicted criminals (Junker, 1993; Kinard, 1991). This result could be due to a tendency of criminals to exaggerate their coping resources. In a study of military personal (Seitz, 1989), the Random Response indicator revealed that 10% of the soldiers randomly responded to the

CRIS. In Junker's study, 17 of the 122 inmate participants (13.9%) had invalid CRIS profiles because of random guessing. In both studies the random guessers were eliminated from data analyses as their scores would contribute to error variance; thus making finding patterns in the data more difficult. These results indicate the importance of using validity scales when assessing coping resources.

Research in Progress

In a veterans' hospital, a 3-year research study (Kimani & Aguayo, 1996) is under way to study the quality of life of patients with the lung disease sarcoidosis. To date, over 40 patients from the Sarcoidois Center have completed the CRIS, the Perceived Stress Scale, and the Daily Hassles Scale. These scales will be analyzed in conjunction with extensive medical data. Kirkscey, Carlson, and Brack (1996) are examining the construct of leadership from within (Palmer, 1994) as it relates to coping resources as measured by the CRIS. Other investigations using the CRIS that are currently in progress include a study of stress-coping resources relative to the progression of treatments for allergies and cross-cultural studies in England, the Ivory Coast, Portugal, and Russia.

Uses of the Instrument

The CRIS is used widely in psychotherapy and training. Clinicians find it useful to assess the resources available to clients, for these resources determine in large measure whether life demands will be viewed as routine tasks, challenges, or stressors. The large number of items and high reliabilities for each scale constitute a strong endorsement for the clinical use of the CRIS. The broad spectrum of coping resources measured by the CRIS renders it useful in predicting how clients will deal with stressful situations. Therapists customarily use the two-paged Score Report in interpreting results to clients within the therapy session. The Interpretive Report is given to the client to read as a homework assignment between sessions. No sophisticated understanding of psychological concepts is necessary on the part of clients to understand the report. The Interpretive Report addresses validity concerns, points out strengths and weaknesses across each of the 15 scales, offers recommendations for treating deficits, and suggests reading materials for clients wishing to learn more about their deficit resources.

The CRIS is used effectively in seminars and workshops dealing with themes such as stress management, marriage adjustment, communication difficulties, and performance failure. In these workshops break-out groups consisting of participants with the same deficit resources have been used to allow the content to be adjusted to their needs. The CRIS has been used in a wide variety of settings. For example, it currently is being used in officer training by the U.S. Air Force, in recovery centers for wounded healers, in mental hospitals and drug addiction units, and in college and university counseling centers. Typically participants take the CRIS early in the workshop and their protocols are faxed to the scoring service. Within minutes results are returned electronically.

Our research suggests that the coping resources of children differ somewhat from those of adults. Consequently, a companion instrument to the CRIS, named the Coping Resources Inventory Scales for Educational Enhancement (CRISEE) was developed. The CRISEE is appropriate for grades 3 through 10 and has a reading level of 1.5. The CRISEE is a 99-item true/false instrument that measures six coping resources and 18 stressors. It has an optional 40 item behavior checklist that the teacher can fill out for each student. The scales on the CRISEE are Academic Confidence, Social Confidence, Family Support, Peer Acceptance, Behavior Control, and an experimental scale named Responsibility. The K-R20 reliabilities of these scales range from .81 to .85. Five types of reports are provided by the PC-CRISEE software: a one-page individual report (two pages if teacher data on the student's behavior is included), a classroom summary report, a grade-level report, a school-level report by grades, and a school system report. When the CRISEE is employed outside the school for individual counseling, only the individual report is generated. Unlike the CRIS, interpreting a CRISEE report is not as involved as interpreting a CRIS report.

Interpreting a CRIS Score Report

The CRIS Score Report is the two-page summary of scores (see Table 3). Clinicians typically choose to work from this summary in presenting the results to clients in the therapy session, and recommended steps for the proper use of the report are then presented.

Step 1: Check the Social Desirability Centile Rank. Go to the back page of the Score Report and look at Social Desirability Centile Rank. Scores above the 90th centile suggest respondents may have a tendency to present themselves in a socially desirable manner. Scores above the 98th centile suggest the scores likely are not representative of the respondent's resources.

Step 2: Check the Infrequency Centile Rank. Go to the back page of the Score Report and look at the Infrequency Centile Rank. The Infrequency scale consists of 24 items indicative of undesirable conditions or practices that less than 20% of the normative sample answered in the undesirable direction. Centile ranks 90 and above could suggest a tendency to fake bad responses or to be excessively harsh in regard to self-evaluation.

Step 3: Check the Random Response indicators. The back page of the Score Report also includes two random response indicators. Both indicators should read "Unlikely" in order for the reports to be considered valid. If the report says "Likely," there is evidence for random guessing. Research indicates that only 3 times in 1,000

Table 3: A Sample CRIS Score Report

The Coping Resources Inventory for Stress
CRIS
(Side One)

NAME: John Doe   DATE: February 13, 1997
ID NUMBER: 236-33-1606

PRIMARY SCALES:	PERCENT	CENTILE	68%	BAND
1. Self-Disclosure	70.0	53	44	64
2. Self-Directedness	75.0	71	57	86
3. Confidence	55.0	30	23	42
4. Acceptance	80.0	85	74	96
5. Social Support	85.0	59	42	86
6. Financial Freedom	80.0	59	47	75
7. Physical Health	75.0	46	29	68
8. Physical Fitness	50.0	54	46	62
9. Stress Monitoring	90.0	71	57	99
10. Tension Control	50.0	43	30	56
11. Structuring	95.0	94	72	99
12. Problem Solving	70.0	43	30	57
COMPOSITE SCALES:				
13. Cognitive Restructuring	62.0	47	35	61
14. Functional Beliefs	86.0	91	80	99
15. Social Ease	68.0	45	32	59
Coping Resource Effectiveness	65.0	66	58	74

Continued on next page

Table 3 (*Continued*)

The Coping Resources Inventory for Stress
CRIS
(Side Two)

WELLNESS INHIBITING ITEMS
(Conditions/Practices Which Interfere With Optimal Health)

ITEM INDICATES	YOUR RESPONSE (0 = No Response, 1 = Yes, 2 = No)
Life Threatening Illness	2
Physical Handicap	2
Seriously Overweight	2
Eating Disorder	2
Frequent Headaches	1
Breathing Problems	2
Sleeping Problems	2
Frequently Anxious	2
Frequently Depressed	1
Often Angry	2
Smoking	2
More Than 3 Caffeine Drinks per Day	2
More Than 2 Alcoholic Drinks per Day	2
Tranquilizers or Sleeping Pills	2
Medicine for Health Problem	2
Crash Diets	2

SCORE VALIDITY

Social Desirability	Percent Score = 15.0	Centile Rank = 12
Infrequency	Percent Score = 0.0	Centile Rank = 17
Random Response (X - Zero):	Unlikely	
Random Response (X - 100):	Unlikely	

Fewer Than Three Items Were Omitted On Any Subscale

---

will a person answering honestly be falsely accused of random guessing.

Step 4: Check the Wellness Inhibiting items. Glance at the 16 Wellness Inhibiting items on the back page of the Score Report and note any wellness inhibiting conditions or practices indicated. The Interpretive Report presents discussions of these scales after the coping resource scales. It should be noted that each Wellness Inhibiting item is based on the respondent's answer to only one item and consequently merely serves as a stimulus for further discussion. Before interpreting the coping resource scales, look for a yes response to the item "Medicine for Health Problems." Check out the medications being taken by respondents, for they may have affected their responses.

Step 5: Now review the Coping Resource Effectiveness score. Discuss first the overall score for the test, the CRE, for it is based on 260 of the 280 test items. The Percent Correct score is the percentage of items the respondent answered in the keyed direction. Thus, a score of 80 indicates that the respondent answered 208 of the 260 items in the keyed direction. The Centile Rank indicates where a person stands in relation to a representative sample of the U.S. population. Hence, a Centile Rank of 75 indicates that the respondent has the same amount (or more) of coping resources as 75% of the normative sample.

Step 6: Next review the 15 Coping Resource scores. When interpreting the individual resource scores, the focus initially should be on the person's strengths to establish a positive context within which to frame deficit scores. It may help also to point out that low scores on some coping resources can be compensated for by higher scores on others.

Step 7: Examine the 68% Band Centiles. You should keep the 68% Band Centiles in mind when interpreting the 15 coping resource scales. These bands are only reported on the Score Report for they would be difficult to understand by the reading public. When any two 68% Band Centiles overlap, then the person's scores are not statistically different from each other. That is, the difference could be accounted for by various errors in the measurement process (e.g., the person's feelings on the day he or she took the CRIS or the misinterpretation of an item). When the 68% Band Centiles do not overlap, then the amount of the person's resources on the two scales is believed to be different.

Future Directions

The CRIS has been translated into Spanish, Russian, French, and Vietnamese and is currently being translated into Portuguese. Presently, it is being used in Russia, Paraguay, French Equatorial Africa, Singapore, and Portugal. Research is being conducted in these centers to examine the necessity for item revision to accommodate differences in cultural values. Ultimately, the test constructors plan to conduct international comparative studies of the mean coping resources of participating countries.

Chapter References

Antonovsky, A. (1979). *Health, stress and coping.* San Francisco: Jossey-Bass.

American Educational Research Association, American Psychological Association, & National Council on Measurement in Education. (1985). *Standards for educational and psychological testing.* Washington, DC: American Psychological Association.

Aycock, D. W., & Matheny, K. B. (1985). *Assessment of stress coping resource modifiability through psychoeducational training.* Unpublished manuscript. Georgia State University, Atlanta.

Bono, J. D. (1995). *The effects of a first time cooperative education work experience on maturity, self-esteem, and problem solving skills*. Unpublished doctoral dissertation, Georgia State University, Atlanta.

Brock, D. D. (1991). *The effects of nutrition on coping with stress*. Unpublished doctoral dissertation, Georgia State University, Atlanta, Georgia.

Buchanan, L. P. (1993). *Coping resources, personality and research design in eating disorder subgroups*. Unpublished doctoral dissertation, Georgia State University, Atlanta.

Buzzell, V. M. (1991). *The effects of stress coping resources, race, and parental history of hypertension on cardio-vascular reactivity to mental stressors*. Unpublished doctoral dissertation, Georgia State University, Atlanta.

Cannella, K. A. S. (1987). *The effectiveness of stress coping interventions: A meta-analysis with methodological implications*. Unpublished doctoral dissertation, Georgia State University, Atlanta.

Carver, C. S., Scheier, M. F., & Weintraub, J. K. (1989). Assessing coping strategies: A theoretically based approach. *Journal of Personality and Social Psychology, 56*(2), 267–283.

Coddington, R. D. (1972). The significance of life events as etiologic factors in the diseases of children. *Journal of Psychosomatic Research, 16*, 17–18.

Curlette, W. L., Aycock, D. W., Matheny, K. B., Pugh, J. L., & Taylor, H. F. (1990). *Coping Resources Inventory for Stress Manual*. Atlanta, GA: Health Prisms.

Davis-Johnson, L. (1991). *The effects of psychological type on stress coping resources and professional burnout*. Unpublished doctoral dissertation, Georgia State University, Atlanta.

Derogatis, L. R. (1980). *The Derogatis Stress Profile (DSP)*. Baltimore, MD: Clinical Psychometric Research.

Dohrenwend, B. S., & Dohrenwend, B. P. (Eds.). (1974). *Stressful life events: Their nature and effects*. New York: Wiley.

Donovan, D. M., & Chaney, E. F. (1985). Alcoholic relapse prevention and intervention: Models and methods. In G. A. Marlatt & J. R. Gordon (Eds.), *Relapse prevention: Maintenance strategies in the treatment of addictive behaviors* (pp. 351–416). New York: Guildford.

Ellsworth, P. C., & Smith, C. A. (1988). Shades of joy: Patterns of appraisal differentiating pleasant emotions. *Cognition and Emotion, 2*(4), 301–331.

Fleishman, J. A. (1984). Personality characteristics and coping patterns. *Journal of Health and Social Behavior, 25*(2), 229–244.

Folkman, S., & Lazarus, R. S. (1980). An analysis of coping in a middle-aged community sample. *Journal of Health and Social Behavior, 21*, 219–239.

Granade, J. (1990). *Patterning of coping resources among alcoholics.* Unpublished manuscript.

Hammer, A. L. (1988, April). *Type and coping resources.* Paper presented at the annual conference of the Association for Psychological Type, Boulder, CO.

Hobfoll, S. E. (1988). Conservation of resources: A new attempt at conceptualizing stress. *American Psychologist, 44*(3), 513–524.

Holmes, T. H., & Rahe, R. H. (1967). The Social Readjustment Rating Subtest. *Journal of Psychosomatic Research, 11*, 213–218.

Houtman, I. L. (1990). Personal coping resources and sex differences. *Personality and Individual Differences, 11*(1), 53–63.

Hughes, J. D. (1993). *Coping resources and human immunodeficiency virus (HIV).* Unpublished doctoral dissertation, Georgia State University, Atlanta.

Junker, G. (1993). *An assessment of multiple intervention strategies for changing addiction-related expectations and coping resources within an incarcerated population.* Unpublished doctoral dissertation, Georgia State University, Atlanta.

Kanner, A., Coyne, J., Schaefer, C., & Lazarus, R. (1981). Comparison of two modes of stress measurement: Daily hassles and uplifts versus major life events. *Journal of Behavioral Medicine, 4*, 1–39.

Kern, R., Gfroerer, K., Summers, Y., Curlette, W., & Matheny, K. (1996). Lifestyle, personality, and stress coping. *Journal of Individual Psychology, 52*(1), 72–81.

Kimani, A., & Aguayo, S. (1996). *The Emory Sarcoidosis Center Research Program: Phase I.* Atlanta, GA: Veterans Affairs Medical Center.

Kinard, R. (1991). *Profiling the stress coping resources of arrested domestic batterers.* Unpublished doctoral dissertation, Georgia State University, Atlanta.

Kirkscey, M. L., Carlson, M. H., & Brack, G. (1996, August). *The construct leadership from within as related to coping resources: Implications for organization consultants.* Paper presented at the annual conference of the American Psychological Association, Toronto.

Laygo, R. M. (1996). *The power of competing cognitive theories of emotions, stress coping, and their interactions in predicting emo-*

tional reactions to stressful events. Unpublished doctoral dissertation, Georgia State University, Atlanta.

Lazarus, R. (1966). *Psychological stress and the coping process.* New York: McGraw-Hill.

Lazarus, R. (1981). The stress and coping paradigm. In C. Eisdorfer, D. Cohen, A. Kleinman, & P. Maxim (Eds.), *Models of clinical psychopathology* (pp. 177–214). New York: Spectrum.

Longine, L., Cannella, K. S., Gilead, M. P., & Mulaik, J. S. (1995). Addicted patients' attitudes, beliefs, and responses to touch. Nursing Research Workshop sponsored by the Research Constituency Center, Nursing Services, Veterans Affairs Medical Center, Atlanta, GA.

Marlatt, G. A., & Gordon, J. R. (Eds.). (1985). *Relapse Prevention.* New York: Guilford Press.

Matheny, K. B., Aycock, D. W., Curlette, W. L., & Junker, G. (1993). The Coping Resources Inventory for Stress: A measure of perceived coping resources. *Journal of Clinical Psychology, 49*(6), 815–830.

Matheny, K. B., Aycock, D. W., Pugh, J. L., Curlette, W. L., & Cannella, K. A. S. (1986). Stress coping: A qualitative and quantitative synthesis with implications for treatment. *The Counseling Psychologist, 14*(4), 499–549.

Matheny, K. B., Curlette, W. L., Aycock, D. W., Pugh, J. L., & Taylor, H. F. (1987). *The Coping Resources Inventory for Stress.* Atlanta, GA: Health Prisms.

Matheny, K. B., & Weatherman, K. E. (1998). Predictors of smoking cessation and maintenance. *Journal of Clinical Psychology, 54*(2), 222–235.

McCarthy, C., Lambert, R., & Brack, G. (1996, August). *A structural model of coping appraisals, emotions, and relationship loss.* Paper presented to Division 12 at the annual convention of the American Psychological Association, Toronto.

Messick, S. (1995). Validity of psychological assessment: Validation of inferences from person's responses and performances as scientific inquiry into score meaning. *American Psychologist, 50*, 741–749.

Miranda, A., Hill, J., & Timberlake, M. (1993, August). *American acculturation by Hispanic immigrants.* Paper presented at the annual conference of the American Psychological Association, Toronto.

Moos, R. H., Cronkite, R. C., Billings, A. B., & Finney, J. W. (1985). *Health and Daily Living Form.* Palo Alto, CA: Social Ecology Laboratory.

Palmer, P. J. (1994). Leading from within: Out of the shadows, into the light. In J. A. Conger (Ed.), *Spirit at work* (pp. 19–40). San Francisco: Jossey-Bass.

Pearlin, L., & Schooler, C. (1978). The structure of coping. *Journal of Health and Social Behavior, 19,* 2–21.

Peeler, J. S. (1991). *Coping resources: Medical patients who are/are not prescribed psychotropic medications by primary care physicans.* Unpublished doctoral dissertation, Georgia State University, Atlanta.

Pugh, J. (1984). *The factors underlying coping resources: An empirical verification.* Unpublished doctoral dissertation, Georgia State University, Atlanta.

Rabkin, J. G., & Struening, E. L. (1976). Life events, stress, and illness. *Science, 19*(4), 1013–1020.

Rollant, P. D., & Curlette, W. L. (1994). A comparison of the effects of interventions on stress coping resources of beginning associate degree nursing students. Paper presented at the annual conference of the American Educational Research Association, New Orleans.

Roseman, I. J., Spindel, M. S., & Jose, P. E. (1990). Appraisals of emotion-eliciting events: Testing a theory of discrete emotions. *Journal of Personality and Social Psychology, 59,* 899–915.

Sarason, I., Johnson, J., & Siegel, J. (1978). Assessing the impact of life changes: Development of the Life Experiences Survey. *Journal of Consulting and Clinical Psychology, 46,* 932–946.

Seitz, M. L. (1989). *Utilizing coping resources and hypochondriasis to explain illness behavior in military personnel.* Unpublished doctoral dissertation, Georgia State University, Atlanta.

Sineath, N., Curlette, W. L., & Brack, G. (1995, August). Relationship of the CRIS to family of origin functionality. Paper presented to the annual conference of the American Educational Research Association, San Francisco, California.

Stewart, G. (1991). *Effectiveness of a psychoeducational intervention for mid-life adults with parent-care respiratory responsibilities (family care givers).* Unpublished doctoral dissertation, University of Florida, Gainesville.

Stone, A., & Neale, J. (1984). New measure of daily coping: Development and preliminary results. *Journal of Personality and Social Psychology, 46,* 892–906.

Walker, M. M. (1991). *The impact of career orientation on relationship support and conceptual stress: A cross-racial study.* Unpublished doctoral dissertation, Georgia State University, Atlanta.

Wedl, L. C. (1986). *Stress coping resources and their relationship to life satisfaction among older persons.* Unpublished doctoral dissertation, Ohio University, Athens.

Wheaton, B. (1983). Stress, personal coping resources, and psychiatric symptoms: An investigation of interactive models. *Journal of Health and Social Behavior, 24,* 208–229.

Wheeler, M., Kern, R., & Curlette, W. (1993). *BASIS-A Inventory.* Highlands, NC: TRT Associates.

The Daily Life Stressors Scale

Christopher A. Kearney and Bonnie L. Horne,
Department of Psychology, University of Nevada,
Las Vegas

■ Instrument Names

Daily Life Stressors Scale
DLSS

■ Developers

Christopher A. Kearney, Ph.D., Department of Psychology, University of Nevada, Las Vegas; Ronald S. Drabman, Ph.D., University of Mississippi Medical Center; and Julie F. Beasley, Ph.D. Department of Psychology, University of Nevada, Las Vegas

■ Contact Information

Dr. Christopher A. Kearney, Department of Psychology, University of Nevada, Las Vegas, 4505 Maryland Parkway, Las Vegas, NV 89154-5030
Telephone: (702) 895-3305; fax: (702) 895-0195

Description and History of the Instrument

The Daily Life Stressors Scale (DLSS; Kearney, Drabman, & Beasley, 1993) was developed in response to the burgeoning need for a measure that targeted everyday life stress in both children and adolescents. Although a great deal of research has been conducted about the effects of major life stressors (e.g., parental divorce, sexual abuse) on youngsters, less work has been done regarding the effects of day-to-day stressors such as going to school or interacting with one's parents at home. The paucity of research into daily life stressors in youngsters, especially with respect to assessment, is unfortunate given that stress has been linked to a variety of internalizing and externalizing behavior problems as well as physiological difficulties (see Arnold, 1990).

Some previous scales have been designed to measure daily life stress in youngsters but carry with them some key conceptual problems. For example, stress is often thought of as (a) an aversive event and/or (b) subjective discomfort. Unfortunately, previous scales of daily life stress focus primarily on the former and not the latter. Second, many items of daily life stress scales for youngsters have been derived from parent reports of their own, or their child's, stress. However, adult memories of stress in childhood are often distorted or inaccurate, and adults are often poor predictors of stress in children (Klein, 1991). Third, daily life stressor scales in children sometimes contain items that occur only occasionally (e.g., pet died, best friend no longer wants to be friendly). Fourth, no scales have been designed for young children, despite evidence that children as young as 6 years can identify their own stressors and coping strategies (Band & Weisz, 1988; Kearney et al., 1993). Finally, previous scales have suffered from methodological drawbacks such as unclear reliability, low sample size in establishing norms, and inadequate length.

The Daily Life Stressors Scale (DLSS) was developed in response to these concerns and designed to measure the degree of daily life stress in youngsters aged 6 to17 years. Specifically, the DLSS is a 30-item measure of the severity of aversive daily life events and negative affectivity. The scale is completed by a child usually in 5 minutes or less. Items are scored on a 5-point Likert-type scale from 0 to 4, with zero being "not at all stressful," 1 being "a little stressful" 2 being "some stressful," 3 being "a lot stressful," and 4 being "very much stressful." Items are arranged in the chronological order of a typical day (e.g., morning activities rated first, school items next, evening items last). Children rate each item, after which a total score (from 0 to 120) is computed. Higher scores thus represent greater stress severity. If an event did not occur for that particular day (e.g., no homework on a Sunday), then a 0 is recorded.

In a subsequent study of parent-child agreement, parent versions of the DLSS were formed (see Beasley & Kearney, 1996). The first parent version was identical to the child DLSS, but parents were asked to complete the scale to *predict* their child's ratings (DLSS-PRE). The second parent version included reformatted items so that parents could *rate* what they felt their child's actual stress level to be (DLSS-RAT; e.g., "My child finds it hard to get up in the morning." In this way, child DLSS scores were compared with parent predictions and ratings to examine informant variance between children and parents. Items for each of these parent versions are scored identically to the child DLSS.

Underlying Assumption and Objective

The underlying assumption of the Daily Life Stressors Scale is that stress in children may be conceptualized as both external life events and internal negative affectivity. The latter refers to a general feeling of dread, nervousness, anxiety, or malaise (see King, Ollendick, & Gullone, 1991). Items from the DLSS were thus designed to reflect both actual stressful events that a child confronts almost every day as well as negative affectivity, or feelings of discomfort about general stimuli. For example, stressful event items from the child DLSS include "My parents yell at me in the morning," "Teachers pick on me," and "I have trouble going to sleep at night." Negative affectivity items from the child DLSS include "I am uncomfortable at lunchtime," "My feelings get hurt and I often want to cry," and "I feel tense or nervous at the dinner table."

The primary objective of the Daily Life Stressors Scale,

therefore, is to accurately measure the severity of everyday stress in youngsters, as the stress relates to both objective external events and subjective internal discomfort. In addition, the scale has been formatted to examine informant variance between children and parents. The DLSS-PRE and DLSS-RAT allow clinicians to examine the accuracy of perceptions regarding internalizing symptoms in youngsters.

Summary of Research Regarding Psychometrics

Psychometric data for the child Daily Life Stressors Scale were derived from three groups of youngsters. A complete description may be found elsewhere (Kearney et al., 1993), but a synopsis is presented here. The first group consisted of 567 students in regular classroom settings (257 males, mean age = 9.94 years; 310 females, mean age = 9.60 years; range, 7–15 years). The second group consisted of 145 youngsters placed in special facilities because parental abandonment, abuse, neglect, or criminal behavior (85 males, mean age = 13.44 years; 60 females, mean age = 11.70 years; range, 6–17 years). The third group consisted of 80 youngsters placed in foster care homes (33 males, mean age = 15.23 years; 47 females, mean age = 15.52 years, range = 13–18 years). Data from these groups were used to examine the test-retest reliability as well as construct and concurrent validity of the child DLSS. Normative values and developmental changes from childhood to adolescence were also examined.

With respect to test-retest reliability, 97 youngsters from the first group completed the DLSS at the time of assessment and 1 week later. Total scores were reliable ($r = .74, p < .001$), as were 29 of the 30 items (range = .28–.71, $p < .01$). Item 21, "It is hard for me to come home from school," was not reliable. With respect to construct validity, it was expected that child DLSS scores would be significantly higher for the second and third (i.e., alternative-setting) groups than the first (i.e., regular-setting) group. This was the case, particularly so for females and older males. Overall, 23 child DLSS items (76.7%) were scored higher by the alternative-setting group than the regular-setting group.

With respect to concurrent validity, total child DLSS scores were correlated with total scores of several other dependent measures thought to be associated with child stress (see Kearney et al., 1993). As expected, child DLSS scores were significantly correlated with depression, hopelessness, state and trait anxiety, low self-esteem, and external locus of control. Normative and developmental data were also generated from these samples. Item-by-item values are presented in the original article, but total score values are presented in Table 1.

Significant differences were found between the regular-setting and alternative-setting groups on DLSS scores for the total sample, total females, total aged 7 to 11 years, total aged

Table 1: **Means and Standard Deviations for the Regular-Setting and Alternative-Setting Groups**

Demographic Group	Regular Setting	Alternative Setting
Total males (n = 257/85)	34.05 (17.04)	34.98 (16.29)
Total females (n = 310/60)	31.20 (17.13)	44.88 (17.86)
Total aged 7---11 years (n = 478/50)	32.36 (17.24)	38.18 (17.20)
Total aged 12+ years (n = 89/95)	33.21 (16.63)	39.55 (17.87)
Males aged 7---11 years (n = 201/25)	34.96 (17.48)	31.92 (16.12)
Males aged 12+ years (n = 56/60)	30.82 (36.25)	36.25 (16.32)
Females aged 7---11 years (n = 277/25)	30.48 (16.85)	44.44 (16.19)
Females aged 12+ years (n = 33/35)	37.27 (18.51)	45.20 (19.19)
Total (n = 567/145)	32.50 (17.14)	39.08 (17.59)

Note: Figures represent means; figures in parentheses in setting columns represent standard deviations.

12 + years, and females aged 7 to 11 years. A significant gender by age interaction was also found. Younger males reported more stress than younger females, whereas older females reported more stress than older males.

Finally, preliminary test-retest data for the parent versions of the DLSS, the DLSS-PRE and DLSS-RAT, have been reported (Beasley & Kearney, 1996). A sample of 27 parents completed each scale at the time of assessment and 1 week later. Reliability figures were significant for the DLSS-PRE ($r = .65, p < .01$) and for the DLSS-RAT ($r = .93, p < .01$).

Conditions for Use

The child version of the Daily Life Stressors Scale is most useful for youngsters suspected of having internalizing disorders. Such youngsters may include those with anxiety or depressive disorders, somatic complaints, trauma, or sudden changes in academic or other behavior. DLSS item scores reported by these children may be compared with normative values to see which areas of the day are most troublesome. The child DLSS may also serve as an accurate dependent measure for treatment outcome or for research into stress-related problems. Parent versions of the DLSS have been designed to investigate informant variance and may be used for this purpose in general clinical or research practice. Overall, the DLSS is a versatile, compact, and psychometrically sound scale that can be easily used by persons of various training.

We emphasize, however, that the Daily Life Stressors Scale should only be used as part of a comprehensive assessment package for internalizing problems. Such a package should include structured or unstructured interviews, other child self-report measures, parent/teacher checklists, behavioral observations, and/or physiological measurements such as heart rate or blood pressure. With respect to structured interviews, for example, we recommend the Anxiety Disorders Interview Schedule for DSM-IV: Parent and Child Versions (Silverman & Albano, 1997). This interview contains various sections that address DSM-IV anxiety disorders as well as related physical symptoms and acting-out problems.

With respect to other child self-report measures, we recommend the Negative Affectivity Self-Statement Questionnaire (Ronan, Kendall, & Rowe, 1994), the Fear Survey Schedule for Children-Revised (Ollendick, 1983), the State-Trait Anxiety Inventory for Children (Spielberger, 1973), the Revised Children's Manifest Anxiety Scale (Reynolds & Paget, 1981), the Children's Depression Inventory (Kovacs, 1992), and the Piers-Harris Children's Self-Concept Scale (Piers, 1984), among others. With respect to parent/teacher checklists, we recommend the Child Behavior Checklist and Teacher's Report Form (Achenbach, 1991a, 1991b) as well as the Conners Parent and Teacher Rating Scales (Conners, 1990). In addition, we recommend that clinicians directly observe behaviors that are often linked to internalizing problems related to stress, such as avoidance, clinging, reassurance seeking, trembling, and noncompliance.

Case Example

We present here a case example that illustrates the use of the Daily Life Stressors Scale. Actual names are not used. Jennifer was a 10-year-old female referred for general anxiety. Upon transfer to a new school setting in January, Jennifer began to experience severe symptoms of worry, physiological symptoms (especially stomachaches), and overall restlessness. She was reportedly adjusting well both socially and academically, but her constant worrying and reassurance seeking were taking its toll on her and her parents, Mr. and Mrs. D.

In the assessment session, Jennifer reported that she felt several unpleasant physical symptoms during the course of the day, but particularly in classes where some performance or new interaction was required. Thus, her level of anxiety tended to fluctuate from day to day. Specifically, Jennifer worried that other people would judge her harshly and was concerned about her appearance, her talking and writing in front of others, and her conversations with strangers. Although a social person who readily interacted with others, Jennifer did report that she continually worried about making mistakes and about how people might react to such mistakes. She demonstrated some cognitive distortions, including catastrophization and minimization of her own accomplishments.

Jennifer's parents essentially confirmed these reports but said their greater concern was their daughter's constant need for reassurance. Jennifer apparently had a habit of asking the same "What if" questions over and over. Commonly asked questions included "What if everyone laughs at me?" "What if I miss the bus?" "What if the teacher doesn't like me?" and "What will happen if I make a mistake?". The asking and answering of these questions often took up to 2 hours per day and was beginning to drain Mr. and Mrs. D. They also expressed concern over Jennifer's somatic complaints, saying that a pediatrician had ruled out any medical cause.

Both Jennifer and her parents were administered respective versions of the Daily Life Stressors Scale. On the child DLSS, Jennifer rated items involving morning and evening activities relatively low but items involving school-related activities relatively high. In particular, scores of 3 ("a lot stressful") or 4 ("very much stressful") were reported for items such as "I feel tense or nervous when I walk into class," "It is hard for me to talk to other people at school," "My classmates tease me," "It is important to be a member of the 'in' group," "I feel uncomfortable at lunchtime," "I am tired in the afternoon," "I am tense or nervous when I have to answer a question in class," "It is hard for me to stay in my seat at school," "My teacher makes me feel uncomfortable," "Teachers pick on me," "It is hard for me to do well in school," and "My feelings get hurt and I often want to cry." Overall, Jennifer's total DLSS score was 52, which is substantially higher than the normative score for her age and gender group (i.e., 30.48).

Jennifer's parents, in completing the DLSS-PRE and DLSS-RAT, reported scores that mirrored their daughter's, although some school-related items were perceived by the parents as less stressful compared with Jennifer's report.

In addition to the interviews and the Daily Life Stressors Scale, the therapist asked Jennifer and her parents to complete questionnaires described in the previous section with respect to fear, general and social anxiety, depression, self-esteem, and overall internalizing and externalizing behaviors. These forms revealed a variety of problematic behaviors, but particularly those related to worry and physiological anxiety. In addition, the therapist conducted a surreptitious behavioral observation of Jennifer's performance in the classroom. The therapist noted that Jennifer generally performed well with others and with respect to academic requirements. However, the therapist also noted that Jennifer, compared with the other students, was spending an inordinate amount of time speaking with the teacher. Later reports from the teacher confirmed that Jennifer was asking many unessential questions about details regarding her schoolwork.

Treatment for Jennifer focused on relaxation training to control some of her physiological symptoms, cognitive therapy to address unneccessary worry, and parent/teacher contingency management to control excessive reassurance seeking. With respect to the latter, for example, Jennifer's parents and teacher were asked to (a) answer a particular question from Jennifer only once per hour, and (b) answer a total of only three questions from Jennifer per hour. If Jennifer asked the same question within an hour or began to ask more than three questions in an hour, then she was ignored. If Jennifer adhered to the schedule of questions, she was allowed to stay up an extra hour at night. Gradually, this schedule was reduced to one question every 2 hours. Following 10 weeks of treatment, Jennifer's level of overall functioning was determined to be good.

Benefits and Limitations

The primary benefit of the Daily Life Stressors Scale (DLSS) is that the measure is a simple, cost-effective, and psychometrically sound method of assessing the severity of daily life stress in children and adolescents. The DLSS can provide a straightforward and useful clinical picture of a child's current level of stress. Many practitioners, educators, and other professionals are faced with youngsters with a variety of stressors, and the DLSS may help identify areas that are most problematic and organize treatment targets. In addition, parent versions of the DLSS can help professionals assess for discrepancies in child and parent reports, a phenomenon inherent to many cases of youngsters with internalizing or stress-related disorders.

The main limitation of the DLSS is that the instrument remains in development. Thus, other items in the future may be found to be more predictive of a child's daily life stress. As a result, we recommend that the DLSS be integrated with a comprehensive assessment protocol. Future research will explore revisions of the scale, usefulness with various clinical samples, whether DLSS scores are related to specific long-term health concerns, and whether DLSS scores are predictive of therapeutic outcome.

The Daily Life Stressors Scale is an effective measure of overt stressful events and covert discomfort that youngsters experience on a day-to-day basis. Given the well-known serious and aversive effects of such everyday stress, the development of accurate assessment devices for this problem should be a high priority for researchers. We invite any questions or comments from readers regarding the DLSS.

Chapter References

Achenbach, T. M. (1991a). *Manual for the Child Behavior Checklist/4-18 and 1991 profile.* Burlington: University of Vermont Department of Psychiatry.

Achenbach, T. M. (1991b). *Manual for the Teachers Report Form and 1991 profile*. Burlington: University of Vermont Department of Psychiatry.

Arnold, L. E. (1990). *Childhood stress*. New York: Wiley.

Band, E. B., & Weisz, J. R. (1988). How to feel better when it feels bad: Children's perspectives on coping with everyday stress. *Developmental Psychology, 24*, 247–253.

Beasley, J. F., & Kearney, C. A. (1996). Source agreement in assessing internalizing symptoms of youth: New evidence for an old problem. *Journal of Anxiety Disorders, 10*, 465–475.

Conners, C. K. (1990). *Manual for Conners' Rating Scales*. North Tonawanda, NY: MultiHealth Systems.

Kearney, C. A., Drabman, R. S., & Beasley, J. F. (1993). The trials of childhood: The development, reliability, and validity of the Daily Life Stressors Scale. *Journal of Child and Family Studies, 2*, 371–388.

King, N. J., Ollendick, T. H., & Gullone, E. (1991). Negative affectivity in children and adolescents: Relations between anxiety and depression. *Clinical Psychology Review, 11*, 441–459.

Klein, R. G. (1991). Parent-child agreement in clinical assessment of anxiety and other psychopathology: A review. *Journal of Anxiety Disorders, 5*, 187–198.

Kovacs, M. (1992). *Children's Depression Inventory manual*. North Tonawanda, NY: Multi-Health Systems.

Ollendick, T. H. (1983). Reliability and validity of the Revised Fear Survey Schedule for Children (FSSC-R). *Behaviour Research and Therapy, 21*, 685–692.

Piers, E. V. (1984). *Piers-Harris Children's Self-Concept Scale: Revised manual 1984*. Los Angeles: Western Psychological Services.

Reynolds, C. R., & Paget, K. D. (1981). Factor analysis of the Revised Children's Manifest Anxiety Scale for blacks, whites, males, and females with a national normative sample. *Journal of Consulting and Clinical Psychology, 49*, 352–359.

Ronan, K. R., Kendall, P. C., & Rowe, M. (1994). Negative affectivity in children: Development and validation of a self-statement questionnaire. *Cognitive Therapy and Research, 18*, 509–528.

Silverman, W. K., & Albano, A. M. (1997). *The Anxiety Disorders Interview Schedule for Children for DSM-IV, child and parent versions*. New York: Psychological Corporation.

Spielberger, C. D. (1973). *Manual for the State-Trait Anxiety Inventory for Children*. Palo Alto, CA: Consulting Psychologists Press.

The Derogatis Affects Balance Scale

A Measure of Affective Balance and Disregulation

Leonard R. Derogatis, Clinical Psychometric Research Inc.
Amy B. Palmer, Loyola College in Maryland

■ Instrument Names

The Derogatis Affects Balance Scale
The Derogatis Affects Balance Scale: A Measure of Affective
Balance and Disregulation
DABS

■ Developers

Leonard R. Derogatis, Ph.D., Clinical Psychometric Research
Inc., Towson, MD

■ Contact Information

The DABS and all related materials are distributed exclusively
by Clinical Psychometric Research Inc., Suite 302, 100 W.
Pennsylvania Ave., Towson, MD 21204.
Telephone: (410) 321–6165; fax: (410) 321–6341

Description and History of the Instrument

In science, the nature of the theories proposed often dictates
the nature of the operational definitions developed to delin-
eate various constructs and, through this mechanism, imposes
some degree of structure upon the nature of measurement.

Stress, when considered as a scientific construct, is no exception to this precept; however, because of the confusing and often contradictory array of stress theories, stress measurement has tended to evolve in an irregular fashion. As described in more detail elsewhere (Derogatis, 1982; Derogatis & Coons, 1993), theories of stress have generally been separated into three types:

■ stimulus oriented
■ response oriented
■ interactional/transactional

Stimulus theories focus on the capacity of events occurring in the environment to induce stress in the individual, while response-oriented theories use the nature and magnitude of the organism's *response* to environmental events to define stress. Interactional theories emphasize personal attributes and characteristics of the individual as important intervening mechanisms that mediate the perception of environmental stimuli and shape the responses they elicit. Consistent with their fundamental premises, each theoretical posture has given rise to distinct measurement approaches.

The best-known measures to arise from stimulus-oriented theory have been the variety of "life events" measurement scales (e.g., Holmes & Rahe, 1967; Horowitz, Wilner & Alverez, 1979; Rahe, Meyer, Smith, Kjaer, & Holmes, 1964). Interactional stress theory has also produced its share of measuring instruments (e.g., Derogatis, 1987b; Derogatis & Fleming, 1997; Jenkins, Rosenman, & Friedman, 1967, Jenkins, Zyzanski, & Rosenman, 1976). The instrument described in the present chapter, the Derogatis Affects Balance Scale (DABS), derives from response-oriented theory. Like most response-oriented measures, it reflects the central underlying tenet that well-being and stress are essentially incompatible states and that to the extent that stress is present, personal well-being is impaired. The most sensitive indicator of impaired well-being has consistently been shown to be affective disregulation, and affects balance is the central measurement construct of the DABS.

Development of the DABS was initiated in the early 1970s, and derived from two major origins:

- a convincing series of studies that demonstrated that positive and negative affects were relatively uncorrelated dimensions of affectivity (Beiser, Feldman, & Egelhoff, 1972; Bradburn, 1969; Gaitz & Scott, 1972; Ware & Wall, 1975); and
- clinical observations made by the author during therapeutic trials that suggested that ultimate therapeutic response was more highly correlated with levels of positive affectivity than with negative affectivity.

Interestingly, this finding has been recently affirmed in a rather compelling fashion (Garamoni, Reynolds, Thase, Frank, & Fasiczka, 1992). At that time, few if any clinical mood scales systematically addressed positive affectivity, and none was designed to rigorously measure affects balance. These events led to the initial publication of the DABS, which was completed in 1975 and originally termed the Affects Balance Scale (ABS) (Derogatis, 1975). The instrument's name was later changed to DABS to avoid confusion with Bradburn's (1969) popular 10-item survey instrument of the same name.

Conceptual Structure of the DABS

In a series of experiments that have systematically related empirical observations and research to theoretical formulations concerning the basic structure of affectivity, a number of investigators (e.g., Watson & Clark, 1988; Watson & Tellegen, 1985) have strongly contributed to the development of what has become known as the *two-factor theory* of affectivity. In the two-factor model, positive affect (PA) and negative affect

(NA) are conceptualized as two fundamental, essentially un-correlated dimensions that represent the cardinal dimensions of human emotional experience. Both state and trait forms of PA and NA are represented in the model, with trait versions corresponding in essence to Extraversion and Neuroticism, respectively (Eysenck & Eysenck, 1968). In the two-factor paradigm, positive affect is described as being associated with feelings of high energy, enthusiasm, and animation, with the capacity for focused concentration and a pleasurable engage-ment with the environment. Negative affect is portrayed as a construct of general psychological distress, subsuming the common dysphoric mood states (e.g., anxiety, depression, anger). At the trait level, NA is characterized as a broadly based, recurrent tendency to experience life circumstances in the context of a dysphoric emotional tenor, which also ex-tends to cognitive style and self-concept. Clinically, the dys-phoric triad of negative affects, ineffective coping, and deni-grated self-concept are frequently observed in formal psychiatric disorders. Trait PA, on the other hand, is charac-terized as a persistent tendency to respond to environmental demands with an active, enabling posture that signals a general sense of competence, mastery, and general well-being. In ad-dition to its correspondence with extraversion, PA is also anal-ogous to Meehl's (1975) concept of high hedonic capacity, which is represented as a constitutional capacity for construc-tive engagement with the environment. Watson and his col-leagues have demonstrated systematic relationships between PA and NA and stress, perceived health status, and anxiety and depressive disorders (Watson, 1988; Watson & Clark, 1988).

Although conceived prior to the emergence of contempo-rary two-factor theory, the conceptual structure of the DABS (Derogatis, 1975) is highly congruent with the two-factor par-adigm. Positive and negative affectivity, and the balance be-tween them, are the paramount constructs that the DABS was designed to operationalize and measure, with the resulting values representing quantitative operational definitions of self-perceived well-being.

A Descriptive Profile of the DABS

The DABS is a multidimensional mood and affects inventory composed of 40 adjective items that measures affectivity and affects balance via eight primary affect dimensions and five global scores. The 40 items of the DABS are scored on a 5-point scale ranging from 0 = "not at all" to 4 = "extremely." The four positive affects dimensions are labeled joy, contentment, vigor, and affection. The negative affects dimensions are anxiety, depression, guilt, and hostility. The five global scores are as follows:

- the Positive Affects Total (PTOT),
- the Negative Affects Total (NTOT),
- the Affects Balance Index (ABI),
- the Affects Expressiveness Index (AEI), and
- the Positive Affects Ratio (PAR).

Recently, a brief form of the DABS, the DABS-SF, has been introduced (Derogatis, 1995), which is composed of only 20 items. The DABS-SF is scored on the same five global scores as the parent test; however, there is no dimensional scoring of the brief form.

The positive affects measured by the DABS are as follows:

- *Joy* is a core dimension of positive affectivity, and reflects a central facet of the emotional state termed happiness. It is an active component of self-perceived well-being and reflects exhilaration, excitement, and elation. Joy ranges in intensity from euphoria at one extreme to cheerfulness and normal pleasure at the other.
- *Contentment* expresses more of a cognitive component of self-satisfaction in addition to positive affective status.

Serenity, peace, and a sense of emotional tranquility are reflected in this dimension, along with feelings of pleasure and well-being.

- *Vigor* is the third positive affects dimension of the DABS, representing the action component of positive affectivity. Vigor demonstrates an enabling energy source that sustains the individual's productive engagement with the environment. High levels of vigor are customarily associated with a positive investment in life and multiple manifest accomplishments.

- *Affection* is the fourth positive affects dimension and refers to an individual's capacity to engage in positive emotional correspondence with other people. Affection demonstrates the universal need to express attachment and receive the love and affection of others. Scores on affection will be high to the extent the individual is able to fulfill this fundamental human need.

Turning to the negative affects constructs:

- *Anxiety* is very much a central component of negative affectivity that appears to have its origins in basic neurobiological "fight-flight" mechanisms. Events that provoke the perception of threat tend to elicit anxiety. Anxiety represents a fear-based, future-oriented affective state, characterized by increased tension, nervousness, and heightened vigilance. Anxiety usually has a pronounced cognitive component, characterized by thoughts of worry and apprehension, and multiple autonomically mediated somatic manifestations.

- *Depression* is also an essential core component of negative affectivity and like anxiety, has its origins in basic neurobiological mechanisms. As an affect state, depression is characterized by sadness, apathy, and dejection. Life events that involve loss, either tangible or symbolic, often elicit depressed affect. The depth of depressive affect may range from mild unhappiness and disaffection, to profound anhedonia, with feelings of hopelessness and despair. The characteristic cognitive pattern that accompanies depressed affect usually involves pessimism, self-deprecation, and self-doubt.

■ *Guilt* is a complex affect state associated with an individual's perception that he or she has failed to properly assume the basic principles of an important personal responsibility imposed upon them by a significant societal agent. Guilt emanates from assumed culpability and blame for failure to comply with prescribed societal standards. The affective dimension of guilt is characterized by sorrow and regret, while cognitive aspects include ruminations concerning the offending action or inaction represented as a personal weakness or inadequacy.

■ *Hostility* is also a negative affect state that has its origins in the basic mammalian fight-flight system. Events that are perceived as threatening or demeaning often evoke hostility. This affect derives from conflicts with individuals, organizations, or institutions and is represented by feelings of resentment and malice toward the conflict's source. Expressions of hostility cover an extremely broad behavioral range, extending from mild irritability and sarcasm to physical confrontation and assault.

As mentioned earlier, the DABS summarizes affective status in terms of five global scores in addition to its eight primary dimension scores. The global scores are intended to serve as operational definitions of broader affective constructs (e.g., self-perceived well-being, emotional balance, and affective equilibrium). The Positive Affects Total (PTOT) is defined as the sum of all scores on the four positive affects dimensions of joy, contentment, vigor, and affection, whereas the Negative Affects Total (NTOT) is represented as the sum of scores on the four negative dimensions of anxiety, depression, guilt, and hostility. The Affects Balance Index (ABI) is defined as PTOT-NTOT/20 and represents the central global measure of affectivity on the DABS. The Affects Expressiveness Index

(AEI) is defined as the sum total of affective expression, regardless of valence (i.e., regardless of positive or negative direction). It represents an attempt to measure the individual's affective "charge" or total affectivity. The Positive Affects Ratio (PAR) illustrates a different approach to measuring global affectivity, in that it is designed to communicate the proportion of total affective expression that is positive. It is defined as the ratio of positive affectivity to total affectivity (i.e., positive plus negative affectivity) on the DABS. The PAR reflects the proportion of affective expression due to positive emotions.

Administration, Scoring, and Norms

A brief introduction to the DABS/DABS-SF, reviewing its nature and purpose, is required in administering the scale, along with a brief set of instructions on completing the test items. The test administrator should always maintain a professional "clinical assessment posture" during the administration of the DABS/DABS-SF, since the respondent will take his or her cues as to the value and importance of the assessment from the examiner's posture. The DABS/DABS-SF should always be introduced to the respondent in a positive and informed manner, thereby communicating the value and significance of the assessment in achieving desired evaluative and therapeutic goals.

In usual administration contexts, the DABS/DABS-SF is introduced to the respondent by a clinician, clinical interviewer, or research technician. Although only 2 minutes is required to effectively introduce the DABS with most individuals, particular care should be exercised when introducing the test to elderly or physically compromised persons. The examiner should be prepared to repeat instructions several times, until he or she is convinced that the respondent clearly understands the nature of the task.

The DABS is available for administration in either paper-and-pencil form or via the computer program, ADMIN-

DABS 4.0. The DABS-SF is available in only paper-and-pencil format. The large majority of respondents complete the DABS in 3 to 5 minutes, while the DABS-SF usually requires 2 to 3 minutes. The standard time referent for the DABS/DABS-SF is *"the past 7 days including today."* The instruments may be used with other time referents (e.g., "2 weeks," "1 month"); however, interpretations of scores relative to the DABS norms will become more tentative.

In scoring the DABS, only the arithmetic operation of addition is used to calculate the eight primary affects dimensions. The scores for each of the five items that comprise each dimension are simply summed to arrive at a raw dimension score. The calculation of the DABS globals is equally straightforward, involving addition, subtraction, and division. PTOT and NTOT are arrived at by simply summing the scores for the 20 positive items and negative items respectively. Once this is accomplished, the difference between PTOT and NTOT is calculated and divided by the constant 20, to arrive at the Affects Balance Index (ABI). The AEI is simply the sum of the 40 item scores, regardless of valence, and the Positive Affects Ratio (PAR) equals the ratio of positive affectivity (PTOT) to total affectivity (PTOT + NTOT).

Currently three published norms are available for the DABS, as well as a single norm that has been published for the DABS-SF (Derogatis, 1996). Published norms for the DABS include a *Community Population Norm* ($N = 480$), an *Inpatient Depression Norm* ($N = 339$), and a *Medical Outpatient (Asthma) Norm* ($N = 100$). The norm for the DABS-SF is based on 270 community adults. All DABS/DABS-SF norms are constructed in terms of *area* T-scores, which are normalizing, standardized transformations that have true centile equivalents associated with them.

Psychometric Characteristics

Reliability and Validity

Reliability is primarily involved with the precision or *accuracy* of measurement, whereas validity addresses the *essence* of what is being measured. Demonstrations of reliability are typically achieved through relatively specific sets of operations, while validation is a highly programmatic endeavor, requiring multiple experiments and research studies. Whereas reliability is established through a highly prescribed set of exercises, the validation process is enduring, expanding, and redefining the limits of generalizability (i.e., valid application) of the psychological measuring instrument involved.

Reliability of the DABS

Since the DABS is a self-report inventory, two forms of reliability are relevant: internal consistency and test-retest. Internal consistency reliability is a measure of homogeneity or consistency of item selection; it reflects the degree to which the items chosen to operationalize the test or subtest in question are drawn from the same population of items. Test-retest reliability is a measure of temporal stability; it measures the degree to which scores achieved at a particular time of assessment correlate with scores achieved on subsequent assessment occasions. In general, there is an inverse relationship between the duration of the period between assessments and test-retest reliability.

In Table 1 both internal consistency and test-retest coefficients are provided for the dimensions and globals of the DABS. Alpha coefficients (α) were based on a sample of 355 psychiatric inpatients, while the test-retest coefficients (r_{tt}) were developed from a small sample of 16 primary breast cancer patients, with 1 week separating the two assessment occasions. Both sets of coefficients are well within the acceptable range and suggest that the DABS is a reliable measure of mood and affects.

Validation of Dimensional Structure

An important demonstration in the construct validation of a multidimensional psychological test involves the verification

Table 1: DABS Internal Consistency and Test-Retest Reliability Coefficients

DABS Measure	Coefficient α ($n = 355$)	Test-Retest r_{tt} ($n = 16$)
Positive Affects		
Joy	.92	.84
Contentment	.85	.80
Vigor	.85	.83
Affection	.84	.81
Negative Affects		
Anxiety	.79	.78
Depression	.85	.82
Guilt	.82	.79
Hostility	.84	.80
Global Scores		
PosTot	.94	.84
NegTot	.93	.81

of dimensional structure. The operational definitions (i.e., dimensions) of the primary hypothesized constructs of the test must be confirmed in terms of real world data. In the case of the DABS, validation requires verification at two distinct levels of structure. At the most basic level, the eight hypothesized primary affects dimensions of the test require confirmation. At a broader conceptual level, the higher-order constructs of positive and negative affectivity require corroboration.

To achieve a verification of dimensional structure, DABS completed at admission by 355 psychiatric inpatients at a private psychiatric hospital were scored and subjected to principal components analysis with an orthogonal varimax rotation. Six factors or dimensions were recovered that met the Scree criterion (Cattell, 1966) and accounted for approximately 70% of the variance in the correlation matrix. Three factors emerged that clearly reflected positive affects dimensions: a combined joy/contentment dimension, an affection dimension, and a vigor dimension. Concerning negative affects, the largest factor represented a combined depression/guilt factor, with two additional components clearly reflecting anxiety and hostility. Although this analysis did not achieve a perfect recovery of the hypothesized eight-factor structure, it did confirm the majority of the constructs hypothesized. The fusing of the positive dimensions of joy and contentment, and the negative dimensions of depression and guilt, is not totally unexpected, considering that the respondents were seriously ill psychiatric patients assessed at time of admission to hospital. In such a situation, affect and mood states would almost certainly have a tendency to become blurred, in a manner not inconsistent with the results of this analysis.

To verify the higher-order factors of positive and negative affectivity, the primary dimension correlation matrix was also subjected to principal components analysis with orthogonal varimax rotation. As anticipated, two principal components were identified that accounted for 72.2% of the variance. The factor structure derived from this analysis is reproduced in Table 2 and represented graphically in Figure 1.

Predictive Validity: The Clinical Utility of a Test

The form of validity that most clinicians and researchers are interested in regarding psychological tests is predictive validity. Predictive validity addresses the utility of a test for specific predictive purposes: for example, how effectively does it identify positive cases, can it discriminate effective from ineffective treatments, and is it capable of distinguishing treatment responders from nonresponders. In the fol-

Table 2: Factor-Loading Coefficients Describing Two
Higher-Order Dimensions of Positive and Negative
Affectivity Underlying DABS Subscales

DABS Dimension	Factor I	Factor II
Joy	.851	-.340
Contentment	.767	-.426
Vigor	.869	-.037
Affection	.798	-.081
Anxiety	-.210	.793
Depression	-.430	.672
Guilt	-.195	.817
Hostility	-.003	.844

lowing sections, we have provided a review of applications
of the DABS as a primary outcomes measure in a variety of
clinical and research contexts in which stress is a major outcomes determinant. In some instances stress is a specifically
identified construct of interest; in others, it is more of an im-
plied variable.

A number of studies with the DABS have focused explicitly
on stress or stress-related states, using contemporary stress
theory as their theoretical base, Wolf, Elston, and Kissling
(1989) used the DABS to establish the affective status of a
sample of freshman medical students. Their goal was to investigate the relationship among hassles, uplifts, life events, and
psychological well-being across a 9-month period. Results of
the study indicated that while hassles was a better predictor
of concurrent and subsequent negative affects states (i.e.,
NTOT), life stress was found to be a better predictor of subsequent positive affectivity and well-being (i.e., PTOT, ABI).
Subsequently, this research team reported a second study on
this issue, in which psychological changes during the first year

Figure 1: Rotated Principal Components from Analysis of DABS Primary Affects Dimensions

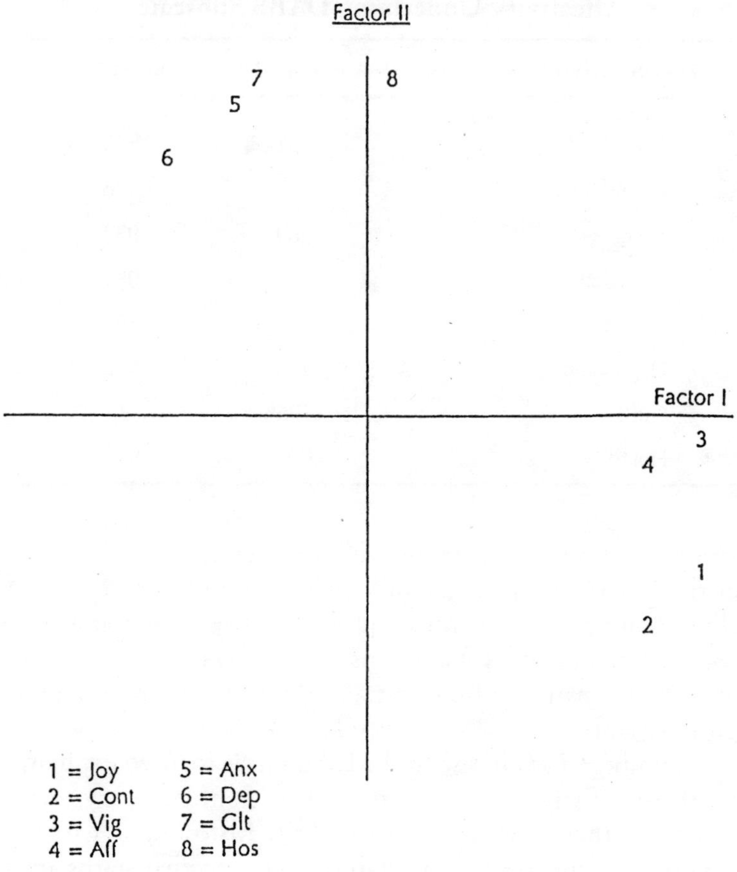

Factor II

7
5

6

Factor I

3
4

1

2

1 = Joy	5 = Anx
2 = Cont	6 = Dep
3 = Vig	7 = Glt
4 = Aff	8 = Hos

of medical school were determined (Wolf, von Almen, Faucett, Randall, & Franklin, 1990). They observed substantial reductions in positive affectivity over the interval, concomitant with elevations in negative affectivity. During the same period, hassles were significantly increased while uplifts and self-esteem were significantly reduced. Correlations among measures, at both baseline and terminal assessment, indicated significant relationships between DABS global scores and both self-esteem and health locus of control.

Although less clearly a stress study per se, a study of the relationship between androgens and depression in hirsute women used the DABS (Derogatis, Rose, Shulman, & Lazarus 1993). Among androgens evaluated, only unbound fractions of testosterone (i.e., biologically active and free testosterone) were found to correlate significantly with the DABS depression score ($r = .60$; $p < .01$). The unbound fractions also showed significant inverse correlations with measures of positive affectivity ($r = -.51$; $p < .05$) and the ABI ($r = -.49$; $p < .05$). Results suggested that depression among hirsute women may be more etiologically related to a deranged neuroendocrine mechanism than to psychological stressors.

Several groups have used the DABS in research focused on the stresses arising from coping with personal loss. Rabins, Fitting, Eastham, and Fetting (1990) used the DABS to contrast the coping effectiveness of caregivers working with Alzheimer's patients with the coping of caregivers involved with cancer patients. Although no noteworthy differences were observed between the two groups, they identified correlates of positive and negative adjustment for both sets of caregivers. Principal among these was the DABS Positive Total score (PTOT), which correlated significantly with a number of social contacts, family cohesiveness, extraversion, and strength of religious faith. Quinn and Strelkauskas (1993) also completed a trial in which they employed the DABS with a sample of recently bereaved individuals under treatment with therapeutic touch. Very substantial changes were noted on all DABS measures from baseline to posttreatment. Positive affectivity was significantly enhanced and negative affectivity was substantially reduced across the treatment period.

Because of the high prevalence, morbidity, and mortality associated with cancer, as well as the relatively noxious consequences deriving from many cancer treatments, cancer illnesses are seen almost universally as high-stress states. The

DABS has been used often with cancer patients and has proven to be a sensitive indicator of well-being status. Many investigators have utilized the DABS to document the affective and emotional dimensions of cancer illnesses and the effectiveness of various coping and adjustment strategies. One of the earliest studies using the DABS (Derogatis, Abeloff, & Melisaratos, 1979) involved research on coping styles and length of survival in a sample of metastatic breast cancer patients. This study explored the role of affective elements in cancer morbidity and mortality. Results showed that DABS negative affect measures significantly discriminated "long" from "short" survivors in this sample. In a related study, Levy, Lee, Bagley, and Lippman (1988) evaluated survival hazards across a 7-year follow-up interval in a sample of first recurrent breast cancer patients. Using a Cox proportional hazards model, these investigators found that disease-free interval, the DABS Joy scale, physician's prognosis, and number of metastatic sites were significant predictors of length of survival. Using other prediction models, the investigators also found that in general, longer survival was associated with positive mood states and concluded that such states represented a measure of resilience or hardiness in dealing with the stresses of cancer. In another similar study, Edwards, DiClemente, and Samuels (1985) used the DABS within a battery of psychological measures with the goal of identifying a pretreatment survival marker for patients with testicular cancer. Twenty-six patients participated in the study, with 19 (long survivors) living to 7 years postassessment and 7 (short survivors) dying during the first year. With results similar to those of Derogatis and Meyer (1979), analysis of DABS profiles revealed that long survivors had significantly higher levels of anxiety, hostility, and depression than did short survivors. The authors interpreted the high levels of negative affectivity as indicators of a successful coping style relative to the disease and its treatment.

Also working with breast cancer patients, Ayers and her colleagues (1994) evaluated the factors involved in predicting compliance with chemotherapy regimen. High scores on DABS measures of Vigor, Anxiety, and Depression and the "fighting spirit" subscale of the Mental Adjustment to Cancer Scale (MAC) predicted good adherence, while high DABS Guilt and Hostility scores predicted poor compliance. A discriminant function analysis correctly assigned 86% of the sample relative to compliance using the above measures. Northouse and Swain (1987) also used the DABS with primary breast cancer patients and their spouses, immediately after mastectomy and subsequently 1 month postsurgery. They found a concordance of affect status between husbands and wives. Both patients and spouses showed a significant decrement in positive affect status immediately postsurgery, which returned to normative levels within a month. There were no significant differences between spouse and patients ABIs at either time of assessment. Carter, Carter, and Prosen (1992) also recently reported a study comparing affects profiles of breast cancer patients and their spouses on the DABS. Consistent with Northouse and Swain (1987), these investigators found few differences between husbands and wives in affective status, with both scoring within normative limits. DABS scores were further analyzed to establish whether distinct patterns of emotional expression might characterize different personality types. Results revealed significant differences in affective expression as measured by the DABS across five personality/gender types.

In the eyes of many professionals, anxiety and stress are synonymous constructs with little to distinguish between them. A number of researchers have utilized the DABS in evaluations of treatments for anxiety-related disorders. Hoehn-Saric (1983) used the DABS within a battery of psychological measures to profile the affective status of chronically anxious patients. Results of the study showed that patients with mixed anxiety-depression had more negative affects profiles than patients suffering from anxiety disorders alone. The negative affects balance was due to both reductions in positive affects and enhancements or elevations in negative affectivity. In further comparisons, the author compared the DABS profiles of patients suffering from generalized anxiety disorder with those of a "mixed" group of anxiety patients, suffering from panic disorder, agoraphobia, and obsessive-compulsive disorder. Profiles were comparable, with the exception that the GAD group had significantly higher scores on the DABS anxiety dimension. This study also compared the affective profiles of patients scoring high on introversion versus those with high extroversion scores. As would be predicted from theory, the extroverted subgroup revealed significantly higher positive affects, and significantly lower negative affectivity.

Sangal, Coyle, and Hoehn-Saric (1983) also used the DABS in a drug trial with anxiety disorders, in an attempt to discriminate treatment responders from treatment nonresponders. Those independently judged improved demonstrated both reduced negative affectivity on the DABS and increased positive affects scores. Looking at both anxiety and depression, Holland and her colleagues (1991) compared alprazolam with progressive relaxation in the treatment of anxious and depressive symptoms in cancer patients. DABS measures of depression and anxiety showed significant reductions across the course of treatment for both drug and behavioral interventions. However, findings revealed a significant advantage for alprazolam over relaxation in both time and magnitude of therapeutic efficacy.

Depression has also been recognized as closely linked to high levels of stress, particularly when stress is chronic and unremitting as opposed to episodic in nature. Garamoni et al. (1991) reported on a study of depressed outpatients and an approximately equal number of healthy controls in which they tested the validity of their States of Mind (SOM) model using the DABS. The primary study hypothesis predicted that the depressive sample would show an affects balance in the negative dialogue range, while healthy controls would demonstrate a balance characterized as positive dialogue. Results showed the patients' affects balance to be precisely in the range predicted (mean = .35; SD = .14), while controls showed a somewhat higher balance than anticipated (mean = .78; SD = .10). The difference between group means was highly significant statistically ($p < .0001$), with almost no overlap between distributions of scores. As predicted, affects balance values were negatively correlated with measures of symptomatic distress.

This research team also reported another investigation (Garamoni et al., 1992) with depressed outpatients who participated in a 20 to 24 session trial of cognitive behavior therapy (CBT). Upon conclusion of the study, patients were assigned to either "responder" or "nonresponder" status based on independent clinical judgments of depression severity. Predictions based on SOM theory were upheld, in that responders shifted their affects balance into the optimal range by the completion of treatment, while nonresponders remained in the negative dialogue range. The authors postulated a corollary hypothesis that responders would achieve their therapeutic movement primarily by reducing negative affectivity, with little alteration in positive affectivity. Results of the study contradicted this hypothesis, in that responders clearly increased positive affectivity significantly over the course of treatment at a rate significantly higher than their rate of negative affects reduction. The authors suggest that this effect may be specific to depressed patients, since research on cognitive balance using anxious patients supported their original hypothesis. These researchers also used the DABS to examine the relationship between affects intensity and phasic REM sleep, pre- and posttreatment with CBT (Nofzinger et al., 1994). Forty-five depressed males and 43 healthy male controls were evaluated with regard to the relationship between affectivity levels and measures of REM sleep. Among depressed patients, there was a significant correlation ($r = .42$, $p < .005$) between REM latency and REM density and the affective expression index (AEI) (which these investigators refer to as "affective intensity"), both prior to and subsequent to treatment. No such relationship was observed in the male controls. The authors suggest that the persistence of the relationship between measures of affectivity and REM sleep, even after effective treatment, may be a signal of persistent vulnerability for disturbed affective processing in certain predisposed depressed individuals.

The DABS has also been used extensively in the area of sexual medicine where stress-induced sexual dysfunctions, as well as stress associated with biogenically based disorders, are firmly established phenomena. In a series of studies, Derogatis and his colleagues have profiled a number of the major sexual diagnostic subgroups with the DABS. In their initial study the affects status of men and women suffering from common sexual dysfunctions (e.g., male erectile disorder, hypoactive sexual desire) were profiled (Derogatis & Meyer, 1979). Individuals affected with these disorders demonstrated ABI's a full standard deviation below the normative mean, in approximately the 15th centile of the norm. Profiles of the sexually dysfunctional showed substantial elevations of negative affectivity ($p < .001$), with concomitant suppression of positive affectivity ($p < .001$) compared with healthy controls.

DABS profiles have also been established for gender dysphoric individuals—that is, male (Derogatis, Meyer, & Vasquez, 1978) and female (Derogatis et al., 1981) transsexuals, who suffer from dramatic stress arising from perceived gender-anatomy dissonance. Male gender dysphorics were characterized by strikingly negative affects balances; positive affectivity was profoundly suppressed compared with the healthy controls ($p < .001$), and dramatic elevations in negative affectivity were also apparent. The authors characterized the male gender dysphorics as suffering from "a pervasive anhedonia." In the female gender dysphoric cohort (Derogatis et al., 1981), affective disequilibrium was not as dramatically evident. Significant suppression of positive affects was observed, but only modest elevations in depression and anxiety were apparent.

In addition to studies using the DABS to evaluate stress in individuals with diagnosed sexual disorders, preliminary results have recently been reported from a study investigating the relationship between affectivity and quality of sexual functioning in healthy community normals (Derogatis, Sudler, Appelgate, & Fleming, 1997). Approximately 250 community men and women from various professions agreed to participate in a brief anonymous survey of quality of sexual functioning and feelings of well-being. Quality of sexual functioning was assessed via the Derogatis Interview for Sexual Functioning (DISF) (Derogatis, 1987a, Derogatis, 1997), and affectivity and well-being were measured via the DABS. Significant correlations were observed between all positive affects measures of the DABS, including PTOT and the ABI, and all domain and global scores of the DISF. Similar findings were absent regarding negative affectivity, with significant correlations being observed only on the DISF Orgasm scale. The findings were interpreted as supporting the premise that positive affectivity is a more sensitive indicator of well-being and functional status than negative affectivity and symptomatic distress, particularly in nonpsychiatric populations.

Case Example

The case example described here explicitly illustrates the proposition introduced in our previously discussed research study on sexual functioning—namely, that affectivity is a more sensitive indicator of perceived well-being in nonpsychiatric populations than is symptomatic distress. Affective dysregulation is almost always in evidence prior to formal psychological symptoms, and relative to recovery, affects balance is usually one of the earliest indicators that stress has substantially abated or effective coping has been initiated.

The patient, Ms. S, was a 31-year-old white, professional woman who was referred from the pulmonary service of a large metropolitan medical center for psychological evaluation. Ms. S had a history of asthma dating back to her junior year of college, but the course of the disorder was atypical and episodic, and the patient's response to treatment was inconsistent, leading the pulmonary specialist to believe that psychological issues might be playing a role in the patient's condition. Ms. S presented as a very attractive and highly articulate professional who freely verbalized her frustration and confusion over her episodic asthma attacks and the failure of various medication regimens to control her problems. Ms. S indicated that she had never sought help or counseling for a psychological problem in the past and had no awareness of any major psychological conflicts at the time of evaluation. As a routine part of the evaluation Ms. S was administered a series of psychological tests, among them the DABS and the DSI, a self-report symptom inventory that is a variant of the SCL-90-R® (Derogatis, 1994).

Ms. S was the youngest daughter of a very successful professional (in her profession) with considerable resources. She reported that she was also her father's favorite, which created some disaffection and rivalry from her siblings, who were also professionals. She had earned very high standing in her graduate training and had a very desirable position at a prestigious firm; however, a powerful "old boy" network was making her life "somewhat difficult" at work. The patient's father argued that this was simply another reason that she should leave her current position and come to work for him. Recently, a man who she had been dating and cared for very much had proposed to her, but she was concerned she had "badgered him into it" and that he really did not wish to marry her of his own accord. Ms. S's parents did not approve of her boyfriend, characterizing him as "a mediocre product" and someone "after her money." Her friends told her "she was too good for him."

Ms. S's DSI Psychological Symptom Profile and DABS Affects Profile appear below in Figures 2 and 3, respectively. From the perspective of symptomatic distress, Ms. S is clinically unremarkable, revealing an absence of elevations on any primary symptom dimensions or global summary scores of

Figure 2: Psychological Symptom Profile of Ms. S

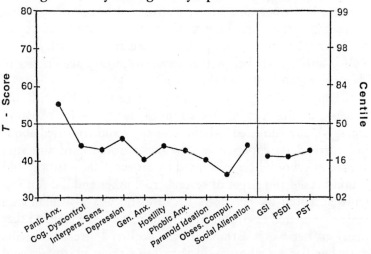

Figure 3: DABS Affectivity Profile of Ms. S

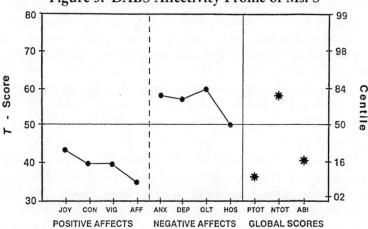

the test. There is a very slight elevation on Panic Anxiety, but this is very typical of asthmatics who sometimes experience a sense of panic during their attacks. The patient's affects profile tells a different story, however. All measures of positive affects are suppressed by 0.5 to 1.5 standard deviations, and her PTOT, the positive affects summary, falls at about the 8th centile. Concerning negative affects, although none of her scores fall in the clinical range, Ms. S shows notable elevations on Anxiety, Depression, and Guilt measures. Overall, Ms. S's ABI is about 1 SD below the normative mean, placing her in about the 16th centile of the norm.

In the context of reviewing these test results with the patient, a different appreciation of her current situation emerged. She admitted to being unhappy and confused about her current life experiences. She had worked hard and succeeded at school, been rewarded by an excellent position, but found herself the target of several cruel jokes and did not feel truly accepted by her peers because she was a woman in a male-dominated environment. Upon review, she realized that many of her worst asthma attacks occurred after arguments with her fiancé, who would then leave their apartment and stay with friends. She would subsequently be "rescued" by her parents, who would take her home with them to recover. By going home with her parents, she would receive love and nurturance but felt like a "dependent little girl" who was incapable of successfully sustaining an adult relationship with a man or being an independent adult woman. It also occurred to Ms. S that her very first asthma attacks occurred while she was studying in Europe for a semester, ostensively having a very rewarding experience but far away from her family and normal supports.

The patient recognized in a fragmentary fashion that she was suffering from substantial dependency conflicts. She was the favorite child in a family of professionals who were all very accomplished and independent, except perhaps for her. She also recognized that since she was the youngest and the last child, her parents probably had an unrecognized investment in maintaining her dependence on them. While at an intellectual level she was aware of her need to grow through these conflicts and accept the challenges of full adulthood, emotionally she feared loss of her parents' love and special place in the family if she became truly independent. She also felt guilty about her special place as the favored child relative to her siblings and that she was unable to definitively solve her conflicts and become an independent adult.

A recommendation was made to Ms. S that she enter into a brief course of insight-oriented psychotherapy focused on more fully understanding and resolving her dependency conflicts. The patient accepted the recommendation, completed the brief treatment regimen, and when last interviewed, was handling her interpersonal relationships with much more awareness and confidence. She no longer retreated to her parents home after arguments with her fiancé, and although the frequency of her asthma attacks did not decrease, she reported considerable reduction in their severity.

The importance of completing an affective profile on this patient cannot be overstated. On presentation Ms. S appeared as a highly accomplished individual, intelligent and physically attractive, with enormous personal and material resources at her disposal. Symptom-oriented assessment indicated a clinically unremarkable profile, as did personality assessment. By learning of an affective disequilibrium from the DABS, we were able to explore the underlying basis of her disaffection and gain substantial insight into a significant series of conflicts blocking her personal growth and compromising treatment for her medical condition. By learning of the potential existence of these problems through an assessment of her affects profile, effective psychological and medical interventions were ultimately delivered.

Conclusion

A central question in interpreting the data presented here concerns the distinction between cause and effect. Do high levels of positive affects reflect a constitutional characteristic, equivalent to Meehl's (1975) notion of "hedonic capacity," which to some degree is genetically determined, or are positive affects more accurately represented as responses, "effects," determined by and indicative of more fundamental biological and psychosocial processes? A definitive answer to this question awaits further study. Whichever posture is taken concerning the basic nature of the relationship between positive affectivity and health and well-being, affects balance has clearly been shown to have substantial associations with multiple health indicators. Just as certain personality constellations are believed to represent markers for the "disease-prone personality" (Friedman & Booth-Kewley, 1987), it is equally possible that positive affects balance represents a reliable marker for disease and stress resistance. The DABS is a brief, reliable, and valid measure of the primary constructs of affectivity, affects balance, and well-being. It is designed to address questions in both clinical and research modalities, and measure affective responses to stress in a sensitive and effective manner.

Chapter References

Ayres, A., Hoon, P. W., Franzoni, J. P., Matheny, K. B., Cotanch, P. H., & Takayanagi, S. (1994). Influence of mood and adjustment to cancer on compliance with chemotherapy among breast cancer patients. *Journal of Psychosomatic Research, 38*(5), 393–402.

Beiser, M., Feldman, J. J., & Egelhoff, C. S. (1972). Assets and affects: A study of positive mental health. *Archives of General Psychiatry, 27,* 545–549.

Bradburn, N. M. (1969). *The structure of well-being.* Chicago: Aldine.

Carter, R. E., Carter, C. A., & Prosen, H. A. (1992). Emotional and personality types of breast cancer patients and spouses. *American Journal of Family Therapy, 20*(4), 300–309.

Cattell, R. B. (1966). The Scree Test for number of factors. *Multivariate Behavioral Research, 1,* 245.

Derogatis, L. R. (1975). *The Affects Balance Scale.* Baltimore, MD: Clinical Psychometric Research.

Derogatis, L. R. (1982). Self-report measures of stress. In L. Goldberger & S. Breznitz (Eds.), *Handbook of stress: Theoretical and clinical aspects* (pp. 270–294). New York: Mcmillan.

Derogatis, L. R. (1987a). *Derogatis Interview for Sexual Functioning (DISF)*. Baltimore, MD: Clinical Psychometric Research.

Derogatis, L. R. (1987b). *The Derogatis Stress Profile (DSP)*. Baltimore, MD: Clinical Psychometric Research.

Derogatis, L. R. (1994). *SCL-90-R®: Admistration, scoring and procedures manual* (3rd ed.). Minneapolis, MN: National Computer Systems.

Derogatis, L. R. (1995). *Derogatis Affects Balance Scale—Short form (DABS-SF)*. Baltimore, MD: Clinical Psychometric Research.

Derogatis, L. R. (1996). *Derogatis Affects Balance Scale (DABS): Administration, scoring and procedures manual.* Baltimore, MD: Clinical Psychometric Research.

Derogatis, L. R. (1997). The Derogatis Interview for Sexual Functioning (DISF): An introductory report. *Journal of Sex and Marital Therapy, 23(4)*, 291–303.

Derogatis, L. R., Abeloff, M. D., & Melisaratos, N. (1979). Psychological coping mechanisms and survival time in metastatic breast cancer. *JAMA, 242*, 1504–1508.

Derogatis, L. R., & Coons, H. L. (1993). Self-report measures of stress. In L. Goldberger & S. Breznitz (Eds.), *Handbook of stress: Theoretical and clinical aspects* (2nd ed., pp. 200–233). New York: Mcmillan.

Derogatis, L. R., & Fleming, M. P. (1997). The Derogatis Stress Profile (DSP): A theory driven approach to stress measurement. In C. P. Zalaquett, & R. J. Wood (Eds.), *Evaluating stress: A book of resources.* Lanham, MD: Scarecrow.

Derogatis, L. R., & Meyer, J. K. (1979). A psychological profile of the sexual dysfunctions. *Archives of Sexual Behavior, 8(3)*, 201–223.

Derogatis, L. R., Meyer, J. K., & Boland, P. (1981). A psychological profile of the transexual: II. The female. *Journal of Nervous & Mental Disease, 169(3)*, 157–168.

Derogatis, L. R., Meyer, J. K., & Vazquez, N. (1978). A psychological profile of the transsexual: I. The male. *Journal of Nervous & Mental Disease, 166(4)*: 234–254.

Derogatis, L. R., Sudler, N., Appelgate, C., & Fleming, M. (1997 March). *Affectivity and quality of sexual functioning.* Paper presented at the 22nd Annual Meeting of the Society for Sex Therapy and Research (SSTAR), Chicago.

Derogatis, L. R., Rose, L. I., Shulman, L. H., & Lazarus, L. A. (1993). Serum androgens and psychopathology in hirsute women.

Journal of Psychosomatic Obstetrics and Gynaecology, 14, 269–282.

Edwards, J., DiClemente C., & Samuels, M. L. (1985). Psychological characteristics: A pretreatment survival marker of patients with testicular cancer. *Journal of Psychosocial Oncology, 3*(1), 79–94.

Eysenck, H. J., & Eysenck, S. B. G. (1968). *Eysenck Personality Inventory.* San Diego: Educational and Industrial Testing Service.

Friedman, H. S., & Booth-Kewley, S. (1987). The disease-prone personality. *American Psychologist, 42,* 539–558.

Gaitz, C. M., & Scott, J. (1972). Age and the measurement of mental health. *Journal of Health & Social Behavior, 13,* 55–67.

Garamoni, G. L., Reynolds, C. F., Thase, M. E., Frank, E., & Fasiczka, A. L. (1992). Shifts in affective balance during therapy of major depression. *Journal of Consulting & Clinical Psychology, 60,* 260–266.

Garamoni, G. L., Reynolds, C. F., Thase, M. E., Frank, E., Berman S. R., & Fasiczka, A. L. (1991). The balance of positive and negative affects in major depression: A further test of the states of mind model. *Psychiatry Research, 39,* 99–108.

Hoehn-Saric, R. (1983). Affective profiles of chronically anxious patients. *Hillside Journal of Clinical Psychology, 5*(1), 43–56.

Holland, J. C., Morrow, G. R., Schmale, A., Derogatis, L. R., Stefanek, M., Berenson, S., Carpenter, P. J., Breitbart, W., & Feldstein, M. (1991). A randomized clinical trial of alprazolam versus progressive muscle relaxation in cancer patients with anxiety and depressive symptoms. *Journal of Clinical Oncology, 9*(6), 1004–1011.

Holmes, T. H., & Rahe, R. H. (1967). The Social Readjustment Rating Scale. *Journal of Psychosomatic Research, 11,* 213–218.

Horowitz, M. J., Wilner, N., & Alvarez, W. (1979). Impact of event scale: A measure of subjective stress. *Psychosomatic Medicine, 41,* 209–218.

Jenkins, C. D., Rosenman, R. H., & Friedman, M. (1967). Development of an objective psychological test for the determination of the coronary-prone behavior pattern in employed men. *Journal of Chronic Diseases, 20,* 371–379.

Jenkins, C. D., Zyzanski, S. J., & Rosenman, R. H. (1976). Risk of new coronary infarction in middle-aged men with manifest coronary heart disease. *Circulation, 53,* 342–347.

Levy, S. M., Lee, J., Bagley, C., & Lippman, M. (1988). Survival hazards analysis in first recurrent breast cancer patients: Seven-year follow-up. *Psychosomatic Medicine, 50,* 520–528.

Meehl, P. E. (1975). Hedonic capacity: Some conjectures. *Bulletin of the Meninger Clinic, 39,* 295–307.

Nofzinger, E. A., Schwartz, R. M., Reynolds, C. F., Thase, M. E., Jennings, J. R., Frank, E., Fasiczka, A. L., Garamoni, G. L., & Kupfer, D. J. (1994). Affect intensity and phasic REM sleep in depressed men before and after treatment with cognitive-behavior therapy. *Journal of Consulting & Clinical Psychology, 62*(1), 83–91.

Northouse, L. L., & Swain, M. A. (1987). Adjustment of patients and husbands to initial impact of breast cancer. *Nursing Research, 36*(4), 221–225.

Quinn, J. F., & Strelkauskas, A. J. (1993). Psychoimmunologic effects of therapeutic touch on practitioners and recently bereaved recipients: A pilot study. *Advances in Nursing Science, 15*(4), 13–26.

Rabins, P. V., Fitting, M. D., Eastham, J., & Fetting, J. (1990). The emotional impact of caring for the chronically ill. *Psychosomatics, 31*(3), 331–336.

Rahe, R. H., Meyer, M., Smith, M., Kjaer, G., & Holmes, T. H. (1964). Social stress and illness onset. *Journal of Psychosomatic Research, 8,* 35–44.

Sangal, R., Coyle, G., & Hoehn-Saric, R. (1983). Chronic anxiety and social adjustment. *Comprehensive Psychiatry, 24*(1), 75–78.

Ware, P., & Wall, T. (1975). *Work and well-being.* Harmondsworth, England: Penguin.

Watson, D. (1988). Intraindividual and interindividual analyses of positive and negative affect: Their relation to health complaints, perceived stress and daily activities. *Journal of Personal & Social Psychology, 54,* 1020–1030.

Watson, D., & Clark, L. A. (1988). Positive and negative affectivity and their relation to anxiety and depressive disorders. *Journal of Abnormal Psychology, 97,* 346–353.

Watson, D., & Tellegen, A. (1985). Toward a consensual structure of mood. *Psychological Bulletin, 98,* 219–235.

Wolf, T. M., Elston, R. C., & Kissling, G. E. (1989, Spring). Relationship of hassles, uplifts and life events to psychological well-being of freshman medical students. *Behavioral Medicine,* 37–45.

Wolf, T. M., von Almen, T. K., Faucett, J. M., Randall, H. M., & Franklin, F. A. (1991). Psychological changes during the first year of medical school. *Medical Education, 25,* 174–181.

The Global Inventory of Stress (GIS)

A Comprehensive Approach to Stress Assessment*

Charles L. Sheridan, University of Missouri–Kansas City
Sally A. Radmacher, Missouri Western State College

■ Instrument Names

The Global Inventory of Stress (GIS), Part I of the
Comprehensive Scale of Stress Assessment
The Global Inventory of Stress (GIS): A Comprehensive
Approach to Stress Assessment
The Global Inventory of Stress: A Comprehensive Approach
to Stress Assessment
The GIS

■ Developer

Charles L. Sheridan, Ph.D., University of Missouri–Kansas
City, 5319 Holmes, Kansas City, MO 64110
Telephone: (816) 235-1069; e-mail: csheridan@cctr.umkc.edu

■ Contact Information

Charles L. Sheridan, Ph.D. (contact information above)
Sally A. Radmacher, Ph.D., Missouri Western State College,
4525 Downs Dr., St. Joseph, MO 64507
Telephone: (816) 271-4445;
e-mail: radmache@griffon.mwsc.edu

---

*The Global Inventory of Stress is copyrighted (1986) by Charles L.
Sheridan.

Description and History of Instrument

The Global Inventory of Stress (GIS) is one of the measures in a stress assessment battery called the Comprehensive Scale of Stress Assessment (CSSA). The CSSA was designed to measure the major dimensions of stress, which includes stressors, stress resistance, and stress symptoms. Many modifications have been made in the battery over the years stimulated by new developments in the measurement of stress and by a range of studies utilizing all or parts of the CSSA. The GIS is the first inventory of the CSSA and can be used as a stand-alone instrument to provide a generic, overall measure of the respondent's status on the major dimensions of stress. The remaining components of the CSSA may also be used as stand-alone inventories when a measure of a specific dimension of stress is needed. The entire CSSA is used when a comprehensive assessment of the global and specific dimensions of stress is desired. A description of the components of the CSSA, other than the GIS, follows:

- The Inventory of Stressors (IOS) is an 80-item yes/no inventory indicating stressors ranging from minor hassles to major life events.
- The Inventory of Stress Resistance Resources (ISRR) is an 83-item yes/no inventory of resources derived from an extensive search of the literature on factors that buffer against stressors or make individuals more vulnerable to stress. (This inventory served as the basis for a measure of stress resiliency, The Personal Style Inventory, which is described in another chapter.)
- The Inventory of Stress-Related Symptoms (ISRS) is a 70-item checklist inventory of an array of symptoms that have a particularly close relationship to stress.

This comprehensive approach to stress measurement was born from the recognition that stress is an extremely complicated construct with multiple dimensions and intervening variables. Social and physical environmental stressors, appraisal and perception of stressors, and a wide variety of internal and external coping resources all interact to determine an individual's response to stress. Most measurements assess just one of these facets of stress and often that facet is measured only partially—for example, stressors may be assessed with respect only to major life events (Holmes & Rahe, 1967) or minor daily hassles (Kanner, Coyne, Schaefer, & Lazarus, 1981). The various contexts of an individual's life in which the stressors are experienced are not considered. For example, people may find their work environment stressful but not their home environment. The different facets of stress in major contexts such as the primary relationship, the work environment, and the social environment should be included in the assessment. Measures of resources for managing stress may include only social supports (Krause & Markides, 1990) or psychological coping skills (Folkman & Lazarus, 1980). In fact, many more kinds of resources may be called upon in managing stress. As Antonovsky (1979) notes, resources for managing stress cover a variety of categories, including material, physical, and cultural resources.

The GIS takes a global approach to stress by including all of the dimensions of stress just mentioned, but it does so briefly and generically. It is a generic scale in the sense that it is not tied to specific stressors, resources, or symptoms. This generic property of the GIS circumvents a problem encountered in most inventories—omission of unique or unusual stressors. The most common method of measuring stress involves inclusion of items that are believed to be representative of the dimension being measured. Yet, there is generally no assurance of this representativeness. Furthermore, a given group or individual may be impacted by some highly unusual or unique stressor. For example, a widow experienced a unique stressor of great magnitude when plans were announced to locate a corporate hog farm that would produce tons of manure a day within a half mile of her home. Obviously this is not the kind of event that she would have been able to check on most inventories of stressors.

Conceptual Structure of the GIS

The GIS is a 22-item self-report measure based on an interactive model that views stress as a construct that is composed of the basic dimensions of stress: (a) stressors, (b) stress-coping resources, and (c) strain. It also includes the major environmental settings in which stress is likely to occur. The GIS uses the dimensions of pleasure (hedonic value), control, and arousal to assess stress in settings. These dimensions have been identified in extensive, systematic investigations as essential factors that emerge consistently in describing environments (Mehrabian & Russell, 1974).

The model underlying the GIS was heavily influenced by work of Antonovsky (1979, 1987), who has argued that stressors are managed through generalized resistance resources that include individual coping skills and resources from the larger social and physical environments. If resources are sufficient to neutralize the stressors, the individual will experience health benefits or eustress. If the demands created by the stressors exceed the individual's resources, then health breakdown or distress will occur. This model is consistent with the work of Dohrenwend, et al. (1978), which also emphasizes an interactive approach to stress, with strain being determined by the interaction between stressors and resources. In addition, her social stress model includes stress—coping resources that cover a very broad range of categories. Although the GIS was developed before the work of Lazarus and Folkman (1984) was known to Sheridan, the assessment of primary and secondary appraisals is also included in the measurement.

The GIS is a comprehensive assessment of stress that includes the following:

- the frequency and intensity of stressors,
- an appraisal of the effectiveness of the respondent's *stress-coping resources*,
- the frequency and intensity of feelings of *strain*, and
- an assessment of the respondent's *primary relationship, work situation,* and *social relationships* along the dimensions of *pleasure, arousal,* and *control.*

The advantages of the GIS are that it provides separate inventories for quantifying each of the dimensions of stress and affords a means to identify stressors that are unique to each respondent and his or her assessment of them.

Definitions of Basic Dimensions of Stress

The term *stressor* was introduced by Selye (1978) to distinguish the cause (stressor) from the effect (stress). We are using the term to describe situations or events that exceed an individual's coping abilities. *Stress-coping resources* are all of the things that people have at their disposal to manage stressors. They encompass a broad range of categories that include the following:

- material resources, having the sufficient assets to obtain life's necessities;
- physical resources, being strong, healthy, and attractive;
- intrapersonal resources, attributes like ego integrity and self-esteem;
- informational and educational resources; and
- social support.

Antonovsky (1979, 1987) suggests that experience with these coping resources during childhood and adolescence results in the development of a personal *sense of coherence,* which acts as a major source of resistance to stress that is effective in very toxic environments. *Strain* is the reaction individuals have when they are exposed to stressors that tax their stress coping resources. Strain is what most people mean when they say they are "feeling stressed." Selye (1978) admits that had he been more proficient in English at the time, he would have called the phenomenon of "stress" the "strain reaction." *Strain* manifests itself in a variety of symptoms including tense muscles, irritability, and headaches.

Administration, Format, and Scoring

The GIS is a 22-item self-report inventory developed to measure the broad spectrum of dimensions underlying the concept of "stress." It is appropriate for use with adolescents and adults with at least a seventh-grade reading level. The inventory takes about 15 minutes to complete, with an occasional respondent taking somewhat longer. The GIS provides definitions for *stressors, stress coping resources, strain, arousal,* and *primary relationships,* then instructs respondents to indicate where they stand on a 5-point scale. The following example shows the definition for *stressors* and one of the related items:

BEFORE ANSWERING, BE SURE TO READ THE FOLLOWING *DEFINITION*

A: "Stressors" are situations or happenings for which we don't have an automatic reaction; that require us to react and make adjustments to them; that sometimes make us feel a sense of stress; and that can sometimes go beyond what we can cope with or handle.

1. Given this meaning of the word "stressor," please estimate how frequently you are stressed currently.

( ) Much more than average.
( ) Somewhat more than average.
( ) About average.

( ) Somewhat less than average.
( ) Much less than average.

Within the stressor dimension, other items ask respondents to indicate the intensity and quantity of stressors they have experienced. It then moves on to the stress-coping resources dimension by providing a definition and assessing various facets of those resources. An example follows:

BEFORE ANSWERING, BE SURE TO READ THE FOLLOWING *DEFINITION*

B: "Stress-coping resources" are all the things that help me deal with stressors (including personal characteristics such as attitudes, habits, affiliations with other individuals and groups, and material resources).

2. Assuming this is the meaning of "stress coping resources," my stress coping resources during the past six months would be rated
( ) Much more than average.
( ) Somewhat more than average.
( ) About average.
( ) Somewhat less than average.
( ) Much less than average.

Each of the items in the GIS is scored on a 5-point scale with nine reverse-keyed items. The GIS yields a total stress score that is obtained by summing scores for all of the items. It also provides subtotals for the three dimensions of stress (stress, stress-coping resources, strain) and the three major settings (primary relationships, work situations, social relationships). Normative data for the GIS22-G, GIS22-C, and GIS7-C are shown in Table 1.

Modifications to the GIS

The original version of the GIS (GIS28-G) consisted of 28 items designed to assess various dimensions of stress in the person's life from the present through the past 6 months.

Table 1: Normative Data from Studies Using Various Forms of the GIS

Study	Samples	n	Mean	SD
GIS22-C				
Baich (1988)	College students	124	36.94	10.83
Beauchamp-Turner & Levinson (1992)	College students			
Schmidt & Sheridan (1994)	Heterogeneous controls	30	38.53	13.58
	Heterogeneous chronic patients	32	40.38	12.50
	Chronic fatigue syndrome patients	126	45.78	13.79
GIS7-C				
Baich (1988)	College students	124	13.07	
Schmidt & Sheridan (1994)	Heterogeneous controls	30	14.50	4.90
	Heterogeneous chronic patients	32	14.66	4.68
	Chronic fatigue syndrome patients	32	16.78	4.85
Snow & Sheridan (1996)	Chronic pain patients	61		
LaMar (1991)	Heterogeneous	83	11.56	3.77
GIS22-G				
Baich (1988)	College students	124	40.03	11.73
Radmacher & Sheridan (1989)	College students	307	41.85	11.31
Ingersoll (1990)	Hypertensive patients	60	33.67	13.50
	Normotensive patients	60	29.78	14.32
LaMar (1991)	Heterogeneous	83	37.60	11.17
Sherk (1991)	College students	163	39.00	10.94
GIS28-G				
Kolenc, Hartley, & Murdock (1990)	College students	227	47.14	13.68

Note: The higher the score is, the greater the perceived stress.

High internal consistency and a strong correlation with avowed health status for this version have been reported (Sheridan & Smith, 1987). The GIS also discriminated between groups expected to have different stress levels (single versus married mothers) in that study six items were removed that appeared to be redundant to respondents (Radmacher & Sheridan, 1989), resulting in the present 22-item scale (GIS22). The items were in fact not redundant but attempted to draw distinctions that seemed too subtle for most respondents to recognize. Baich (1988) initiated a second modification by changing the wording of GIS items so that respondents were asked to assess their current stress, instead of stress from the present through the past 6 months. This version is identified as GIS22-C. Baich then compared the GIS22-G with the GIS22-C with respect to prediction of symptoms and affect. The GIS22-C proved to be a better predictor of stress-related symptoms and of dysphoria than the original version. The superiority of the predictive power of the GIS22-C needs to be replicated in other samples and with other outcome measures, but it may be preferable for many applications. To avoid confusion, the form of GIS under discussion will be identified by adding a number reflecting the number of items, and either a "G" when the form asks for responses covering "now and the past 6 months" or "C" for the form that asks for ratings of current stress.

Psychometric Characteristics

Reliability

Reliability is the extent to which a test score is stable and free from error. Basically, it is an index of test consistency. There are two types of reliability: test-retest reliability (temporal stability) and internal consistency. Test-retest refers to the degree that the results of measures are stable over time. Internal consistency refers to the extent to which the test items are measuring one construct. This reliability is usually established with a coefficient alpha of .70 or greater. With a sample of 209 women and 98 men college students, assessed the internal consistency and temporal stability of the GIS22-G was assessed (Radmacher & Sheridan, 1989). A coefficient alpha of .86 was obtained, which indicates an adequate internal consistency. A test-retest over a two-week period yielded an r of .89 which indicates that the GIS22-G also has adequate temporal stability. LaMar (1991) obtained a test-retest reliability over 28 days of .87. The internal consistency of the GIS remains adequate even on the brief version. A coefficient alpha of .82 was obtained for the GIS7-C administered to 64 chronic disease patients and 30 nonpatient controls (Schmidt & Sheridan, 1994). The GIS7-C is a seven-item scale that combines the stressor and stress-coping resources subscales using the form that asks for ratings of current stress.

Criterion-Related Validity

Anastasi (1988) defines validity as "the degree to which the test actually measures what it purports to measure" (p. 28). Criterion validity is the extent to which a test is effective in predicting some criterion that is an independent measure of what the test is supposed to predict. A number of empirical studies have been conducted that establish the criterion-related validity of the various forms of the GIS as valid measures of the interactive dimensions of perceived stress.

From the data obtained from the college students mentioned earlier, evidence for the validity of the GIS22-G has been provided by correlating it with the following criteria (Radmacher & Sheridan, 1989): (a) student grade point average (GPA); (b) the Social Readjustment Rating Scale (SRRS; Holmes & Rahe, 1967); (c) the anxiety subscale of the Multiple Affect Adjective Checklist (MAACL; Zuckerman & Lubin, 1985); and (d) the Orientation to Life Questionnaire (OTL; Antonovsky, 1987). (The OTL is Antonvosky's measure of sense of coherence.) The GIS22-G correlated .36 with the SRRS, −.67 with the OTL, .56 with MAACL anxiety subscale, and −.15 with GPA. All of these correlations were statistically significant and in the predicted direction. Partial correlations indicated that GIS22-G and OTL, although highly correlated, made independent contributions to outcome predictions. Although the correlation between GIS22-G and GPA was low, it was statistically significant ($p < .005$), and none of the shared variance between the two can be accounted for by similarity of measures.

Williams (1990) provides further evidence for the criterion-related validity of the GIS22-G in a study of 162 women critical care nurses. In addition to the GIS, her study included (a) the SRRS, (b) the OTL, (c) the Personal Views Survey (a third-generation hardiness test), and (d) the Seriousness of Illness Rating Scale (Wyler, Masuda, & Holmes, 1968). The correlations between each of these measures and the GIS22-G were statistically significant and in the predicted direction.

Neubauer (1992) reports analyses of other measures taken on the same set of adult female nurses just described, including measures of illness frequency, absenteeism, and job satisfaction. Using canonical correlation, she combines these variables into a single measure of work effectiveness, satisfaction, and health with predictors including the previously mentioned measure of hardiness (PVS), the Work Environment Scale (Moos & Insel, 1974), and several measures reflecting aspects of the work environment (e.g., type of shift, rate of turnover). She concludes that the GIS22-G had the strong relationship of all the variables to the combined criterion variable. In particular, those with lower GIS22-G scores reported less illness and greater job satisfaction.

LaMar (1991) gave the entire CSSA, which includes the GIS22-G, to 83 volunteers, then asked them to record the GIS stressor and stress coping resources subscales (GIS7-C) daily for 28 days along with a short measure of daily health status. The correlations of the GIS22-G were statistically significant with the average of daily GIS7-C ($r = .79$) and with each of the other health measures, including the average of the daily health status, two measures of stress related symptoms, and an inventory of health status, all taken 28 days after the initial GIS22-G was completed. The averaged daily GIS7-C proved, in most instances, to be a better predictor of health measures than the full GIS22-G given on one occasion. The GIS7-C will be discussed later in this chapter.

Evans (1994) gave the GIS28-G, the OTLI scale, the State-Trait Anxiety Scale (Spielberger, Gorsuch, & Lushene, 1970) and the Well-Being Scale (WBS-25; Schlosser, 1990) to a group of nontraditional students (142 women and 32 men) enrolled in a presumably stressful summer session. Strong and statistically significant correlation coefficients were found in the expected direction between the GIS28-G and the OTL scale (−.65), State Anxiety (.60), Trait Anxiety (.71), and Well-Being (−.56). When combined, GIS and OTL made independent contributions to the prediction of the two measures of anxiety and of Well-Being. In contrast with earlier findings (Radmacher & Sheridan, 1989), neither GIS nor OTL predicted grade point average in this sample. It may be that this group of nontraditional students had developed coping strategies that allowed them to perform well under stress.

In a sample of college students (101 women and 62 men), Sherk (1990) used gender, the GIS22-C, the OTLI, and the Situational Humor Response Questionnaire (SHRQ; Martin & Lefcourt, 1983) as predictors, and the Cohen-Hoberman Inventory of Physical Symptoms (Cohen & Hoberman, 1983) as the outcome measure. GIS22-C, OTL, and gender were all statistically significant predictors of physical symptoms. Sherk performed a multiple regression with GIS22-C forced into the equation first, followed by stepwise entry of gender, OTL and SHRQ. Only the OTL made a significant additional contribution to the prediction of symptoms.

Using the method of contrasted groups (Anastasi, 1988), Beauchamp-Turner and Levinson (1992) gave the GIS22-C to 62 people who identified themselves as frequent meditators and 60 people who indicated that they either did not meditate or meditated infrequently. The participants also completed the CSSA Inventory of Stress-Related Symptoms and the MAACL. They found that the GIS22-C scores were significantly lower for the frequent meditators compared with the nonmeditators. The correlations between GIS22-C and Stress-Related Symptoms were high and statistically significant for both frequent and infrequent mediators. However, the correlation between GIS and the dysphoria subscale of the MAACL was significant only for infrequent meditators. The authors attributed the absence of a GIS-dysphoria linkage in frequent meditators to the stress-buffering effects of meditation.

Ingersoll (1990) gave the GIS22-G and the Social Desirability Scale (Crowne & Marlow, 1960) to 60 male patients under treatment for hypertension and 60 nonhypertensive patient controls. Each group was evenly divided according to whether they were over or under 60 years of age and whether they were obese or nonobese. Because of extremely low participation of African Americans who were invited, the study was limited to white participants. Ingersoll argued on the basis of prior literature that hypertension in older and obese patients might be less influenced by stress than in younger, nonobese patients because it appears that hypertension is more influenced by sympathetic arousal in the latter group. He found that the GIS22-G scores were indeed higher in the nonobese hypertensive patients and highest for the young, nonobese hypertensive group. These relationships were especially clear when social desirability scores were held constant.

Cloud (1995), after several pilot studies with African Americans, adapted the GIS and OTL to improve compliance and administered them to 152 African Americans and 80 white Americans. She also administered a brief measure of social desirability that had previously been shown to correlate highly with the Crowne-Marlowe Scale (Bigham, Martin & Sheridan, 1994). Cloud found that both the OTL and the GIS differentiated between hypertensives and nonhypertensives when social desirability was used as a covariate.

In another study, the entire CSSA, including the GIS22-C,

was administered to 64 patients diagnosed with chronic disease and 30 nonpatient controls (Schmidt & Sheridan, 1994). Thirty-two of the patients had received the diagnosis of chronic fatigue syndrome (CFS), and the remaining patients had miscellaneous diagnoses of chronic disease, not including CFS. In addition to the CSSA, the following measures were administered:

- Fatigue Severity Scale (FSS; Krupp, LaRocca, Muir-Nash, & Steinberg, 1989);
- The Inventory of Health Status (IHS; Mulhern, 1994); and
- The Personal Style Inventory (PSI), an inventory of stress vulnerability that included a measure of negative affect (Bigham, Sheridan, & Martin, 1994; Martin & Sheridan, 1994).

Fatigue severity scores correlated significantly with GIS22-C ($r = .42, p < .0001$). The IHS, a well-validated self-report measure of general somatic health status, provides two separate measures of health status, the first of which assesses medical diagnosis and range of sick-role behaviors (IHST) and the second of which identifies symptoms reflecting somatic health status (SYM). Strong and statistically significant correlations in the expected direction were found between the GIS22-C and the IHST ($r = .47, p < .001$) and SYM ($r = .54, p < .001$). With the items for the short form extracted from the original data, significant correlations were also found between the GIS7-C and the FSS ($r = .39, p < .0001$), and the IHST and SYM ($r = .45, p < .0001$).

Negative Affectivity and the GIS

There is a perspective that the relationships between stress and health measures are exaggerated because of a common influence of negative affectivity (NA; Costa & McCrae, 1987; Watson & Pennebaker, 1989). More recently, some research has provided strong evidence that both stress and negative affectivity have an influence on health when the health measure is not subject to distortions in self-reporting. For example, Cohen, Tyrrell, and Smith (1993) have shown in well controlled studies that a measure combining NA and perceived stress predicts occurrence of the common cold when rhinoviruses have been experimentally planted in the nasal passages of volunteers. Negative affectivity has been viewed not as a nuisance variable but as an early effect of stress which might evolve into somatic disease if ignored (Sheridan & Smith, 1987). Still, the high correlations between anxiety and the GIS require us to take seriously the possibility that GIS responses are secondary to NA. (It is worth mentioning that NA may be an early indicator of the impact of stress and at the same time influence reporting of stress and health.)

To assess the role of NA in GIS scores, a measure of NA was included in the data of Schmidt and Sheridan (1994) as part of the measure of stress vulnerability. Mulhern (1994) had previously shown that this measure, called the PSINA, correlated with more familiar measures of NA (Costa & McCrae, 1987; Tellegen, 1982) as highly as they correlated with each other, with correlations in the .70 range. Multiple regressions were done with the measures of fatigue and health status described earlier as the criterion variables. PSINA was forced into the equation first, and then the GIS22-C was allowed to enter according to the SPSS default criteria for stepwise regression. In each instance, GIS22-C scores alone made a statistically significant contribution in the final equations. An identical procedure was applied to the GIS7-C and the same outcomes measured. Results were essentially the same as those for the GIS22-C. Both the GIS22-C and the GIS7-C predicted the criteria independently of NA.

Case Example

A case study is described here to illustrate the GIS as a screening device in a medical setting. Mr. B was a 34-year-old man referred to a multidisciplinary reconditioning and work-readiness program with a referring diagnosis of postrepair nonunion left tibial shaft. While working on his road construction job, he was injured, sustaining a closed head injury, blunt chest trauma, and fractures of both legs. The patient had two surgeries on the left lower leg and was wearing a brace. He had been unable to work for 18 months.

His first assessment and treatment was by a physical therapist who concluded that his case seemed uncomplicated by psychological factors. Nevertheless, he underwent psychological evaluation as a routine part of the rehabilitation program. This evalution included administration of the GIS-22C and several other inventories, including a measure of affect (MAACL; Zuckerman & Lubin, 1985). These assessments were integrated with a clinical interview.

In the interview, Mr. B acknowledged feeling distressed but reported that he was taking action to cope and doing "pretty well." His total GIS-22C score was modestly elevated (approximately one standard deviation above the mean), but this was in part due to his experiencing a low amount of stress in social relationship other than his marriage and job. GIS test results indicated much more than an average number of stressors that were intense in nature. The typical level of strain the patient avowed was approximately two standard deviations above the mean. He affirmed a fair number of somatic symptoms and many psychological symptoms of overload. Sources of stressors included the marital relationship and a very unpleasant job situation. His scores of these dimensions contrasted sharply with those pertaining to nonprimary social relationships, which were quite modest. During the interview Mr. B elaborated on the GIS findings, confirming the impression provided by the GIS. It became evident that he was highly distressed from pressure from his wife to return to work with a concomitant high frequency of arguments. Financial concerns were also very significant, along with worry over the possibility that his employer would find an excuse to dismiss him.

The GIS findings were consistent not only with the interview results but also with the MAACL affect scores, which indicated moderately severe to severe levels of depression, anxiety, and hostility. GIS results were also consistent with assessment of his personal stress resistance as revealed in his responses on the Personal Style Inventory (described in another chapter). These indicated less than effective stress coping skills, resources, and approaches to stressors, which appeared to be ineffective and perhaps even stress amplifying. The patient was referred to counseling.

Benefits and Limitations

The GIS indicates whether problems are focused on stressors, resources, or symptoms and provides separate assessments of primary and social relationships and work situations. It can be used when the major aspects of stress should be measured and identification of specific stressors, resources, or symptoms is unnecessary. The concept behind the CSSA is that one can do a quick general assessment with the GIS, and this is often all that is needed. If more details are required, one can use the more specified assessments provided by the remaining instruments of the CSSA, inquiring about the specifics underlying a high score in a given category.

Compelling evidence indicates that the GIS in its various forms is a reliable instrument with criterion-related validity. Since its predictions of health outcomes has been shown to be largely independent of negative affectivity, we can also affirm its discriminant validity. In addition, the modest demands made by the GIS on reading skills and its generic nature make it applicable to a wide range population. The GIS has been shown to predict a variety of dependent measures, including academic performance, work satisfaction, dysphoria, fatigue, and various measures of illness, sick-role behaviors, and symptoms. When it has been combined with other measures of stress and stress resistance, it has consistently accounted for more variance in health status when compared with the other measures. The reliability and validity of the GIS has been established in many heterogeneous samples, thus allowing the conclusion that it is applicable to diverse populations.

Use of the GIS is limited to adolescents and adults with at least a seventh-grade reading level. It takes at least 15 minutes, with an occasional respondent taking somewhat longer.

Chapter References

Anastasi, A. (1988). *Psychological testing* (6th ed.). New York: Macmillan.

Antonovsky, A. (1979). *Health, stress, and coping.* San Francisco: Jossey-Bass.

Antonovsky, A. (1987). *Unravelling the mystery of health.* San Francisco: Jossey-Bass.

Baich, S. (1988). *The assessment of current stress.* Unpublished master's thesis, University of Missouri-Kansas City.

Beauchamp-Turner, D., & Levinson, D. (1992). Effects of meditation on stress, health, and affect. *Medical Psychotherapy: An International Journal, 5*, 123–131.

Bigham, S., Martin, D. M., & Sheridan, C. L. (1994). Validation of a comprehensive measure of stress vulnerability. *First World Conference on Stress, No. 19. Program and Abstracts* (p. 40). Bethesda, MD: International Society for the Investigation of Stress.

Cloud, L. D. (1995). *Psychosocial life-style stressors and the African-American hypertensive.* Unpublished doctoral dissertation, University of Missouri–Kansas City.

Cohen, S., & Hoberman, H. (1983). Positive events and social supports as buffers of life change stress. *Journal of Applied Social Psychology, 13*, 99–125.

Cohen, S., Tyrrell, D. A., & Smith, A. P. (1993). Negative life events, perceived stress, negative affect, and susceptibility to the common cold. *Journal of Personality and Social Psychology, 64*(1), 131–140.

Costa, P. T., & McCrae, R. R. (1987). Hypochondriasis, neuroticism, and aging: When are somatic complaints unfounded? *American Psychologist, 40*, 19–28.

Crowne, D., & Marlowe, D. (1960). A new scale of social desirability independent of psychopathology. *Journal of Consulting Psychology, 24,* 349–354.

Dohrenwend, B., Krosnoff, L., Askenasy, A., & Dohrenwend, B. (1978). Exemplification of a method for scaling life events: The Peri-Life Events Scale. *Journal of Health and Social Behavior, 19,* 205–229.

Folkman, S., & Lazarus, R. (1980). An analysis of coping in a middle-aged community sample. *Journal of Health and Social Behavior, 21,* 219–239.

Holmes, T., & Rahe, R. (1967). The social readjustment rating scale. *Journal of Psychosomatic Research, 11,* 213–218.

Ingersoll, W. (1990). *Differential grouping of psychological and physiological characteristics in essential hypertension.* Unpublished doctoral dissertation, University of Missouri–Kansas City.

Kanner, A. D., Coyne, J. C., Schaefer, C., & Lazarus, R. S. (1981). Comparison of two modes of stress measurement: Daily hassles and uplifts versus major life events. *Journal of Behavioral Medicine, 4,* 1–39.

Kolenc, K., Hartley, D., & Murdock, N. (1990). The relationship of mild depression to stress and coping. *Journal of Mental Health Counseling, 12,* 76–92.

Krause, N., & Markides, K. (1990). Measuring social support among older adults. *The International Journal of Aging and Human Development, 30,* 37–53.

Krupp, L. B., LaRocca, N. G., Muir-Nash, J., & Steinberg, A. D. (1989). The fatigue severity scale: Application to patients with multiple sclerosis and systemic lupus erythematosus. *Archives of Neurology, 46,* 1121–1123.

LaMar, L. (1991). *A study of the relationship of illness onset to daily stress levels.* Unpublished doctoral dissertation, University of Missouri–Kansas City.

Lazarus, R. S., & Folkman, S. (1984). *Stress, appraisal and coping.* New York: Springer.

Martin, R., & Lefcourt, H. (1983). Sense of humor as a moderator of the relations between stressors and moods. *Journal of Personality and Social Psychology, 45,* 1313–1324.

Martin, D. M., & Sheridan, C. L. (1994). Stress, health, and borderline personality organization. *First World Conference on Stress, No. 152. Program and Abstracts* (p. 62). Bethesda, MD: International Society for the Investigation of Stress.

Mehrabian, A., & Russell, J. (1974). *An approach to environmental psychology*. Cambridge, MA: MIT Press.

Moos, R. N., & Insel, P. M. (1974). *Family, work, and group environment scale manual*. Palo Alto, CA: Consulting Psychologists Press.

Mulhern, M. (1994). *The validation of the inventory of health status*. Unpublished doctoral dissertation, University of Missouri–Kansas City.

Neubauer, P. (1992). The impact of stress, hardiness, home and work environment on job satisfaction, illness, and absenteeism in critical care nurses. *Medical Psychotherapy: An International Journal, 4*, 109–122.

Radmacher, S. A., & Sheridan, C. L. (1989). The global inventory of stress: A comprehensive approach to stress assessment. *Medical Psychotherapy: An International Journal, 2*, 75–80.

Schlosser, B. (1990). The assessment of subjective well-being and its relationship to the stress process. *Journal of Personality Assessment, 54*(1–2), 128–140.

Schmidt, S. A., & Sheridan, C. L. (1994). Avowed fatigue and symptom range as a function of stress in Chronic Fatigue Syndrome patients with reporting distortions controlled. In *Proceedings of the Annual Scientific Conference of the American Association for Chronic Fatigue Syndrome*, p. 67.

Selye, Hans (1978). *The stress of life*, revised ed. New York: McGraw-Hill.

Sheridan, C. L., & Smith, L. K. (1987). Toward a comprehensive scale of stress assessment: Norms, reliability, and validity. *International Journal of Psychosomatics, 34*, 48–54.

Sherk, L. (1990). *The use of sense of coherence and humor when coping with stress*. Unpublished masters thesis, University of Missouri–Kansas City.

Snow, D. L., & Sheridan, C. L. (1996). [Perceived stress in chronic pain patients]. Unpublished raw data.

Spielberger, C. D., Gorsuch, R. L., Lushene, R. E. (1970). *Manual for the State-Trait Anxiety Inventory*. Palo Alto, CA: Consulting Psychologist Press.

Tellegen, A. (1982). *Brief manual for the differential personality questionnaire*. Unpublished manuscript, University of Minnesota, Minneapolis.

Watson, D., & Pennebaker, J. W. (1989). Health complaints, stress, distress: Exploring the central role of negative affectivity. *Psychological Review, 96*, 234–254.

Williams, S. (1990). The relationship among stress, hardiness, sense of coherence, and illness in critical care nurses. *Medical Psychotherapy: An International Journal, 3*, 171–186.

Wyler, A. R., Masuda, M., & Holmes, T. H. (1968). Seriousness of illness rating scale. *Journal of Psychosomatic Research, 11*, 363–375.

Zuckerman, M., & Lubin, B. (1985). *Manual for the MAACL-R: The multiple affect adjective checklist revised.* San Diego: Educational and Industrial Testing Service.

The Hilson Career Satisfaction/Stress Index

Robin Inwald, William Traynor, and Vicki Favuzza, Hilson Research Inc.

■ Instrument Names

The Hilson Career Satisfaction Stress Index[1]
HCSI

■ Developer

Robin Inwald, Ph.D., Hilson Research Inc.

■ Contact Information

For information regarding the Hilson Career Satisfaction/ Stress Index or other Hilson Research tests, contact Hilson Research Inc., P.O. Box 150239, 82-28 Abingdon Road, Kew Gardens, NY 11415.

Telephone: (800): 926-2258; fax: (718) 849-6238

Description and History of the Instrument

The Hilson Career Satisfaction/Stress Index (HCSI) is a 161-question true/false inventory that was developed to aid in the identification of employee stress symptoms, performance difficulties, negative attitudes toward work, antisocial attitudes, and/or substance abuse difficulties. Since at least a minimal level of employee job satisfaction is integral to the success of any organization, the HCSI is designed to help both adminis-

---

1. The HCSI was developed by Robin Inwald and is a registered trademark of Hilson Research Inc.

trators and personnel identify job dissatisfaction and stress patterns that may lead to increased employee frustration and decreased productivity. The HCSI can be used for both clinical and/or self-development purposes. In a counseling situation, a clinical report can be generated to aid psychologists or other mental health professionals in making recommendations for treatment or follow-up. In an employee assistance setting, a self-development report can be generated to provide direct feedback to the individual. Employers of individuals in high risk occupations also use the HCSI as an aid in "fitness-for-duty" evaluations (Girodo, 1991a, 1991b). It also can be used to assess perceived stress and/or negative feelings about work for specific groups of employees.

Items and Scales

The HCSI contains 161 items grouped into three main scales (Stress Patterns, Anger/Hostility Patterns, and Dissatisfaction with Career) and one validity measure (Defensiveness). Items in each scale consist of specific questions that relate to the scale's content. For example, the Stress Patterns scale contains the following questions:

"I often feel dizziness, rapid heart beat, or very shaky feelings because of the pressure of this job"
"Bad dreams have been bothering me lately"
"After a bad day at work, I really feel the need for a drink to relax"

Individuals are asked to respond true or false to each item with the answer that best fits how they "usually feel."

Each of the main scales consist of various content areas. The Stress Patterns scale contains the following content areas: Stress Symptoms, Drug/Alcohol Abuse, and Interpersonal Support. High scores in these areas suggest the presence of physical stress symptoms, lack of a strong social support network in times of stress, and/or a tendency to use alcohol or drugs to relieve pressures. The Anger/Hostility Patterns scale consists of the Disciplinary History, Excusing Attitudes, and Aggression/Hostility content areas. These content areas measure the level of hostility and anger as expressed in antisocial behaviors or antagonistic attitudes relating to the workplace. The third main scale, Dissatisfaction with Career, contains the Dissatisfaction with Supervisor, Relationship with Co-Workers, and Dissatisfaction with Job content areas. These areas measure how well individual work-related goals have been met. High scores in these areas indicate dissatisfaction with career progress, supervisors, and/or co-workers.

For all scales, the greater number of endorsed items, the greater the indication of specific job dissatisfaction, anger/frustration, defensiveness, and/or stress patterns for the individual tested. A technical manual is available to help users of the instrument understand and interpret results (Inwald & Jaufman, 1989).

Administration, Scoring, and Interpretation

Administration

The HCSI can be administered individually or in a group setting. Each individual is given an HCSI test booklet and an answer sheet. The questions are printed in the test booklet, and each individual marks their true/false responses on the computer scorable answer sheets. Conditions of administration for the HCSI should be that of "reasonable comfort and with minimal distractions" as suggested by the APA *Standards for Educational and Psychological Tests* (American Psychological Association, 1985). These standards suggest that "noise, disruption, extremes of temperature, inadequate work space, illegible materials and so forth are among the conditions that should be avoided in testing situations" (ibid.).

Items on the HCSI have been calculated to be at a fifth-grade reading level. If during testing an individual has questions about the definitions of words, the examiner may answer them. No additional coaching, however, may be provided regarding the interpretation of items. If an individual is having particular difficulty with an item, it may be omitted. Testing takes approximately 20 to 30 minutes.

Scoring

The HCSI is completely computer scored, which eliminates the type of accidental errors that are often the result of hand scoring. Computerized scoring of the HCSI also allows a much greater quantity of information to be provided to the test user. Another advantage of computer scoring is the ability to store all test data for later retrieval, rescoring, and/or analysis.

Three scoring services currently are available for the HCSI. It can be scored using an in-house computer and modem with the Hilson Research Remote System Software (2- to 3-second on-line scoring time per test), by the Hilson Research Fax Service (same day service), or by the Hilson Research Mail-In Service (same-day processing).

HCSI Printout Interpretation

HCSI test results are printed in an easy-to-read computer printout that groups item responses according to scales. As a result, a large amount of information is available in a logically organized format for quick review or more detailed analysis. The HCSI report consists of eight sections, described next:

Narrative Report. The first section is the HCSI Narrative Report. General summary statements are made about an individual's response style, stress patterns, anger/hostility patterns, and expressed career dissatisfaction. These statements, which are made about tests scores, are constructed to apply to a large number of people and, for this reason, should be used only as a general guide. Users should become comfortable with the raw data in making their evaluations. Information should be verified by conducting follow-up interviews as well as by using other data available to the test administrator (e.g., background checks or other test measures). The HCSI Narrative Report is not intended to be a substitute for an interview or to be used as a sole source for an employee evaluation.

The HCSI contains both a Clinical and Self-Development Narrative Report. The Clinical Narrative Report is a formal report, written in the third person, which is meant to be read by mental health or human resource professionals (such as clinicians, counselors, and/or psychologists). The Self-Development Report is written in the first person and communicates directly to the person who has taken the test.

Critical Items for Follow-up Evaluation. The Critical Item for Follow-up Evaluation section contains a printout of those items that reveal stress symptoms or job dissatisfaction and were endorsed by the individual. These endorsed items, which are printed in their entirety, have been found to be especially useful to clinicians. Critical item endorsements should be used in follow-up interviews and verified by the employee. Very often, one or two items will reveal problems that have been denied elsewhere. In no case, however, should one or two item endorsements on the critical items list be used as the reason for a negative evaluation or for evaluating an employee as abnormally "stressed" or dissatisfied.

Profile Graph (Employee Norms). The Profile Graph provides users with information about how an individual scored in relation to others tested with the HCSI using the Hilson Research HCSI norms. Norms were developed for a group of 1,351 individuals.

When interpreting the results of the HCSI Profile Graph, the Defensiveness (DN) scale should be reviewed first. If the DN score is over 60T, the person may have been unusually defensive or guarded in answering the questions. This type of response style may result in other scales appearing lower than they would normally be if the person had been more candid on this inventory.

The next step is to identify the main HCSI scales with the highest t-scores. Scales exceeding 70T on the graph represent areas where the individual has scored outside the "average range" (or two standard deviations above the mean) compared with others who have been tested previously. Elevated scales suggest areas where the person may have revealed specific problems, and they should be explored further. T-scores over 60 indicate slight elevations (one standard deviation above the mean) and also may indicate areas for further exploration. Scores from 41T to 59T are within the average range for the norming group. Finally, any scores below 41T provide some indication that the problem areas measured by these scales do not apply to this individual and/or have been denied.

Profile Graph (Promotional Norms). The HCSI Promotional Norms Graph indicates how the tested individual scored in relation to employees who were candidates for promotion. This graph is interpreted in the same way as the HCSI Employee Norm Graph. However, t-scores for the tested individual will often be markedly higher when compared with promotional candidates than when compared with employee norms. This result may be due to population differences or to the fact that the promotional candidates tended to be more defensive than the general employees and were less willing to admit to minor shortcomings.

Local Norms Profile Graph. Individual organization, local, or specific occupational norms also can be provided for the HCSI. Once an organization has administered the HCSI to a sufficient number of individuals, local norms can be generated. In this profile, an individual's scores are compared with those of his or her own organization or occupation. The results are then interpreted in the same manner as are the other profile graphs.

Scale/Content Area Descriptions. Each report contains a complete list of all HCSI scales and content areas (e.g., SY—

Stress Symptoms). Users can easily refer to these descriptions when interpreting the profile graphs.

True/False Item Endorsements. This section contains a listing of the individual's responses so that the accuracy of the computer's reading of the answer sheet can be verified. A "T" represents a true endorsement, an "F" represents a false endorsement, and a "_" indicates that the person either left the item blank or filled in both true and false on the answer sheet.

Item Tag Words. This is the last section of the HCSI report. Abbreviations are listed for all scales, and beneath each are the individual item numbers for all of the items included in a particular scale score. Each item is followed by the individual's response ("T" or "F") and a brief tag word referring to the content of the item. For example, 10T WORKDONE, means that the individual responded true to question 10, "I have always gotten my work done on time."

Psychometric Characteristics

Norms

The HCSI was administered to 1,351 individuals. Norms, including means and standard deviations, were developed for each HCSI scale for 1,130 male and 221 female participants. The sample was composed of 80% white, 13% black, and 4% Hispanic individuals, with the remaining 3% indicating "other" on the answer sheet. "Critical" scores (defined by the researchers as scores falling two standard deviations above the mean) were calculated to aid in identifying those candidates who scored significantly higher than their peers on specific scales.

Reliability

HCSI item responses were examined to determine the reliability of individual scales for 1,351 individuals. For each of the main scales, alpha coefficients ranged from .83 to .94 (see Table 1). The average of these four main scales was .86.

Concurrent Validity

Two samples were used for computing correlations between the HCSI and the Hilson Personnel Profile/Success Quotient (HPP/SQ). The first group was a sample of 36 state employees, and the second was a group of 198 city employees. There were many negative correlations between the two tests. This finding was expected since the HPP/SQ is a test that identifies positive qualities in an individual, whereas the HCSI reflects stress and dissatisfaction patterns.

In both groups, the Defensiveness (DN) scale on the HCSI correlated negatively with the Candor (CA) scale on the HPP/SQ at −.96 and −.90, respectively. Thus, those who were candid in answering questions on the HPP/SQ also were willing to admit to shortcomings on the HCSI. In the group of 198 city employees, there were several significant correlations between the HPP/SQ scales (measuring social skills, work ethic, etc.) and the HCSI Stress Patterns scale (ST). This suggests that achievement and initiative are inversely related to stress symptoms. It may be that individuals with increased stress symptoms are likely to have less initiative and be less "goal oriented." Again, this outcome might be expected since the two tests measure opposing personality characteristics.

Table 1: Reliability

Scale	Alpha	N
AP	.84	1,304
ST	.85	1,271
DC	.94	1,298
DN	.83	1,333

There also was a negative correlation $(-.27)$ between the Drive (DR) scale on the HPP/SQ and the Dissatisfaction with Career (DC) scale on the HCSI. This suggests some relationship between an individual's tendency to "go the extra mile" and his or her perceived recognition, career opportunity, and potential for advancement. It may be that highly driven individuals, who tend to work harder than their peers and who may demonstrate workaholic tendencies, are most likely to believe they are receiving sufficient emotional rewards on the job.

Predictive Validity

All current employees in a municipal agency $(N = 196)$ were administered the HCSI and the Hilson Personnel Profile/Success Quotient (HPP/SQ) during in-service training sessions. Six months after testing, a global rating was assigned by the supervisor as to whether each member's performance was "exceptional" $(N = 19)$, "average" $(N = 158)$, or "poor" $(N = 19)$. When "exceptional" members were compared with all others using discriminant function analysis, the HPP/SQ and HCSI scales correctly identified 70.9% as to group membership. When "poorly" performing members were compared with all others, 71.4% of the members were correctly classified. T-tests revealed that "exceptional" members showed lower scores on four HCSI scales, Dissatisfaction with Career (DC), Dissatisfaction with Job (DJ), Anger/Hostility Patterns (AP), and Total Score (TS) $(p < .01)$. Those rated as "poor" performers showed higher scores on the HCSI Dissatisfaction with Career (DC) and Dissatisfaction with Job (DJ) scales $(p < .05)$.

Construct Validity

Factor Analysis. To identify the factors measured by the HCSI, a factor analysis was performed using the HCSI scales for a sample of 1,351 employees from various occupations.

Findings suggest that the four main HCSI scales comprise a single factor, perhaps described as "stress and dissatisfaction with career," that accounts for 59.3% of the variance (see Table 2).

Scale Correlations. To assess the degree to which the HCSI scales correlate with each other, intercorrelations were calculated for 1,351 employees (see Table 3). The defensiveness scale, as expected, showed a highly negative correlation with the other major scales. This suggests that the more defensive individuals are in their responses, the lower their scores will be on the HCSI.

Application

The HCSI has proven to be a useful tool in various occupational and clinical settings. It has been used as one part of

Table 2: Factor Analysis

HCSI Scales	Factor Matrix
DN	-.37
ST	.86
AP	.89
DC	.84

Table 3: Scale Intercorrelations

	DN	ST	AP	DC
DN	----			
ST	-.21	----		
AP	-.27	66	—	
DC	-.11	61	.66	—

fitness-for-duty evaluations, as well as for promotional and/ or counseling purposes. The HCSI has aided employers and individuals in identifying job dissatisfaction and stress patterns that may lead to increased frustration and decreased productivity.

In addition to the HCSI, another inventory relating to stress, the Hilson Life Stress Questionnaire (HLSQ), is currently in development. This questionnaire is intended for use with senior populations and focuses on issues such as Assertive Coping Style, Accommodating Coping Style, Fear of Memory Loss, and Fear of Death.

Benefits and Limitations

The HCSI can help both employers and employees identify stress patterns and expressed job dissatisfaction that can lead to increased employee frustration and decreased productivity. Not only does the HCSI include information about an employee's attitude toward his or her job, but it also provides normative data regarding that individual's coping skills. For example, the HCSI may assist in differentiating between a disgruntled/generally angry (high AP score) employee, whose negative attitude would be present toward any job owing to that person's own personality orientation, as opposed to an employee whose dissatisfaction is primarily related to actual conditions on the job (low AP score).

As with all self-report inventories, the HCSI is limited to an individual's admissions of difficulties. The results, therefore, should be verified using information from other sources.

Chapter References

American Psychological Association. (1974). *Standards on Educational and Psychological Tests.* Washington, DC.

American Psychological Association. (1985). *Standards on Educational and Psychological Tests.* Washington, DC.

Girodo, M. (1991a). Drug corruption in undercover agents: Measuring the risk. *Behavioral Sciences and the Law, 9,* 361–370.

Girodo, M. (1991b). Personality, job stress, and mental health in undercover agents: A Structural Equation Analysis. *Journal of Social Behavior and Personality, 6*(7), 375–390.

Robin E., Inwald, R. E., & Jaufman, J. C. (1989). *Hilson Career Satisfaction Index technical manual.* Kew Gardens, NY: Hilson Research Inc.

The Inventory of Positive Psychological Attitudes

Measuring Attitudes That Buffer Stress and
Facilitate Primary Prevention Using Constructs
Responsive to Diverse Cultural World Views*

Jared D. Kass, Lesley College

■ Instrument Names

The Inventory of Positive Psychological Attitudes
IPPA-32R, IPPA

■ Developers

Jared D. Kass, Ph.D., Professor of Counseling and
  Psychology, Graduate School of Arts and Social Sciences,
  Lesley College; Director, Behavioral Health Services
  Program, Greenhouse Psychotherapy Associates,
  Cambridge, MA
Richard Friedman, Ph.D., Jane Leserman, Ph.D., Margaret
  Caudill, M.D., Ph.D., Patricia Zuttermeister, M.A., and
  Herbert Benson, M.D., New England Deaconess Hospital,
  Boston, MA

■ Contact Information

Jared D. Kass, Ph.D., Professor of Counseling and
  Psychology, Graduate School of Arts and Social Sciences,
  Lesley College, 7 Mellen St., Cambridge, MA 02138-2790
Telephone: (617) 349-8340; fax: (617) 349-8333;
  e-mail: jkass@mail.lesley.edu

---

*Jared D. Kass, Ph.D, holds the copyright for the IPPA.

Description and History of the Instrument

The Inventory of Positive Psychological Attitudes (IPPA) is a 32-item multidimensional self-report instrument measuring positive attitudinal domains that buffer stress and which facilitate the primary prevention of stress-related psychological and physical disorders. It is composed of two subscales. The first subscale, containing 15 items, measures Self-Confidence During Stress (SCDS). The second subscale, containing 17 items, measures Life Purpose and Satisfaction (LPS). In its entirety, the IPPA measures an individual's Confidence in Life and Self (CLS). These attitudinal constructs were designed to be responsive to the worldviews of culturally diverse populations.

The IPPA was developed for use with adults and adolescents. It takes 15 minutes to complete and requires a sixth-grade reading level. The IPPA can be administered in written form and orally. Using a Likert scale ranging from 1 to 7, individuals report their degree of agreement with 32 different statements. The IPPA can be administered in two formats.

- The standard format is used for research and diagnosis. In this format, the 32 items are presented in a randomized pattern, including reverse ordering of positive directionality on the Likert scales.
- The self-test format is used in psychoeducational settings in which individuals will score their own tests. In this format, statements for each subscale (SCDS and LPS) are grouped together. There is no reverse ordering of the positive dimensions on the Likert scales. In addition, instructions for scoring and an initial interpretation are provided for the individual subject.

I developed the conceptual foundations of the IPPA and the original item pool in 1985–1986. Support for this project was provided by Lesley College through a faculty development grant for research in health psychology.

The refinement of the item pool, validation procedures, and preliminary clinical testing were conducted from 1987 to 1990 in collaboration with Richard Friedman, Ph.D.; Jane Leserman, Ph.D.; Margaret Caudill, M.D., Ph.D.; Patricia Zuttermeister, M.A.; and Herbert Benson, M.D.—all at the Division of Behavioral Medicine, Department of Medicine, New England Deaconess Hospital, Mind/Body Medical Institute, Harvard Medical School, Boston, MA. Results from this validation study are reported elsewhere (Kass et al., 1991). Support for this project was provided by Laurance S. Rockefeller, the Fetzer Institute, and the United States Public Health Service (HL 27227).

The initial format of the IPPA contained 30 items (IPPA-30). At that time, the SCDS subscale contained 13 questions. To further strengthen the construct validity of the SCDS subscale, I have added two questions to this scale. In addition, the wording of five other SCDS questions was clarified (IPPA-32R). The factor structure and reliability of the revised instrument have been tested and are consistent with the factor structure of the IPPA-30 (Kass, 1997).

A self-test format for the IPPA-32R has been developed. Plans are now being developed to translate the IPPA-32R into Spanish. Table 1 presents sample questions from the IPPA-32R in a self-test format.

Underlying Assumptions, Premises, and Objectives

Psychological assessment, within both clinical and health psychology, has tended to focus on the identification of attitudes that contribute to, or are symptomatic of, psychological and physical disorders. This approach is appropriate when clinicians and researchers seek to identify the degree to which individuals are impaired or at risk. This approach is less useful, however, when clinicians and researchers seek to identify the nature and strength of attitudes that contribute to primary prevention and the restoration of psychological and physical health (Antonovsky, 1979).

Table 1: Inventory of Positive Psychological Attitudes (IPPA-32R) Self-Test

SELF CONFIDENCE DURING STRESS:

1. When there is a great deal of pressure being placed on me

| I get tense | 1 | 2 | 3 | 4 | 5 | 6 | 7 | I remain calm |

2. I react to problems and difficulties

| with a great deal of frustration | 1 | 2 | 3 | 4 | 5 | 6 | 7 | with no frustration |

3. In a difficult situation, I am confident that I will receive the help that I need.

| disagree strongly | 1 | 2 | 3 | 4 | 5 | 6 | 7 | agree strongly |

LIFE PURPOSE AND SATISFACTION:

1. During most of the day, my energy level is

| very low | 1 | 2 | 3 | 4 | 5 | 6 | 7 | very high |

2. As a whole, my life seems

| dull | 1 | 2 | 3 | 4 | 5 | 6 | 7 | vibrant |

3. My daily activities are

| not a source of satisfaction | 1 | 2 | 3 | 4 | 5 | 6 | 7 | a source of satisfaction |

4. I have come to expect that every day will be

| exactly the same | 1 | 2 | 3 | 4 | 5 | 6 | 7 | new and different |

In the last three decades, increased attention has been placed on explaining how positive attitudes may contribute to health. These conceptual efforts have focussed on the stress-buffering effects of positive attitudes. Considerable research has demonstrated that frequent activation of the stress response produces chronic hyperarousal as well as dysregulation of neurotransmitter functions related to the sympathetic nervous system–adrenal medulla axis and the hypothalamic-pituitary-adrenal cortex axis of the endocrine system (Gatchel & Baum, 1983; Rose, 1980). As sequelae to hyperarousal and dysregulation of these systems, individuals regularly develop a range of disorders (Gatchel & Blanchard, 1993). These include psychological disorders (characterized by elevated levels of hostility, depression, or anxiety—either individually or in combination) (Gold, Goodwin, & Chrousos, 1988a, 1988b; Krystal et al., 1989; Van Der Kolk, 1988)—and physical disorders (characterized by pathology of the cardiovascular, gastrointestinal, immunological, and neuromuscular systems) (Andersen, Kiecolt-Glaser, & Glaser, 1994; Blascovich & Katkin, 1993; Dorian & Garfinkel, 1987; Taylor, 1986). In addition, individuals under stress regularly develop a range of health-risk behaviors. These behaviors, which may be attempts to regulate the stress response through forms of self-medication, are leading causes of premature morbidity and mortality in the United States. They include cigarette smoking, excessive consumption of high-fat foods, and dependence on alcohol and drugs (Brannon & Feist, 1997; Grunberg & Baum, 1985; Sunderwirth, 1985).

Although stress is recognized to be an inescapable aspect of life, research has begun to suggest that positive attitudes can function as intervening variables that buffer or prevent the stress response (Hafen, Frandsen, Karren, & Hooker, 1992; Lazarus & Folkman, 1984). By contributing to a positive worldview, these attitudes help individuals to be less reactive to, and to cope more successfully with, stressful circumstances and events. Thus, by helping regulate autonomic functions, positive attitudes can help to prevent psychological illnesses, medical illnesses, and health-risk behaviors associated with the stress response.

Two central constellations of positive attitudinal constructs have been hypothesized to contribute to health. The first constellation concerns locus of control. Using Rotter's (1966) model of internalized versus externalized locus of control, Langer and Rodin (1976) demonstrated that internal locus of control contributes to health. Similarly, Seligman has shown that learned helplessness leads to diminished coping and adaptation (Seligman, 1975). Wortman and Brehm (1975) refined this model by showing that expectations of internal locus of control counter helplessness. The second constellation concerns perceived meaning. Using Crumbaugh and Maholick's operational definition (Crumbaugh, 1968; Crumbaugh & Maholick, 1969, Crumbaugh & Maholick, 1964), Stevens, Pfost, and Wessel (1987) demonstrated that purpose in life contributes to improved coping. Using a somewhat different operational definition, Reker has shown that life purpose leads to improved psychological functioning (Reker, Peacock, & Wong, 1987). Additionally, Abby and Andrews (1985) found satisfaction with life to be associated with diminished levels of depression.

Initially, investigations regarding the efficacy of these two constellations remained separate. To some extent, the two constellations may have been seen as competing explanatory hypotheses. Eventually, researchers began to conceptualize these constellations as complementary and to measure them within multidimensional instruments. For example, Kobasa, Maddi, and Kahn (1982) developed the concept of "stress-hardiness" and conceived it as having both control and meaning dimensions. Similarly, Antonovsky (1987) developed the concept of "sense of coherence." This construct was also conceived as containing both control and meaning dimensions.

However, it has become apparent that both the first-generation unidimensional scales and the second-generation multidimensional scales contain limitations in the ways that they conceptualized the control and the meaning dimensions.

These limitations have been articulated from two related perspectives:

- *The multicultural and feminist perspective:* This perspective points out that assessment instruments tend to define psychological health as the attitudes and behaviors that reflect the sanctioned worldview of the dominant cultural group within our society (Brown & Ballou, 1992, Suzuki, Meller, & Ponterotto, 1996). This is a worldview that considers individuals as *isolated* and values *individualism.* Thus, these assessment tools are not responsive to persons from cultural groups that do not share this worldview. Nor are they responsive to the psychological effects on identity formation of the devaluation experienced by those who are not part of the dominant cultural group. These perspectives emphasize that many women and subordinate cultural groups hold a different worldview in which individuals experience themselves, not as isolated, but connected to others. Miller and her colleagues point out that women experience themselves in relational contexts, and that it is from these relational contexts that they derive an empowered sense of self (Jordan, Kaplan, Miller, Stiver, & Surrey, 1991; Miller, 1976). Sue points out that, for cultures whose behavior and attitudes are guided by a worldview of *connectedness,* there are beneficial forms of external locus of control (e.g., family and community) that are not measured in typical locus of control scales (Sue, 1978; Sue & Sue, 1981). Both Miller and Sue, among others, also point out that a primary source of diminished self-confidence for women and individuals from subordinated cultural groups is socially-sanctioned devaluation.
- *The religious-existential perspective:* Existential philosophy has tended to support this society's dominant worldview by suggesting that humans are essentially alone (May & Yalom, 1989; Yalom, 1981). The religious-existential perspective, however, has insisted that, while indi-

viduals must take full responsibility for their lives, they can derive meaning from a relationship with life's spiritual core. Tillich and Frankl have both suggested that a central cause of an individual's most fundamental experience of anxiety is the perception that life lacks intrinsic meaning (Frankl, 1959, 1969; Tillich, 1952). In addition, they have suggested that a central source of psychological strength can be an individual's relationship to a transcendent reality (Frankl, 1966; Tillich, 1952). Thus, meaning in life can be experienced not simply as a functional derivative of one's personal goals or work, but as an ontological attribute of life itself. In this worldview, too, an individual is fundamentally not alone.

These critical perspectives suggest that assessment instruments that operationalize control and meaning dimensions without including attitudes that can emerge from an individual's sense of connection to others or a transcendent reality are inadequate to measure the full potential range of a person's positive attitudinal coping resources. Whether individuals perceive themselves as connected to members of their family, their community, a transcendent reality, or a mixture of these three factors, receiving help from such trustworthy sources can buffer activation of the stress response in substantial ways. In addition, the clinical use of assessment instruments that fail to provide a mechanism for consideration of cultural identity (and the potential effects of devaluation on the formation of positive attitudes) is also inadequate, because such instruments lead to the assumption that there is something wrong with the culturally devalued individual, rather than the devaluing society.

As a third-generation positive attitudinal scale, the IPPA was developed to address these limitations in the conceptualization of the control and meaning dimensions and to provide a mechanism for the consideration of cultural identity during clinical assessment.

Control Dimension: Self-Confidence during Stress (SCDS)

The IPPA is built upon the hypothesis that the stress-buffering aspects of control derive from the perception that stressful events are *under* control, rather than from the perception that the individual is *in* control. Perceptions that events are under control exist on a continuum. The range of this continuum includes perceived internal locus of control, positive forms of external locus of control, and habitually calm responses to stressful situations that reflect perceptions of ontological security. Thus, the Self-Confidence during Stress subscale of the IPPA includes three types of attitudes:

- The first type measures perceived internal locus of control during stressful situations. Examples are "When I need to stand up for myself, I can do it quite easily," "I feel adequate when I am in difficult situations," and "I react to problems and difficulties with no frustration."
- The second type measures positive forms of external locus of control. Examples are "In a difficult situation, I am confident that I will receive the help that I need" and "During times of stress, I do not feel isolated and alone."
- The third type measures habitually calm responses to stressful situations that reflect perceptions of ontological security. Examples are "During stressful circumstances, I am never fearful" and "When there is a great deal of pressing being placed on me, I remain calm."

Although these three types of attitudes are somewhat different from each other, factor analyses suggest that they are related. Thus, the continuum of attitudes measured by the *Self-Confidence during Stress* subscale appears to have structural integrity.

Meaning Dimension: Life Purpose and Satisfaction (LPS)

The second dimension of the IPAA is based on the hypothesis that meaning-based attitudinal resources also exist on a continuum. The range of this continuum includes nonspecific perceptions of life satisfaction, personally constructed forms of meaning, and ontologically derived forms of meaning. Thus, the Life Purpose and Satisfaction (LPS) scale also contains three types of items:

- The first type measures nonspecific life satisfaction. Examples are "My daily activities are a source of satisfaction" and "During most of the day, my energy level is very high."
- The second type measures personally constructed forms of meaning. Examples are "I feel that the work I am doing is of great value," "At this time, I have clearly defined goals in my life," and "I feel that my life so far has been productive."
- The third type measures the ontological dimension of meaning. Examples are: "When I think deeply about life, I feel there is a purpose to it," "When sad things happen to me or other people, I continue to feel positive about life," "Deep inside myself, I feel loved," and "I do not feel trapped by the circumstances of my life."

Although these three types of attitudes are also somewhat different from each other, factor analyses suggest that they are related. Thus, the continuum of attitudes measured by the Life Purpose and Satisfaction subscale appears to have structural integrity.

Unifying Conceptualization: Confidence in Life and Self (CLS)

While the IPPA was designed to be a multidimensional instrument, the subscales within the IPPA were conceptualized as complementary aspects of a positive worldview: Confidence in Life and Self (CLS). Thus, while both SCDS and LPS are hypothesized to contain independent stress-buffering effects, and while an individual's scores on the two subscales can be substantially different, an optimally positive worldview was hypothesized to include strength in both dimensions. The psychometric properties of the IPPA demonstrate a mixture of convergence and divergence between the two subscales that this conceptual model anticipated. Factor analyses have consistently distinguished between the two subscales. At the same time, interscale correlation has been high. In addition, research results suggest that high scores on the total IPPA are often more strongly associated with positive outcomes than high scores on the individual subscales. Thus, there is an aggregate, or complementary, effect between the two subscales. These data lend support to the validity of the hypothesized construct, Confidence in Life and Self, as a reflection of an underlying positive worldview.

Mechanism for the Consideration of Cultural Identity in Clinical Assessment

A full consideration of cultural identity during the collection of research data requires use of a comprehensive cultural identity assessment instrument (Suzuki et al., 1996). The IPPA was not designed for this purpose. However, it was designed to contain a structural item that would promote the consideration of cultural identity in clinical or preventive interventions with individuals and small groups. The LPS subscale contains the item "I wish I were different than who I am: disagree strongly . . . agree strongly." When discussing responses to each IPPA item with a client, the culturally skilled counselor can use this item to investigate salient features of a client' cultural identity: the client's self-perception of her cultural identity, the effect of the client's cultural experience on his or her formation of positive attitudes regarding self and life, and the degree of comfort that the client feels with the counselor, based on differences or similarities in their cultural identities. Culturally skilled use of this open-ended item requires the acquisition of multicultural counseling skills by the clinician.

Such skill acquisition should be considered part of the requisite training for competent administration of the IPPA.

Summary of Research

Multidimensional Structure

Confirmation of the hypothesized multidimensional structure of the IPPA has been obtained using principal components and common factor analyses. In such analyses, an item pool is differentiated mathematically into factors, utilizing data gathered from appropriate samples. If these mathematically obtained factors match the hypothesized theoretical factors, the theoretical structure of the questionnaire is considered sound.

Using a sample of 368 adults (172 outpatients receiving behavioral medicine treatment, 88 undergraduate students, 108 graduate students), principal components analysis with varimax rotation differentiated items on the IPPA-30 into two factors corresponding to the hypothesized theoretical factors SCDS and LPS (Kass et al., 1991). Factor I (eigenvalue = 10.32; variance explained = 34.38%) contained the hypothesized 17 items of the LPS scale. Item loadings ranged from 0.45 to 0.76. Factor II (eigenvalue = 2.29; variance explained = 7.62%) contained the hypothesized 13 items of the SCDS scale. Item loadings ranged from 0.46 to 0.68. Despite clearly differentiated loading patterns, there was also convergence between the factors. One LPS item loaded above 0.4 on the SCDS scale. Similarly, two SCDS items loaded above 0.4 on the LPS scale. This degree of convergence was considered acceptable because these factors are hypothesized to be complementary aspects of an underlying positive worldview.

Further confirmation of this factor structure has been found using a sample of 1,029 adult employees at a large corporation (46% female, 54% male, 90.7% white) (Zuttermeister, Kass, Geiss, & Friedman, 1992). In this study, common factor analysis with varimax rotation was employed. From an initial pool of 54 items, 17 items were selected as Factor I. These items belonged to the hypothesized LPS scale. Additionally, 13 items were selected as Factor II. These items belonged to the hypothesized SCDS scale. A confirmatory common factor analysis was then conducted using only the 30 items. Table 2 reports results from this analysis. Loadings for the LPS factor ranged from 0.403 to 0.739. Loadings for the SCDS factor ranged from 0.391 to 0.648. Once again, despite substantial divergence, there was some convergence. Two LPS items loaded above 0.4 on the SCDS scale. One SCDS item loaded over .4 on the LPS scale. This degree of convergence was again considered acceptable given the hypothesized complementary nature of the two scales.

The factor structure of the IPPA-32R has also been tested (Kass, 1997). Common factor analyses were performed with varimax rotation on response data from a sample of 309 adults (55% female, 45% male, 90% white). An exploratory analysis with an unspecified number of factors differentiated 2 factors, corresponding to the LPS scale and the SCDS scale. The first factor (eigenvalue = 8.89; 27.8% variance explained) included the 17 items of the LPS scale. Factor loadings ranged from 0.432 to 0.815. The second factor (eigenvalue = 6.85; 21.4% variance explained) included the 15 items of the SCDS scale. Factor loadings ranged from 0.391 to 0.759. Once again, despite clear factor differentiation, a degree of convergence was found. One item from the LPS scale loaded above 0.4 on the SCDS scale. Four items on the SCDS scale loaded above 0.4 on the LPS scale. These results suggest that the factor structure of the IPPA-32R is highly analogous to the factor structure of the IPPA-30.

In summary, factor analyses have consistently supported the theorized multidimensional structure of the IPPA. The LPS and SCDS scales are different from each other. At the same time, these analyses show that the two subscales are not fully orthogonal. This convergence suggests that they are complementary aspects of an underlying positive worldview.

Table 2: Multidimensional Factor Structure of the IPPA-30 Common Factor Analysis with Varimax Rotation*

LPS Scale	Factor I	Factor II
Energy level is high	0.403	0.229
Life seems vibrant	0.724	0.161
Daily activities satisfy	0.608	0.135
Every day is new and different	0.617	0.136
Purpose to life	0.459	0.188
My life has been productive	0.607	0.182
My work is valuable	0.588	0.119
I do not wish I were different	0.506	0.402[†]
Clearly defined goals	0.479	0.245
Continue to feel positive about life when sad	0.423	0.502[†]
My life feels worthwhile	0.700	0.292
Present life satisfies me	0.739	0.259
Feel joy in my heart	0.612	0.222
Do not feel trapped by my life circumstances	0.619	0.315
No regrets regarding my past	0.451	0.335
Feel loved	0.507	0.311
Hopeful about solving my problems	0.561	0.331
SCDS Scale		
Calm during pressure	0.137	0.537
React to problems with no frustration	0.225	0.648
No anxiety during stress	0.160	0.545
Can like myself after a mistake	0.286	0.464
No catastrophic worries during stress situations	0.140	0.555
Can concentrate during stress	0.153	0.528
No fear during stressful circumstances	0.159	0.575
Can stand up for myself when I need	0.239	0.431
Feel adequate during difficult situations	0.368	0.520
Able to respond positively during difficulties	0.413[†]	0.492
Can relax during times of stress	0.369	0.391
Remain calm in frightening situations	0.099	0.529
Worry about the future during stress	0.286	0.461
Eigenvalues	6.430	4.770
Total Variance Explained	21.43%	15.90%

*Confirmatory analysis using the 30 items of the IPPA. No restrictions on number of factors.

†Loading above .4 on both factors.

The degree to which Confidence in Life and Self can be considered a structural unit was then assessed through tests of reliability.

Reliability

To determine the reliability of the IPPA scales, their internal consistency (the degree to which each respondent gave consistent answers to scale items) was measured. This criterion of reliability, also called homogeneity, was determined using Cronbach's alpha coefficient of reliability.

In the sample of 368 adults, Cronbach's alpha coefficients were found to be consistently high for each IPPA-30 scale, for both the sample as a whole and for each subgroup within the sample. For the entire sample, Cronbach's alpha coefficients were SCDS, 0.86; LPS, 0.91; Total IPPA (CLS), 0.93. Scores were similar for each subgroup (behavioral medicine outpatients, undergraduate students, graduate students). The range of alpha coefficients was SCDS, 0.80–0.86; LPS, 0.87–0.92; Total IPPA (CLS), 0.88–0.94 (Kass et al., 1991).

In the sample of 1,029 corporate employees, Cronbach's alpha coefficients were found to be consistently high for each IPPA-30 scale, both within the whole sample and within subgroups sorted by gender. For the SCDS subscale, the alpha coefficients were: total group, 0.855; females, 0.842; males, 0.858. For the LPS subscale, the alpha coefficients were: total group, 0.912; females, 0.908; males, 0.914. For the total IPPA (CLS), the alpha coefficients were: total group: 0.930; females, 0.926; males, 0.934 (Zuttermeister et al., 1992).

In the sample of 309 adults (Kass, 1997), Cronbach's alpha coefficients were also found to be high for each IPPA-32 scale. For SCDS, the alpha was 0.917. For LPS, the alpha was 0.942. For CLS (total IPPA), the alpha was 0.957. As anticipated, the revisions in the SCDS scale seem to have strengthened its reliability substantially. In addition, it appears that these revisions may also have strengthened the reliability of the total IPPA (Confidence in Life and Self).

In summary, these data help confirm the structural reliability of the IPPA scales. Both the SCDS and LPS subscales have a high degree of internal consistency. They are different from each other (as shown in the factor analyses), and they each display a high degree of homogeneity. At the same time, the CLS (total) scale also shows a high degree of internal consistency. Although the SCDS and LPS scales are different from each other, they are also related. These findings suggest that Confidence in Life and Self is a unified construct containing complementary aspects.

Construct Validity

Factor analysis and reliability tests evaluate the structural validity of a scale. However, they do not determine whether a scale actually measures its hypothesized attitudinal domains. Such construct validity can be assessed through two lines of inquiry. First, is there a measurable correspondence between the new scale and other scales that are recognized to measure related domains? Second, can this scale differentiate between population samples (whom we know to be different in these attitudinal domains)?

Correspondences between the IPPA and comparable scales. Using a sample of 368 adults, my colleagues and I compared the IPPA with McNair's Bi-Polar Profile of Mood States (McNair, Lorr, & Droppleman, 1981). This scale measures six attitudinal domains:

- Composed/Anxious,
- Agreeable/Hostile,
- Elated/Depressed,
- Confident/Unsure,
- Energetic/Tired, and
- Clearheaded/Confused.

In addition, we compared the IPPA with Bradburn's Affect Balance Scale measuring life satisfaction (Bradburn, 1969),

Rosenberg's Self-Esteem Scale (Rosenberg, 1965), and the UCLA Loneliness Scale (Russell, Peplau, & Ferguson, 1978). Table 3 presents findings from this study. As anticipated, there were positive correlations between the IPPA scales and positive moods, life satisfaction, and self-esteem. There was a negative correlation between the IPPA and loneliness. The strength of the positive and negative correlations ranged from .38 to .79, with most falling in the .50 to .65 vicinity. Correlations were significant at $p < .0001$ (Kass et al., 1991).

Table 3: Construct Validity of the IPPA Correlations between IPPA Scales and Other Attitudinal Measures

	Inventory of Positive Psychological Attitudes			p Value
	SCDS	LPS	CLS Total	
McNair Bi-Polar Profile of Mood States (POMS)*				
Composed/Anxious	.60	.56	.63	< .0001
Agreeable/Hostile	.37	.47	.46	< .0001
Elated/Depressed	.55	.65	.66	< .0001
Confident/Unsure	.65	.67	.72	< .0001
Energetic/Tired	.38	.49	.48	< .0001
Clearheaded/Confused	.51	.56	.58	< .0001
Rosenberg Self-Esteem Scale*	.67	.76	.79	< .0001
Bradburn Affect Balance Scale*	.55	.65	.66	< .0001
UCLA Loneliness Scale*	-.50	-.64	-.63	< .0001
Derogatis Psychiatric Symptom Checklist (SCL- 90-R)†				
Hostility	-.41	-.35	-.41	< .0001
Depression	-.57	-.60	-.64	< .0001
Anxiety	-.54	-.40	-.50	< .0001
Global Severity Index	-.57	-.52	-.59	< .0001

*Kass et al. (1991).
†Zuttermeister et al. (1992).

Using a sample of 1,009 corporate employees, my colleagues and I compared the IPPA to Derogatis' Symptom Checklist-90R (SCL-90R). This measure of psychiatric symptoms contains nine subscales: Hostility, Depression, Anxiety, Phobic Anxiety, Paranoid Ideation, Psychoticism, Obsessive-Compulsivity, Interpersonal Sensitivity, and Somatization. In addition, a Global Severity Index can be derived (Derogatis, 1983). Significant negative correlations, ranging from $r = -.21$ to $r = -.64$ ($p < .0001$), were found between the IPPA and all SCL-90R scales (Zuttermeister et al., 1992). Thus, as anticipated, Confidence in Life and Self (CLS) was negatively related to Hostility, Depression, Anxiety, and Global Severity. These correlations are reported in Table 3.

The data from these studies suggest two conclusions. First, there is a substantial degree of correspondence between the IPPA and the related attitudinal scales. In the social sciences, correlations in the range of $r = .500$ to $r = .600$ are considered to reflect a high degree of similarity. It is reasonable to conclude, then, that the IPPA scales measure positive attitudinal domains related to these other scales. However, it is important to note that if there were complete correspondence between the IPPA and the other attitudinal scales, they would be synonymous. In that event, the IPPA scales could not be considered unique attitudinal constructs. This reasoning leads to the second, and somewhat converse, conclusion. There are substantial divergences between the IPPA scales and the other scales. Correlations in the range of $r = .500$ to $r = .600$ reflect a shared variance (r^2) of 25% to 36%. Thus, the scales also perform with a reasonable amount of difference and cannot be considered synonymous. In conclusion, the IPPA scales tap positive attitudinal domains (Self-Confidence during Stress, Life Purpose and Satisfaction, and Confidence in Life and Self) that are similar to, but distinct from, those tapped by other scales.

Discrimination between differing populations. To test the discriminative validity of the IPPA, my colleagues and I utilized the sample of 368 adults, composed of three different subgroups. We hypothesized that healthy graduate students with defined and attainable career goals would have the highest levels of positive attitudes; that outpatients facing uncertain medical prognoses would have the lowest levels of positive attitudes; and that healthy undergraduates with somewhat less defined career goals would score in between. Scores were compared using an analysis of covariance (ANCOVA) with sex, age, race, and education as covariates. Post hoc comparisons were obtained using Newman-Keuls tests. The results confirmed the hypotheses, with one exception. The graduate and undergraduate students scored significantly higher than the medical outpatients on all three IPPA scales. The graduate students scored significantly higher than the undergraduate students on the LPS and CLS scales. The graduates, however, did not score higher than the undergraduates on SCDS. Although this latter finding did not support the original hypothesis, the differences between the medical outpatients and the student groups suggested that the discriminative powers of the SCDS scale were sufficient. Thus, all three IPPA scales demonstrated a substantial ability to discriminate between differing populations (Kass et al., 1991).

In conclusion, the data from these studies lend strong support for the construct validity of the IPPA scales.

Outcome Research

Research suggests that stress can contribute to psychological and physical illnesses through two pathways. First, through mechanisms of hyperarousal characteristic of the stress response, chronic dysregulation of key neurological and physiological functions produces psychological symptoms (hostility, depression, and anxiety) and medical symptoms in vulnerable functional areas (cardiovascular, gastrointestinal, immunological, and neuromuscular) (Gatchel & Baum, 1983; Taylor, 1986). Second, as a response to (or to cope with) their psychological symptoms, individuals engage in behaviors (cigarette smoking, overeating, use of alcohol and drugs) that can cause physical illness (Brannon & Feist, 1997). Thus, the health-promoting effects of positive attitudes should be observable in three ways:

- reductions in psychological symptoms (hostility, depression, and anxiety);
- reductions in stress-related medical symptoms; and
- reductions in health-risk behaviors.

Ideally, investigations of the impact of positive attitudes should include prospective, long-term research seeking evidence that such attitudes help individuals maintain low levels of psychological symptoms, health-risk behaviors, and stress-related medical illnesses. To date, long-term prospective research has not been conducted with the IPPA. However, short-term research has been conducted that offers evidence that the positive attitudes measured by the IPPA are related to reductions in these areas.

In a sample of 228 outpatients being treated for chronic pain within a 10-week behavioral medicine program (Kass et al., 1991), the IPPA was found to be associated with reductions in psychological symptoms and stress-related medical symptoms. Psychological symptoms were measured by the Global Severity Index (GSI) of the SCL-90R (Derogatis, 1983). Stress-related medical symptoms were measured by the four scales of the Multidimensional Pain Inventory (Kerns, Turk, & Rudy, 1985) and the McGill Pain Questionnaire (Melzack, 1975). Data was gathered before and after treatment. Increases in CLS were associated with decreases in the GSI ($r = -.57$; $p < .01$). Increases in CLS were also associated with decreases in pain severity ($r = -.29$; $p < .01$; MPI-1), interference ($r = -.28$, $p < .01$; MPI-2), affective distress ($r = -.36$; $p < .01$; MPI-4), and the global pain rating index of the McGill Questionnaire ($r = -.20, p < .02$). In addition, increases in CLS were associated with increases in life control ($r = .37$, $p < .01$; MPI-3). These data suggest that increases in CLS contribute to decreases in psychological and medical symptoms among chronic pain patients.

This study also sought to determine whether decreases in pain ratings were better explained by increases in positive attitudes or decreases in psychological symptoms. These opposing variables, though related, are not mirror images. Thus, increases in positive attitudes may be a more useful predictor for decreases in pain than decreases in psychological symptoms. Multiple-regression analyses were performed with the pain scales as dependent variable and the IPPA (CLS) and SCL-90R (GSI) as co-independent variables. These analyses showed the IPPA to be the more effective predictor for pain severity (MPI-1) and pain interference (MPI-2). With life control (MPI-3) and affective distress (MPI-4), the most effective explanatory model was the interaction between CLS and GSI. The GSI was the more effective predictor only on the McGill PRI. Thus, in four of the five pain measures, the IPPA provided superior or necessary explanatory data. These results suggest that increases in CLS can contribute substantively to reductions in chronic pain.

In a related study, Tate (1994) found increases in CLS to be associated with decreases in psychological symptoms and decreases in combined medical-psychological symptoms. This study was conducted at a different behavioral medicine clinic, utilizing 183 adult outpatients in a 9-week program under treatment for a variety of stress-related illnesses. Before and after treatment, at a 6-month follow-up, data were gathered using the IPPA, the SCL-90-R, and Leserman's Medical and Psychological Symptoms Checklist (Borysenko, 1989). The MPSCL measures 33 stress-related medical symptoms on three dimensions (frequency, degree of discomfort, and degree of interference). In addition, the MPSCL measures 13 stress-related behaviors, 14 negative thought patterns, and 15 negative affective states on one dimension (the degree to which the symptoms bother the individual). A global score for these dimensions is obtained (MSP). Spearman rank-order correlations were used to compare relationships between the change scores of these variables.

Tate (1994) found negative correlations between changes in CLS and GSI from pre- to posttreatment ($r = -.504$), from posttreatment to 6-month follow-up ($r = -.394$), and from pretreatment to 6-month follow-up ($r = -.571$). Significance values were $p < .001$. Thus, increases in CLS were strongly associated with reductions in psychological symptoms.

Tate (1994) also found negative correlations between CLS and MPS scores from pre- to posttreatment ($r = -.550$), from posttreatment to 6-month follow-up ($r = -.468$), and from pretreatment to 6-month follow-up ($r = -.625$). Significance values were $p < .001$. The global MPS score does not differentiate between medical, behavioral, and psychoaffective symptom dimensions. However, the strength of these correlations suggests that increases in CLS were associated with decreases in all dimensions, including medical symptoms.

Evidence has also been found suggesting that cigarette smoking among women may be reduced when stress regarding physical appearance is buffered by SCDS (Kass et al., 1994). Hostility is a well-recognized risk factor for cigarette smoking among women and men. However, the causes of hostility in women and men may be different. In this study of 126 adult graduate students (86 women, 40 men), data were gathered on hostility (using the SCL-90R), stress (using an index developed to ascertain perceived degree of stress in five dimensions of daily life: health issues in self and family, physical appearance, relationships, educational studies and career, and daily schedule), family structure during childhood (using a question based on attachment theory), and the IPPA. Results showed that hostility was strongly associated with stress regarding physical appearance for women but not men. This finding was consistent with the recognition that many women smoke to stay thin. The researchers then sought to determine whether positive attitudes buffered stress concerning physical appearance and helped to reduce hostility. A multiple-regression analysis was performed with hostility as the dependent variable. Co-independent variables in the initial model were age, structure of family during childhood, self-confidence during stress, stress concerning physical appearance, and other stress factors (family, educational studies, daily schedule). Using interactive stepwise regression, a best possible model was obtained to explain variance in hostility. This model retained only stress concerning physical appearance (standardized beta = .214) and self-confidence during stress (standardized beta = −.433). The significance value for this model was $p < .001$. Variance explained by this model was 26.7%. This model showed that stress regarding physical appearance contributed to hostility, whereas self-confidence during stress helped to reduce hostility. Thus, SCDS was buffering the effects of stress regarding physical appearance in the hostility level of these women. These findings suggest that self-confidence during stress contributes to the reduction of hostility in women and may, therefore, help prevent women from smoking cigarettes.

In conclusion, this outcome research suggests that positive attitudes measured by the IPPA can reduce stress-related psychological symptoms, health risk behaviors, and medical symptoms. Therefore, continued use of the IPPA may help social scientists to better understand the role of positive attitudes in mental and physical health.

Benefits and Limitations

In addition to its value as a research instrument, the IPPA is useful during clinical treatment and preventive psychoeducational interventions. It offers the clinician and the patient a profile of an individual's positive worldview and his or her attitudinal resources for coping with stressful circumstances and events. Whether these resources are abundant or lacking, the IPPA creates a positive context for interpretation. This approach differs from a focus on negative diagnoses, which can create additional anxiety for vulnerable patients.

The IPPA can be used in a variety of clinical and psychoeducational settings: stress reduction personnel programs, behavioral medicine treatment for stress-related illnesses, school counseling with adolescents, drug and alcohol prevention programs for adolescents and young adults, career counseling for adults in transition, and mental health counseling with adolescents and adults. During primary prevention strategies, in which interventions may take place before illness has developed, the need for a yardstick that focuses on positive attitudes is particularly salient. In these instances, a focus on deficits is rarely as successful as a focus on the development of strengths. Use of the IPPA can provide clinicians and clients with a particularly appropriate tool for assessment and positive developmental change.

The IPPA is not a replacement for measures of psychiatric symptoms. The IPPA is not designed to assess the nature of a patient's psychopathology or the degree to which such psychopathology may place that individual at risk. If, for example, a patient may be suicidal, use of Beck's Hopelessness Scale (Beck, Kovacs, & Weissman, 1975; Beck, Weissman, Lester, & Trexler, 1974) is the appropriate means to assess risk. Similarly, the use of Derogatis's (1983) SCL-90R and other comparable instruments are the appropriate tools for the identification of psychiatric symptoms. Thus, use of the IPPA by a clinician who is not also trained to recognize or assess psychopathology can place a client in danger.

In instances in which the use of psychiatric assessment tools is necessary, it is useful, however, to complement them with the IPPA. Assessment of psychopathology rarely provides a whole picture of a client. Identifying a client's areas of strength, providing a conceptual model of the positive resources that a client needs to develop, and offering a positively oriented yardstick to help a client monitor his or her own growth are key elements in successful diagnosis and treatment.

The case example in the following section exemplifies how the IPPA can be used to situate clinical interventions in a positive context and to provide concrete ways for clients and clinicians to observe and measure positive attitudinal change.

Case Example

Previous work (Kass, 1996a, 1996b) has described clinical methods for helping medical patients cope with the stress of life-threatening illnesses by strengthening their sense of life purpose and self-confidence during stress. The following example describes use of the IPPA to help a patient develop these coping resources.

Mr. M, a 28-year-old male from a lower-middle-class Armenian family and neighborhood, was referred to psychotherapy by his physician for the treatment of anxiety. During intake, Mr. M discussed a previous psychotherapeutic experience in which an anxiety scale had been administered. His score had revealed a pronounced level of anxiety. Although he received positive assurances from the clinician and perceived the clinician as competent, Mr. M began to fear, after the evaluation, that the clinician believed that something was wrong with Mr. M's mind. He also began to fear that this supposed diagnosis was accurate. Afraid to face this possibility, he had not returned to treatment.

Two years later, upon the continued advice of his physician, he again sought counseling. Use of the IPPA during initial assessment helped produce a more positive response to the counseling process. In this instance, the IPPA was administered verbally, with the psychotherapist and client reading each item together to generate as much relaxed conversation as possible. The clinician and Mr. M collaborated to develop and discuss a profile of his positive attitudes. Several insights emerged. First, a high score on the work-related question in the LPS dimension ("The work that I am doing is of great value") led to a lively discussion of Mr. M's career as a computer technician. Mr. M excelled in his area of specialization, network support and maintenance. This conversation had a positive effect on the psychotherapist, who began to see Mr. M as an intelligent and talented individual. It also had a positive effect on Mr. M, who began to see the psychotherapist as someone in whom he could confide without fear of negative labeling.

The conversation deepened further when they discussed the identity item in the LPS dimension ("I wish I were different than who I am: disagree strongly . . . agree strongly"). Mr. M had ambivalent feelings regarding this item that revolved around his cultural identity as an Armenian American. Mr. M was self-conscious about his slight accent and the low opinion he felt that most Americans had for individuals of Armenian descent. Yet he was proud of his heritage and did not want to hide it. As he saw that the counselor understood this issue and did not show evidence of disapproval based on his cultural identity, Mr. M requested a second session to discuss his "problem."

At the second session, Mr. M asked to look again at the inventory of positive attitudes. His problem, he explained, concerned the item, "When a situation becomes difficult, I find myself worrying that something bad is going to happen to me or those I love." This item is in the SCDS dimension. He then explained that he had been engaged to be married for the last 5 years. Each time that he and his fiancée had selected a wedding date, he had had an anxiety attack and canceled the plan. Having grown up in a traditional family, he still lived in his parents' home. It soon became clear that Mr. M was highly dependent up his mother, a widow and a highly dependent person herself. As each wedding date was announced, she had become anxious and ill and had expressed fear that her son's departure would mark the end of her life. As a response to these episodes, Mr. M had grown increasingly fearful that he would cause his mother to have a heart attack and die. The anxiety had now escalated to the point where he telephoned his mother each day from work, no longer took out-of-town vacations, and was considering breaking the engagement completely. Only the growing frustration of his fiancée had convinced him to follow his physician's advice and to seek counseling again.

Mr. M's story made it clear that he was highly anxious and would benefit from counseling, and through the positively oriented context generated by the IPPA, his initial experience of himself in these counseling sessions had been positive. This experience relieved an initial degree of anxiety and freed Mr. M to see the psychotherapist as an ally in whom he could confide.

Using a cognitive-behavioral approach with a family systems perspective, the psychotherapist proceeded to help Mr. M test, and then discard, his irrational schema. At each step in this process, the psychotherapist asked Mr. M to score items on the IPPA that related to his "problem." Through this procedure, Mr. M could observe his gradual growth toward a lack of worry that something bad would happen to those he loved. At the same time, he saw other items moving in more positive directions, too: "When I have made a mistake during a stressful situation, I continue to like myself," "During times of stress, I do not feel isolated and alone," and "I do not feel less than adequate when I am in difficult situations." These concrete ways to measure positive change, coupled with continued reinforcement of the areas in his life where he excelled, helped Mr. M move to a position of greater self-confidence.

Summary

The Inventory of Positive Psychological Attitudes (IPPA) is a 32-item multidimensional self-report instrument measuring positive attitudinal domains that buffer stress and facilitate the primary prevention of stress-related psychological and physical disorders. It is composed of two subscales: Self-Confidence during Stress (SCDS) and Life Purpose and Satisfaction (LPS). In its entirety, the IPPA measures Confidence in Life and Self (CLS). These constructs were designed to be responsive to the worldviews of culturally diverse populations.

Research with the IPPA has yielded positive results. Validation procedures confirmed the multidimensional structure of the IPPA, a high degree of reliability for each subscale, and construct validity. Outcome research suggests that these positive attitudes contribute to lower levels of psychological symptoms, stress-related medical symptoms, and health-risk behaviors. This research also suggests that decreases in stress-related medical symptoms may be explained more adequately by increases in positive attitudes than by decreases in psychological symptoms.

The IPPA can help create a positive context for clinical and preventive interventions. It can help identify attitudinal strengths and provides a conceptual model of positive resources. The IPPA can help clinicians structure conversations with clients regarding areas where they lack positive attitudes, and it provides a mechanism to discuss the potential effects of cultural identity on a client's confidence in life and self. Finally, the IPPA provides a positively oriented yardstick to help clients monitor their own growth. The IPPA is not a replacement for instruments that assess psychopathology. Where psychopathology must be measured, the IPPA should be used as a complementary tool. Research and clinical practice with the IPPA suggests that it can be a valuable assessment instrument during clinical and preventive interventions.

Chapter References

Abby, A., & Andrews, F. (1985). Modeling the psychological determinants of life quality. *Social Indicators Research, 16*, 1–34.

Andersen, B. L., Kiecolt-Glaser, J. K., & Glaser, R. (1994). A biobehavioral model of cancer stress and disease course. *American Psychologist, 49*(5), 389–404.

Antonovsky, A. (1979). *Health, stress, and coping*. San Francisco: Jossey-Bass.

Antonovsky, A. (1987). *Unraveling the mystery of health*. San Francisco: Jossey-Bass.

Beck, A. T., Kovacs, M., & Weissman, A. (1975). Hopelessness and suicidal behavior: An overview. *Journal of the American Psychological Association, 234,* 1146–1149.

Beck, A. T., Weissman, A., Lester, D., & Trexler, L. (1974). The measurement of pessimism: The Hopelessness Scale. *Journal of Consulting and Clinical Psychology, 42,* 861–865.

Blascovich, J., & Katkin, E. S. (Eds.). (1993). *Cardiovascular reactivity to psychological stress and disease.* Washington, DC: American Psychological Association.

Borysenko, J. (1989). *Minding the body, mending the mind.* Boston: Addison-Wesley.

Bradburn, N. (1969). *The structure of psychological well-being.* Chicago: Aldine.

Brannon, L., & Feist, J. (1997). *Health psychology: An introduction to behavior and health.* (3rd ed.). Pacific Grove, CA: Brooks/Cole.

Brown, L., & Ballou, M. (Eds.). (1992). *Personality and psychopathology: Feminist reappraisals.* New York: Guilford.

Crumbaugh, J. C. (1968). Crossvalidation of the Purpose-in-Life test based on Frankl's concepts. *Journal of Individual Psychology, 24,* 74–81.

Crumbaugh, J. C., & Maholick, L. T. (1964). An experimental study in existentialism: The psychometric approach to Frankl's concepts of noogenic neurosis. *Journal of Clinical Psychology, 20,* 200–207.

Crumbaugh, J. C., & Maholick, L. T. (1969). *Manual of instruction for the Purpose in Life test.* Munster, IN: Psychometric Affiliates.

Derogatis, L. R. (1983). *SCL-90-R administration, scoring and procedures manual.* Towson, MD: Clinical Psychometric Research.

Dorian, B., & Garfinkel, P. E. (1987). Stress, immunity and illness: A review. *Psychological Medicine, 17,* 393–407.

Frankl, V. (1959). *Man's search for meaning.* New York: Simon & Schuster.

Frankl, V. (1966). Self-transcendence as a human phenomenon. *Journal of Humanistic Psychology, 6,* 97–106.

Frankl, V. (1969). *The will to meaning.* New York: New American Library.

Gatchel, R. J., & Baum, A. (1983). *An introduction to health psychology.* Reading, MA: Addison-Wesley.

Gatchel, R. J., & Blanchard, E. B. (1993). *Psychophysiological disor-*

ders: Research and clinical applications. Washington, DC: American Psychological Association.

Gold, P. W., Goodwin, F. K., & Chrousos, G. P. (1988a). Clinical and biochemical manifestations for depression: Relation to the neurobiology of stress (part 1). New England Journal of Medicine, 329(6), 348–353.

Gold, P. W., Goodwin, F. K., & Chrousos, G. P. (1988b). Clinical and biochemical manifestations of depression: Relationship to the neurobiology of stress (part 2). New England Journal of Medicine, 329(7), 413–420.

Grunberg, N. E., & Baum, A. (1985). Biological commonalities of stress and substance abuse. In S. Shiffman and T. A. Wills (Eds.), Coping and substance abuse. New York: Academic Press, Inc.

Hafen, B. Q., Frandsen, K. J., Karren, K. J., & Hooker, K. R. (1992). The health effects of attitudes, emotions, relationships. Provo, UT: EMS Associates.

Jordan, J. V., Kaplan, A. G., Miller, J. B., Stiver, I. P., & Surrey, J. L. (1991). Women's growth in connection. New York: Guilford.

Kass, J. (1996a). Coping with life-threatening illnesses using a logotherapeutic approach, Stage I. Health care team interventions. International Forum for Logotherapy, 19(Spring), 15–19.

Kass, J. (1996b). Coping with life-threatening illnesses using a logotherapeutic approach, Stage II. Clinical mental health counseling. International Forum for Logotherapy, 20(Spring), 10–14.

Kass, J. (1997). Positive attitudes and health risk behaviors: New refinements and further validation of the Inventory of Positive Psychological Attitudes (IPPA). Unpublished manuscript.

Kass, J., Burton, L., Ferranti, L., Davis, F., Gawelek, M. A., & Roffman, E. (1994). Reducing risks for cigarette smoking in women: Determinants of, and mediators against, hostility. Paper presented at the annual meeting of the Society for Prevention Research, Palm Beach, FL.

Kass, J., Friedman, R., Leserman, J., Caudill, M., Zuttereister, P., & Benson, H. (1991). An inventory of positive psychological attitudes with potential relevance to health outcomes. Behavioral Medicine, 17(3), 121–129.

Kerns, R. D., Turk, D. C., & Rudy, T. E. (1985). The West-Haven Yale Multidimensional Pain Inventory (WHYMPI). Pain, 23, 245–256.

Kobasa, S., Maddi, S., & Kahn, S. (1982). Hardiness and health: A prospective study. *Journal of Personality and Social Psychology*, *42*(1), 168–177.

Krystal, J. H., Kosten, T. R., Southwick, S., Mason, J. W., Perry, B. D., & Giller, E. L. (1989). Neurobiological aspects of PTSD: Review of clinical and preclinical studies. *Behavior Therapy, 20*, 177–198.

Langer, E. J., & Rodin, J. (1976). The effects of choice and enhanced personal responsibility for the aged: A field experiment in an institutional setting. *Journal of Personality and Social Psychology*, *34*(3), 191–198.

Lazarus, R., & Folkman, S. (1984). *Stress, appraisal, and coping.* New York: Springer.

May, R., & Yalom, I. (1989). Existential psychotherapy. In R. J. Corsini & D. Wedding (Eds.), *Current psychotherapies* (4th ed.) (pp. 363–402), Itasca, IL: Peacock.

McNair, D. M., Lorr, M., & Droppleman, L. F. (1981). *Profile of mood states: Manual.* San Diego: EDITS/Educational and Industrial Testing Service.

Melzack, R. (1975). The McGill Pain Questionnaire: Major properties and scoring methods. *Pain, 1*, 277–299.

Miller, J. B. (1976). *Toward a new psychology of women.* New York: Penguin.

Reker, G. T., Peacock, E. J., & Wong, P. T. (1987). Meaning and purpose in life and well-being: A life-span perspective. *Journal of Gerontology, 42*(1), 44–49.

Rose, R. M. (1980). Endocrine responses to stressful psychological events. *Psychiatric Clinics of North America, 3*(2), 251–276.

Rosenberg, M. (1965). *Society and the adolescent self-image.* Princeton, NJ: Princeton University Press.

Rotter, J. (1966). Generalized expectancies for internal versus external control of reinforcement. *Psychological Monographs, 80*, 601.

Russell, D. L., Peplau, L., & Ferguson, M. (1978). Developing a measure of loneliness. *Journal of Personality Assessment, 42*(3), 290–294.

Seligman, M. (1975). *Helplessness: On depression, development, and death.* San Francisco: W. H. Freeman.

Stevens, M. J., Pfost, K. S., & Wessels, A. B. (1987). The relationship of purpose in life to coping strategies and time since the death of a significant other. *Journal of Counseling and Development, 65*, 424–426.

Sue, D. W. (1978). Eliminating cultural oppression in counseling: Toward a general theory. *Journal of Counseling Psychology, 25,* 419–428.

Sue, D. W., & Sue, D. (1981). *Counseling the culturally different: Theory and practice.* New York: John Wiley.

Sunderwirth, S. G. (1985). Biological mechanisms: Neurotransmission and addiction. In H. B. S. Milkman (Ed.), *The addictions.* Lexington, MA: Lexington Books.

Suzuki, L. A., Meller, P. J., & Ponterotto, J. G. (Eds.). (1996). *Handbook of multicultural assessment: Clinical, psychological, and educational applications.* San Francisco: Jossey-Bass.

Tate, D. (1994). *Mindfulness meditation group training: Effects on medical and psychological symptoms and positive psychological characteristics.* Unpublished doctoral dissertation, Brigham Young University, Provo, UT.

Taylor, S. (1986). *Health psychology.* New York: Random House.

Tillich, P. (1952). *The courage to be.* New Haven, CT: Yale University Press.

Van Der Kolk, B. A. (1988). The trauma spectrum: The interaction of biological and social events in the genesis of the trauma response. *Journal of Traumatic Stress, 1*(3), 273–290.

Wortman, C. B., & Brehm, J. W. (1975). Responses to uncontrollable outcomes: An integration of reactance theory and the learned helplessness model. In L. Berkowitz (Ed.), *Advances in experimental social psychology* (pp. 277–336), New York: Academic Press.

Yalom, I. (1981). *Existential psychotherapy.* New York: Basic Books.

Zuttermeister, P., Kass, J., Geiss, S., & Friedman, R. (1992, April). *Further validation of the inventory of positive psychological attitudes.* Paper presented at the 13th Annual Scientific Sessions of the Society for Behavioral Medicine, New York.

The Multidimensional Scale of Perceived Social Support (MSPSS)

Gregory D. Zimet, Indiana University School of Medicine

■ Instrument Names

The Multidimensional Scale of Perceived Social Support
MSPSS

■ Developers

Gregory D. Zimet, Ph.D., Indiana University School of Medicine; Nancy W. Dahlem, Ph.D.; Sara G. Zimet, Ed.D.; and Gordon K. Farley, M.D., University of Colorado Health Sciences Center

■ Contact Information

Dr. Gregory D. Zimet, Section of Adolescent Medicine, Riley Children's Hospital Room 1740X, 702 Barnhill Drive, Indianapolis, IN 46202
Telephone: (317) 274-8812; fax: (317) 274-0133;
e-mail: gzimet@iupui.edu

Description and History of the Instrument

Over the course of the 1970s, interest grew in the role of social support as a potentially important coping resource. A number of early studies reported findings that higher levels of social support ameliorated the negative emotional effects of stress (Andrews, Tennant, Hewson, & Vaillant, 1978; Gore, 1978;

Lin, Simeone, Ensel, & Kuo, 1979; Schaefer, Coyne, & Lazarus, 1981; Wilcox, 1981). However, it became clear that social support was an extraordinarily broad construct that allowed for multiple, very different operationalizations. In the mid-1980s, Tardy (1985) proposed that social support could be defined along five dimensions:

- Direction—whether support is given or received
- Disposition—is support available and is available support utilized?
- Objectivity/subjectivity—description of support resources or evaluation of satisfaction with support
- Content—what form does the support take? and
- Network—what are the structures of the social systems providing support?

A central issue in social support measurement relates to these definitional issues. To attempt to address all five (or even several) dimensions in a single instrument would result in a complex, lengthy questionnaire, which would be particularly impractical to administer in research studies when multiple measures are being used. An alternative is to clearly specify what aspects of social support are measured in a particular instrument.

The Multidimensional Scale of Perceived Social Support (MSPSS) was designed to be a brief, psychometrically sound measure of the subjective assessment of the adequacy of received emotional social support. The relatively narrow focus enabled us to limit the number of scale items to 12, which is an important pragmatic issue when subject time is limited or multiple measures are being administered at one time, as is often the case. In addition, we designed the MSPSS to evaluate perceptions of support from three important dimensions of individuals' social lives: family, friends, and a significant other. Finally, though the first study on the MSPSS was published in 1988 (Zimet, Dahlem, Zimet, & Farley, 1988), the scale was developed over several years throughout the early and mid-1980s. Multiple pilot studies, which included repeated reliability assessment and exploratory factor analyses, helped refine and simplify the measure and ensured that the final scale would be psychometrically sound.

Description

The MSPSS is a 12-item self-administered questionnaire designed to measure the perceived adequacy of social support from three sources: family, friends, and a significant other. Each of these three dimensions is assessed with four items. Response choices are in the form of a 7-point Likert-type scale (1 = very strongly disagree to 7 = very strongly agree). Items are worded simply and require only a fourth-grade reading level, as assessed by the Flesch-Kincaid formula (Grammatik, 1994). As a result, the MSPSS takes less than five minutes to complete.

Scoring the MSPSS is very straightforward. Total scale scores are derived by summing across the items, then dividing by 12, resulting in a mean total score that can be referenced to the 7-point response scale. In a similar fashion, each of the three subscale scores are calculated by summing across their respective items, then dividing by four. Subscale items are as follows:

- Family (items 3, 4, 8, and 11)
- Friends (items 6, 7, 9, and 12)
- Significant Other (items 1, 2, 5, and 10).

See Table 1 for a list of MSPSS items.

Although the MSPSS has not been normed on a large, population-based sample, it has been administered to demographically diverse groups of subjects across multiple studies. Descriptive data for the MSPSS are available on samples of university undergraduates (Dahlem, Zimet, & Walker, 1991; Kazarian & McCabe, 1991; Zimet et al., 1988), pregnant

Table 1: MSPSS Items and Subscale Membership

Item Number	Subscale
1. There is a special person who is around when I am in need	Significant Other
2. There is a special person with whom I can share joys and sorrows	Significant Other
3. My family really tries to help me	Family
4. I get the emotional help and support I need from my family	Family
5. I have a special person who is a real source of comfort to me	Significant Other
6. My friends really try to help me	Friends
7. I can count on my friends when things go wrong	Friends
8. I can talk about my problems with my family	Family
9. I have friends with whom I can share my joys and sorrows	Friends
10. There is a special person in my life who cares about my feelings	Significant Other
11. My family is willing to help me make decisions	Family
12. I can talk about my problems with my friends	Friends

women (Zimet, Powell, Farley, Werkman, & Berkoff, 1990), pediatric residents (Zimet et al., 1990), psychiatrically hospitalized adolescents (Kazarian & McCabe, 1991), adult psychiatric outpatients (Cecil, Stanley, Carrion, & Swann, 1995), and various groups of adults from Turkey, using a Turkish translation of the MSPSS (Eker & Arkar, 1995). Table 2 summarizes descriptive data for the MSPSS and its subscales from several of these studies.

Psychometric Characteristics

Reliability

The reliability of the MSPSS has been evaluated in terms of stability of responses over time, as well as internal consistency of items. In the first study describing the development of the MSPSS, test-retest reliability was evaluated for a subset of 69 of 275 Duke University undergraduates, who were readministered the scale 2 to 3 months after first completing the MSPSS (Zimet et al., 1988). The test-retest reliability values for the Family, Friends, and Significant Other subscales were .85, .75, and .72, respectively. The lower coefficients for the Friends and Significant Other subscales compared with the Family subscale may simply reflect the more changeable nature of those relationships compared with the relative stability of family relationships. For the whole scale, the test-retest reliability coefficient was .85. These values indicate that the MSPSS has relatively good stability over time.

Assessments of the internal consistency of the MSPSS, via Cronbach's coefficient alpha, have been reported by a number of researchers (Cecil et al., 1995; Dahlem et al., 1991; Eker & Arkar, 1995; Kazarian & McCabe, 1991; Zimet et al., 1988, 1990). Across the 13 subject groups evaluated in these six studies, coefficient alphas for the total scale ranged from .77 to .92 (mean = .87). Coefficient alphas values ranged from .81 to .93 (mean = .87) for the Family subscale, from .78 to

Table 2: Means and Standard Deviations of MSPSS Subscales across Multiple Subject Groups

Subject Group	MSPSS Subscales			
	Family	Friends	Significant Other	Total Scale
Duke University[*]	5.80 (1.12)	5.85 (0.94)	5.74 (1.25)	5.80 (0.86)
University of Western Ontario[†]	5.75 (1.08)	5.84 (0.90)	5.89 (1.21)	5.81 (0.79)
Urban University Denver, CO[¥]	5.31 (1.07)	5.50 (1.25)	5.94 (1.34)	5.58 (1.07)
Psychiatrically hospitalized adolescents[§]	4.86 (1.28)	5.32 (1.67)	5.80 (1.28)	5.33 (1.23)
Adults -- psychiatric outpatients[″]	5.20 (2.00)	4.50 (2.00)	5.20 (1.90)	5.00 (1.60)
Pregnant women[#]	6.02 (1.16)	5.64 (1.27)	6.39 (0.88)	6.01 (0.90)

[*]n = 275; Zimet et al. (1988).

[†]n = 165; Kazarian and McCabe (1991).

[¥]n = 154; Dahlem et al. (1991).

[§]n = 51; Kazarian and McCabe (1991).

[″]n = 144; Cecil et al. (1995).

[#]n = 265; Zimet et al. (1990).

.94 (mean = .88) for the Friends subscale, and from .79 to .98 (mean = .88) for the Significant Other subscale. These results indicate that the MSPSS and its subscales have strong internal consistency across multiple and very diverse subject groups.

Dimensional Structure

Consistent with the findings regarding internal reliability, the three-factor structure of the MSPSS has been empirically confirmed across several studies through the use of exploratory factor analysis (Cecil et al., 1995; Dahlem et al., 1991; Eker & Arkar, 1995; Kazarian & McCabe, 1991; Zimet et al., 1988, 1990). In every case, three factors were extracted that corresponded to the proposed Family, Friends, and Significant Other subscale structure of the MSPSS. Across the seven subject groups evaluated in these six studies, factor loadings for the Family subscale items ranged from 0.74 to 0.91, with cross-loadings of 0.00 to 0.38. Factor loadings for the Friends subscale items ranged from 0.74 to 0.91, with cross-loadings of 0.00 to 0.42. Finally, factor loadings for the Significant Other subscale items ranged from 0.62 to 0.94, with cross-loadings of 0.01 to 0.36. These factor analysis findings suggest that the proposed factor structure of the MSPSS is robust across demographically diverse subject groups.

Validity

Typically, validity (i.e., are we measuring what we think we are measuring?) is more difficult to establish than reliability (i.e., are we measuring something with consistency?). One approach to evaluating validity, construct validity, is to demonstrate that the target measure is associated (or not associated) with another measure, as theory would dictate (see DeVellis, 1991). In the initial study describing the psychometric properties of the MSPSS, construct validity was established by the significant negative correlations of the scale to measures of depression and anxiety (Zimet et al., 1988). In this case the underlying theory that was supported was that higher levels of social support would ameliorate psychological distress.

In subsequent studies, the construct validity of the MSPSS was confirmed further. Kazarian and McCabe (1991) showed that the MSPSS and its subscales were positively correlated with a self-esteem measure and negatively correlated with depression inventories. Cecil et al. (1995) demonstrated that the MSPSS was moderately positively correlated with the Network Orientation Scale (Vaux, Burda, & Stewart, 1986), an instrument that addresses individuals' orientation toward the use of social support networks. Other results (Zimet et al., 1990) addressed the validity of the Significant Other and Family subscales of the MSPSS. Among a group of pediatric residents, those who were married scored significantly higher on the Significant Other subscale than unmarried residents. Their scores on the other two subscales did not differ significantly. Among a group of adolescents living abroad, only the Family subscale was significantly associated with a question regarding the frequency with which concerns were shared with their mothers. These two sets of findings help to establish the validity of two of the MSPSS subscales and suggest that respondents are able to meaningfully discriminate among sources of social support.

Applications

The MSPSS was designed principally for research use, not clinical application. It has been included in a wide variety of studies, including research on children's adjustment following immigration (Short & Johnston, 1997), postsurgical adjustment of older heart surgery patients (Oxman, Freeman, & Manheimer, 1995; Oxman & Hull, 1997), psychosocial predictors of coronary artery disease (Blumenthal et al., 1987), the evaluation of relapse prevention approaches for addiction treatment programs (Graham, Annis, Brett, & Venesoen, 1996), the psychosocial adjustment of battered women (Barnett, Martinez, & Keyson, 1996), adult adjustment related to parental death in childhood (Mireault & Bond, 1992), the prediction of postpartum depression (Powell & Drotar, 1992), self-perceived handicap among Swiss men with hearing loss (Hallberg, Johnsson, & Axelsson, 1993), psychosocial factors related to childhood pedestrian injury (Christoffel et al., 1996), recovery in trauma patients (Glancy et al., 1992), and the receipt of alcohol treatment services among Native American Indian adolescents (Novins, Harman, Mitchell, & Manson, 1996).

The diverse applications of the MSPSS reflected in these studies (diverse in subject groups and in study focus) point to its flexibility, ease of use, and robust psychometric characteristics. It is important to note that social support as measured by the MSPSS was not a statistically significant predictor of outcome in several of these studies (e.g., Christoffel et al., 1996; Glancy et al., 1992; Oxman et al., 1995). However, the MSPSS proved to be an important and statistically significant predictor of the key outcome variables in many of the research investigations cited (e.g., Barnett et al., 1996; Blumenthal et al., 1987; Graham et al., 1996; Mireault & Bond, 1992; Oxman & Hull, 1997; Powell & Drotar, 1992; Short & Johnston, 1997).

Short and Johnston's (1997) study of maternal factors associated with children's adjustment following immigration is an example of one interesting use of the MSPSS. In this study, the sample was composed of Chinese families who had recently emigrated from Hong Kong to British Columbia, Canada. To ensure that the study materials were understandable, all questionnaires, including the MSPSS, were translated into Chinese script. The MSPSS was one of two social support measures included in the study. The other instrument, the Parent Support Scale (PSS), was designed specifically for the study and assessed practical parenting support received from family, friends, and spouse. The authors included the MSPSS, in part, because its simplicity and clarity of wording made translation relatively easy. The internal reliability coefficient for the Chinese translation of the MSPSS total scale was .94, suggesting that the translation resulted in a coherent measure of social support. Initial bivariate correlations indicated that for girls, maternal reports of social support (on both the MSPSS and PSS) were negatively associated with child behavior problems. No such correlations were found for boys. Given the similar pattern of correlations of the two support measures, the authors created a social support composite measure by standardizing scores on the two measures (i.e., creating z-scores), then adding the standardized scores together. In a hierarchical multiple linear regression analysis for the girls, the social support composite measure proved to operate as a significant independent predictor of behavior problems. In a similar analysis for the boys, however, there was no main effect for social support, but there were two significant interactions involving the social support composite (i.e., stress by support and distress by support). The stress by support interaction indicated that the association of maternal stress to child behavior problems decreased with increasing social support. Conversely, the distress-by-support interaction indicated that the relationship of maternal distress to child behavior problems increased with rising social support. The authors discuss in some detail the potential implications of their interesting set of findings involving maternal perceptions of social support and child behavior problems among recent Chinese immigrants to British Columbia. This rather complex study exemplifies the flexibility and utility of the MSPSS in research on stress and psychosocial adjustment.

Conclusion

Across multiple psychometric studies, the MSPSS has demonstrated excellent reliability, a stable factor structure, and good validity. The relatively strong psychometric characteristics of the scale, combined with its brevity, clarity, and simplicity of administration, make it a versatile research instrument for the measurement of subjectively assessed emotional social support received from family, friends, and a significant other. In addition, the MSPSS now has a rather extensive track record of use in studies of stress and adaptation across many different behavioral and medical topics and including demographically diverse subject groups.

Chapter References

Andrews, G., Tennant, C., Hewson, D. M., & Vaillant, G. E. (1978). Life event stress, social support, coping style, and risk of psychological impairment. *Journal of Nervous and Mental Disease, 166,* 307–316.

Barnett, O. W., Martinez, T. E., & Keyson, M. (1996). The relationship between violence, social support, and self-blame in battered women. *Journal of Interpersonal Violence, 11,* 221–233.

Blumenthal, J. A., Burg, M. M., Barefoot, J., Williams, R. B., Haney, T., & Zimet, G. (1987). Social support, Type A behavior, and coronary artery disease. *Psychosomatic Medicine, 49,* 331–340.

Cecil, H., Stanley, M. A., Carrion, P. G., & Swann, A. (1995). Psychometric properties of the MSPSS and NOS in psychiatric outpatients. *Journal of Clinical Psychology, 51,* 593–602.

Christoffel, K. K., Donovan, M., Schofer, J., Wills, K., Lavigne, J. V., & Kids'n'Cars Team. (1996). Psychosocial factors in childhood pedestrian injury: A matched case-control study. *Pediatrics, 97,* 33–42.

Dahlem, N. W., Zimet, G. D., & Walker, R. R. (1991). The Multidimensional Scale of Perceived Social Support: A confirmation study. *Journal of Clinical Psychology, 47,* 756–761.

DeVellis, R. F. (1991). *Scale development: Theory and applications.* Newbury Park, CA: Sage.

Eker, D., & Arkar, H. (1995). Perceived social support: Psychometric properties of the MSPSS in normal and pathological groups in a developing country. *Social Psychiatry and Psychiatric Epidemiology, 30,* 121–126.

Glancy, K. E., Glancy, C. J., Lucke, J. F., Mahurin, K., Rhodes, M., & Tinkoff, G. H. (1992). A study of recovery in trauma patients. *Journal of Trauma, 33,* 602–609.

Gore, S. (1978). The effect of social support in moderating the health consequences of unemployment. *Journal of Health and Social Behavior, 19,* 157–165.

Graham, K., Annis, H. M., Brett, P. J., & Venesoen, P. (1996). A controlled field trial of group versus individual cognitive-behavioural training for relapse prevention. *Addiction, 91,* 1127–1139.

Grammatik 6.0a, WordPerfect Grammar Checker [computer software]. (1994). Orem, UT: Novell.

Hallberg, L. R. M., Johnsson, T., & Axelsson, A. (1993). Structure of perceived handicap in middle-aged males with noise-induced hearing loss, with and without tinnitus. *Audiology, 32,* 137–152.

Kazarian, S. S., & McCabe, S. B. (1991). Dimensions of social support in the MSPSS: Factorial structure, reliability, and theoretical implications. *Journal of Community Psychology, 19,* 150–160.

Lin, N., Simeone, R. S., Ensel, W. M., & Kuo, W. (1979). Social support, stressful life events and illness: A model and an empirical test. *Journal of Health and Social Behavior, 20,* 108–119.

Mireault, G. C., & Bond, L. A. (1992). Parental death in childhood: Perceived vulnerability, and adult depression and anxiety. *American Journal of Orthopsychiatry, 62,* 517–524.

Novins, D. K., Harman, C. P., Mitchell, C. M., & Manson, S. M. (1996). Factors associated with the receipt of alcohol treatment services among American Indian adolescents. *Journal of the American Academy of Child and Adolescent Psychiatry, 35,* 110–117.

Oxman, T. E., Freeman, D. H., & Manheimer, E. D. (1995). Lack of social participation or religious strength and comfort as risk factors for death after cardiac surgery in the elderly. *Psychosomatic Medicine, 57,* 5–15.

Oxman, T. E., & Hull, J. G. (1997). Social support, depression, and activities of daily living in older heart surgery patients. *Journal of Gerontology: Psychological Sciences, 52B,* 1–14.

Powell, S. S., & Drotar, D. (1992). Postpartum depressed mood— The impact of daily hassles. *Journal of Psychosomatic Obstetrics and Gynaecology, 13,* 255–266.

Schaefer, C., Coyne, J. C., & Lazarus, R. S. (1981). The health-related function of social support. *Journal of Behavioral Medicine, 4,* 381–406.

Short, K. H., & Johnston, C. (1997). Stress, maternal distress, and children's adjustment following immigration: The buffering role of social support. *Journal of Consulting and Clinical Psychology*, *65*, 494–503.

Tardy, C. H. (1985). Social support measurement. *American Journal of Community Psychology*, *13*, 187–202.

Vaux, A., Burda, P., & Stewart, D. (1986). Orientation toward utilization of support resources. *Journal of Community Psychology*, *14*, 159–170.

Wilcox, B. L. (1981). Social support, life stress, and psychological adjustment: A test of the buffering hypothesis. *American Journal of Community Psychology*, *9*, 371–386.

Zimet, G. D., Dahlem, N. W., Zimet, S. G., & Farley, G. K. (1988). The Multidimensional Scale of Perceived Social Support. *Journal of Personality Assessment*, *52*, 30–41.

Zimet, G. D., Powell, S. S., Farley, G. K., Werkman, S., & Berkoff, K. A. (1990). Psychometric characteristics of the Multidimensional Scale of Perceived Social Support. *Journal of Personality Assessment*, *55*, 610–617.

The Perinatal Posttraumatic Stress Disorder (PTSD) Questionnaire (PPQ)

Michael T. Hynan, University of Wisconsin–Milwaukee

■ Instrument Names

The Perinatal Posttraumatic Stress Disorder (PTSD)
Questionnaire (PPQ)
PTSD-PPQ

■ Developer

Michael T. Hynan, Ph.D., University of
Wisconsin–Milwaukee

■ Contact Information

Dr. Michael T. Hynan, Psychology Department, University
of Wisconsin–Milwaukee, Milwaukee, WI 53201
Telephone: (414) 229-4746; e-mail: hynan@csd.uwm.edu;
home page: http://www.uwm.edu/~hyman

Description and History of the Instrument

The Perinatal Posttraumatic Stress Discorder (PTSD) Questionnaire (PPQ) is a 14-item, yes/no questionnaire designed
to measure symptoms of PTSD specifically related to childbirth experiences. Parents of newborn infants requiring hospitalization in a neonatal intensive care unit (NICU) have pro-

vided qualitative descriptions of psychological stress related to childbirth (Harrison & Kositski, 1983; Hynan, 1987; Nance, 1982). In addition to reports of general distress, these parents often described symptoms of PTSD including intrusive memories, avoidance symptoms, and increased arousal. I constructed the PPQ to quantify these qualitative reports. The first three items on the PPQ describe symptoms of unwanted intrusions (e.g., "Did you have several bad dreams of giving birth or of your baby's hospital stay?" "Did you have any sudden feelings as though your baby's birth was happening again?"). These next six items describe symptoms of avoidance or numbing of responsiveness (e.g., "Were you unable to remember parts of your baby's hospital stay?" "Did you avoid doing things which might bring up feelings you had about childbirth and your baby's hospital say?" "Did it become more difficult for you to feel tenderness or love for others?"). The last five items describe symptoms of arousal (e.g., "Were you more irritable or angry with others than usual?" "Did you feel more guilt about the childbirth than you felt you should have?" "Did you feel more jumpy?"). Respondents are instructed to answer yes to an item only if the experience last for more than 1 month during the 6 months after a birth. Thus far, research using the PPQ has been limited to the reports of mothers of high-risk infants (defined as infants, whether premature or full-term, that required hospitalization in a NICU) and control mothers of full-term, healthy infants.

The selection of items for the PPQ was based on two sources: (a) the diagnostic criteria for PTSD listed in the *Diagnostic and Statistical Manual of Mental Disorders* (DSM), third edition, revised (American Psychiatric Association, 1987), and (b) a similar questionnaire designed to measure symptoms of PTSD in Israeli combat soldiers (Solomon, Weisenberg, Schwarzwald, & Mikulincer, 1987). The complete PPQ has been published in the Journal of Perinatology (DeMier, Hynan, Harris, & Manniello, 1996).

Underlying Assumptions, Premises, and Objectives

One primary assumption underlying the development of PPQ was that the experience of childbirth followed by hospitalization of the infant in a NICU could be considered as a stressful, even traumatic, event for the infant's parents. The PPQ was developed using the conceptual framework of Lazarus's (1966, 1981) stress theory. Within this framework, the events of pregnancy, childbirth, and an infant's hospitalization are considered to be potential stressors. Parents emotional responses to these stressors are assumed to be determined by (a) the magnitude of the stressors, (b) a variety of mediating variables (e.g., the coping styles of the parents and their level of social support), and (c) the interactions among points a and b and parental distress.

My colleagues and I have used a number of research strategies to evaluate the validity of the PPQ as a measure of PTSD. In this chapter I will describe research on the concurrent and construct validity of the PPQ using criteria such as other measures of PTSD and general distress, including psychotherapy for postpartum distress.

In addition, we have also investigated the relationship between the magnitude of perinatal stressors and the PPQ. A review of the PTSD literature by March (1993) found the stressor magnitude was directly related to the risk of developing PTSD in 16 of 19 studies reviewed. Thus, we expected a positive relationship between the severity of perinatal stressors and the frequency of item endorsement on the PPQ. In quantifying stressor magnitude, we followed a research strategy for structural equation modeling (Anderson & Gerbing, 1988; Hoyle & Smith, 1994) by first specifying a measurement model of perinatal stressors. Once we identified a reliable model, we evaluated its relationship with the PPQ. This strategy has been useful in identifying a measurement model of prenatal stressors that is predictive of birth outcomes, such as gestational age (Lobel, 1994; Lobel & Dunkel-Schetter, 1990; Lobel, Dunkel-Schetter, & Schrimshaw, 1992).

Criterion A of the diagnosis of PTSD involves exposure to a traumatic event (such as a serious threat or harm to one's child) that is accompanied by intense fear, helplessness, or horror (*DSM-IV*; American Psychiatric Association, 1994). Davidson and Foa (1991, p. 346) have referred to Criterion A as "the gatekeeper to PTSD." Without such a stressor, a person cannot be diagnosed with PTSD. We believe that ample evidence indicates that having a newborn child hospitalized in a NICU is a traumatic event for many parents. For example, Affleck, Tennen, and Rowe (1991) interviewed 114 mothers of premature infants, 6 months and 18 months after their infant's birth. Many of these mothers described "an almost constant fear that their baby could die at any moment" (Affleck et al., 1991, p. 5). At both postpartum measurement intervals, large percentages of these mothers described painful memories of both childbirth and their infant's hospitalization on the Impact of Event Scale (IES; Horowitz, Wilner, & Alvarez, 1979). These memories were often intrusive, and many mothers also reported attempts to avoid these painful reminders. Gennaro (1988) reported that mothers of premature infants had elevated levels of depression on the Depression Adjective Checklist (Lubin, 1967) and elevated levels of anxiety on the state scale of the State-Trait Anxiety Inventory (Spielberger, Gorsuch, & Luchine, 1970) when compared with mothers of healthy infants. Thompson, Oehler, Catlett, and Johndrow (1993) reported significant psychological distress on the Symptom Checklist-90-Revised (Derogatis, 1983) in 33% to 48% of mothers of very low-birth-weight infants (depending on the time of postpartum evaluation). Since we view childbirth followed by hospitalization of the infant in a NICU as a stressful event, one of the tasks of our research program was to develop a method of measuring the magnitude of this perinatal stress. Consider the following four scenarios:

- A 600-gram infant is born at 26 weeks gestation to a mother with severe pre-eclampsia. The infant has mechanically assisted ventilation for 6 weeks, developing mild chronic lung disease. The infant also has apnea, bradycardia, and a mild intraventricular hemorrhage during a 10 week hospitalization in a NICU.

■ A 1,600-gram infant is born at 34 weeks gestation. This infant spends 2 weeks in a NICU with no complication worse than successfully treated jaundice.

■ A 4,000-gram infant is born at 40 weeks gestation with low Apgar (Apgar, Holaday, James, Weisbrot, & Berrien, 1958) scores of 2 at 1 minute and 3 at 5 minutes. The infant is given mechanically assisted ventilation and sent to the NICU. The infant is successfully weaned off the ventilator and is discharged in 3 days.

■ A 4,000-gram infant is born at 40 weeks gestation with high Apgar scores of 9 at 1 minute and 9 at 5 minutes. This infant stays with mother in the hospital; both are discharged within 48 hours.

Many observers would agree that the four scenarios differ in the magnitude of stress presented to parents. In an attempt to measure the magnitude of these stressors, my colleagues and I have developed a measurement model of perinatal stressors (DeMier & Hynan, 1994).

In the original report (Hynan, 1991), I identified six potential indices of perinatal stressors that formed a perinatal stress composite. These indices are gestational age of the infant measured in weeks, birthweight measured in grams, Apgar (Apgar et al., 1958) scores at 1 minute and 5 minutes, length of the infant's hospitalization measured in days, and a rating of the severity of the infant's postnatal complications. This postnatal complications rating (PCR; DeMier et al., 1996) is an eight-unit scale that I developed that quantifies the severity of postnatal complications recorded from hospital charts. The PCR was developed by having neonatologists and neonatal nurses rank-order the severity of numerous infant postnatal complications in terms of their perceived impact on parental distress. Therefore, the PCR is not a measure of objective medical risk (although it is very similar to a medical risk scale). Instead, the PCR is a measure of the magnitude of the parents' perception of the danger posed by a postnatal complication. Examples of a variety of complications on the PCR and their respective ranks are:

- no apparent complications—0;
- anemia, jaundice—1;
- apnea, bradycardia—2;
- respiratory distress syndrome (on respirator less than 5 days)—3;
- hydrocephalus, respiratory distress syndrome (on respirator 5 or more days)—5; and
- anencephaly, intraventricular hemorrhage (Grade IV)—7.

The six indices of perinatal stress were highly intercorrelated (Hynan, 1991). A multiple-regression analysis indicated that a linear combination of the six indices accounted for 58.5% of the variance in Blumberg's (1980) neonatal risk scale, which predicted maternal depression, anxiety, and negative perceptions of the infant. Using a principal components factor analysis, I reported a two-factor solution that accounted for 74.7% of the original variance in the six measures.

A subsequent reanalysis of these data by DeMier (1994), using the generalized least-square method of factor analysis, indicated that three factors (not two) best represented the six measures of perinatal stressors. The first factor (labeled Infant Maturity) was represented by gestational age, birth weight, length of hospitalization, and the PCR. The second factor (labeled Apgar scores) was represented by Apgar scores at 1 minute and 5 minutes. The third factor (labeled Complications) was represented by the PCR and length of hospitalization. This measurement model for perinatal stressors is presented in Figure 1.

DeMier, Hynan, Hatfield, Harris, Manniello, and Varner (1997) recently evaluated the utility of this measurement model using confirmatory factor analysis with the EQS pro-

Figure 1: The measurement model for perinatal stressors. Rectangles represent the six measured variables and their associated error variances. Circles represent the three factors. Arrows represent hypothesized relationships among the variables, factors, and error variances.

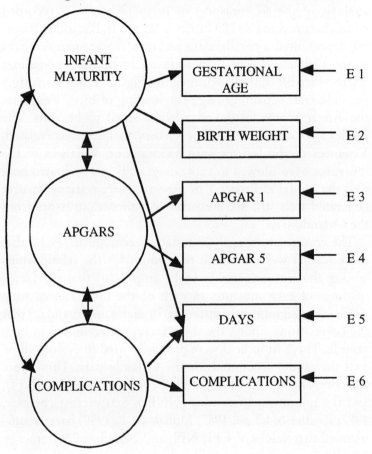

gram (Bentler, 1992). The confirmatory factor analysis was performed on data sets extracted from hospital records of premature births in hospitals in Indianapolis, Indiana, and Orlando, Florida. The confirmatory analysis evaluated how well the model in Figure 1 (obtained from an exploratory factor analysis of the six measures of perinatal stressors recorded from chart reviews of 189 births from the Indianapolis hospital) represented a parallel data set from 165 premature births at the Orlando hospital. In addition to the factor loadings (factor-variable links) identified in Figure 1, all remaining possible factor loadings (e.g., the loading of birth weight on the Apgar scores factor) were constrained to be zero. The model also allowed the three factors to be intercorrelated. Variances of the factors were fixed at one; variances of the measures were allowed to vary. Essentially, we evaluated how well the model in Figure 1 fit the variance/covariance matrix generated from the six measures of perinatal stressors from the Orlando data.

The confirmatory analysis tested three hypotheses: (a) that three factors were sufficient to account for the relationships among the six measures in each sample, (b) that the factor loadings of each measure on each of the three factors were similar (not significantly different) in each sample, and (c) that the correlations among the three factors were similar in each sample. Three fit indices were primarily used to evaluate how well the model accounted for the Orlando data. These were the comparative fit index (CFI), the normed fit index (NFI), and the nonnormed fit index (NNFI). Statisticians (Bentler, 1987; Bentler & Chou, 1987; Muliak et al., 1989) have recommended that values of CFI, NFI, and NNFI ≤ 0.9 (range = 0.0 to 1.0 except for the NFI, which can exceed 1.0) indicate that the model fits the data well. The CFI, NFI, and NNFI were 0.997, 0.995, and 0.996, respectively. We interpreted this outcome as an indication that the measurement model in Figure 1 is a reliable model for measuring perinatal stressors.

Summary of Research

Reliability

DeMier (1994) reports a coefficient alpha of .85 for the PPQ in a sample that contained 92 mothers of high-risk infants and 50 mothers of healthy, full-term infants. Of this sample of 142 mothers, 62 completed the PPQ a second time at intervals of 2 to 4 weeks after the first administration. The test-retest reliability of the PPQ in this subsample was .92.

Validity

DeMier et al. (1996) investigated the relationships among the six indices of perinatal stressors, PPQ scores, and reports of formal counseling or therapy for postnatal emotional distress. Participants were 78 mothers of premature infants, 14 mothers of full-term infants hospitalized in an NICU, and 50 mothers of healthy, full-term infants. High-risk mothers were primarily recruited from mothers attending national or regional meetings of Parent Care, Inc., and from members of parent groups (e.g., Parents of Prematures) in California, Florida, Indiana, Michigan, and Utah. Mothers of healthy infants were primarily recruited from classes at the University of Wisconsin–Milwaukee.

Mothers completed a survey asking them to describe the birth of one of their children along with their emotional reactions during the following 6 months. Mothers who had had only healthy, full-term babies were asked to describe the birth of their first infant. Mothers of premature babies were asked to describe the birth of their most premature infant (or sickest premature baby in cases of multiple births). Mothers of full-term infants who required hospitalization in a NICU were asked to describe the birth of their sick, full-term baby. Descriptions of the births included the six measures of perinatal stressors mentioned previously. In addition, mothers were asked whether they sought help for postnatal experiences from a professional counselor or therapist.

The three groups of mothers differed in the mean number of items endorsed on the PPQ, F (2,139) = 30.7, p < .001. Mothers of premature infants (M = 7.1, SD = 3.4) and mothers of full-term, sick infants (M = 6.0, SD = 3.3) did not differ in their frequency of PPQ responses. Both of these groups of mothers of high-risk infants endorsed more PPQ items (p < .01) than mothers of healthy, full-term infants (M = 2.5, SD = 2.8). A stepwise forward multiple-regression analysis was done to determine the correlation between the six indices of perinatal stressors as predictors and PPQ scores as the criterion. In this analysis, predictors were entered in order of their largest correlation (partial correlation for all predictors after the first one) with the PPQ. The PCR accounted for 29.8% of the variance in PPQ scores, multiple R = .55, $F(1,140)$ = 58.7, p < .001. Gestational age of the infant accounted for an additional 3.0% of the variance, multiple R = .57, $F(2,139)$ = 33.5, p < .001. The last predictor to provide a significant increment in variance (2.2%) was length of stay in the NICU, multiple R = .59, $F(3,138)$ = 24.4, p < .001.

Not one of the mothers of healthy infants reported formal counseling or therapy for their childbirth experiences. We then subdivided the group of mothers of high-risk infants into two groups. The first group answered yes to a configuration of responses on the PPQ that would have qualified for a diagnosis of PTSD (American Psychiatric Association, 1987), if such questions had been asked in a formal diagnostic interview. (This would have required at least six yes responses distributed according to diagnostic criteria.) The second group of high-risk mothers would not have met diagnostic criteria for PTSD but had endorsed four or more questions on the PPQ. Thirty-three percent of the first group of mothers and 18% of the second group of mothers reported that they had sought formal help from a counselor or therapist for their perinatal experiences.

Having found in the DeMier et al. (1996) data that three of the six indices of perinatal stressors accounted for 35% of the variance in PPQ responses (and that the PCR was the strongest predictor of PPQ responses), we attempted to replicate these findings using the measurement model specified in Figure 1 as the predictor of PPQ responses. Specifically, we asked whether a measurement model obtained from hospital records of premature births would predict responses on the PPQ in a new sample of mothers of both high-risk and healthy infants (DeMier et al., 1997).

In this replication study, 99 mothers of premature infants, 69 mothers of healthy, full-term infants, and 21 mothers of full-term infants requiring hospitalization in an NICU answered a questionnaire very similar to the one used by DeMier et al. (1996). The primary data analyses were conducted on the mothers' descriptions of the six measures of perinatal stressors and their PPQ responses. In determining how well our measurement model would predict PPQ responses in this sample of mothers, we decided to modify the model by dropping the Apgar scores and the Apgar factor. Only 109 of the total sample of 189 mothers remembered the Apgar scores of their infant, so dropping these measures allowed us to evaluate the predictability of the PPQ using the full sample.

To evaluate the modified measurement model and the PPQ, mothers' responses to the PPQ were added to the model as a fifth measure with hypothesized links to the two remaining factors. This model is shown in Figure 2. In this revised model, birth weight, gestational age, length of hospitalization, and PPQ scores had loadings on the Infant Maturity factor. Length of hospitalization, PCR scores, and PPQ scores had loadings on the Complications factor. Ten subjects were excluded from the analysis as outliers. This analysis also used raw data input and the maximum likelihood, robust method of extraction because some distributions were nonnormal. This analysis evaluated how well the model specified in Figure 2 fit the variance/covariance matrix generated by the measures

Figure 2: The modified measurement model of perinatal
stressors including symptoms of posttraumatic stress
disorder (PTSD) endorsed on the Perinatal PTSD
Questionnaire. Rectangles represent the five measured
variables and their respective error variances. Circles
represent the two factors. Arrows represent hypothesized
relationships among the variables, factors, and error
variances.

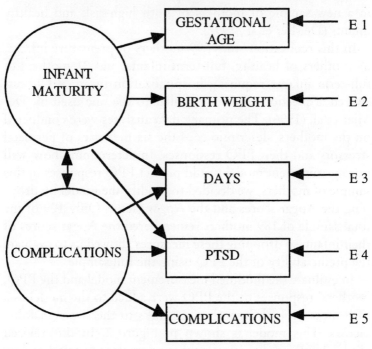

(birth weight, gestational age, length of hospitalization, PCR,
and PPQ) reported by the replication sample of mothers.

The model in Figure 2 fit the mothers' data well. The CFI,
NFI, and NNFI were 0.994, 0.990, and 0.981, respectively.
Additional analyses indicated that reports of PTSD symptoms
were significantly related to both the Infant Maturity factor
(standardized regression coefficient = 0.21) and the Complications factor (standardized regression coefficient = 0.40).

The two factors accounted for 33% of the variance in PPQ reports.

Because the Infant Maturity and Complications factors were significantly correlated (.66), we performed an additions analysis to determine the relationship between the Complications factor alone and the PPQ. This analysis removed the link between the PPQ and Infant Maturity, otherwise the analysis was the same as the previous one. This analysis revealed that the model did not fit the data quite as well as the model that included the Infant Maturity—PPQ link. The CFI, NFI, and NNFI were 0.987, 0.982, and 0.967, respectively. In this last model, 30% of the variance in PPQ reports was accounted for by the complications factor alone.

These findings replicate the results of the DeMier et al. (1996) study, which found that 35.0% of the variance in PPQ reports by mothers was accounted for by the mothers' report of the PCR, gestational age, and length of stay in the NICU. When the measurement model was used as the predictor of PPQ scores (rather than mothers' descriptions of their own infants' births), the validity shrinkage was slight, from 35.0% to 33.0% of the variance. This finding is especially noteworthy because the measurement model was generated from data from premature births only, yet the measurement model still had predictive utility when applied to a group combining mothers of healthy infants, premature infants, and full-term infants hospitalized in a NICU. The findings of both studies are consistent with many studies showing a reliable relationship between the severity of a variety of traumatic events and the development of symptoms of PTSD (March, 1993).

At this point in our research program, we concluded that there was ample evidence that the PPQ was a valid measure of general psychological distress in high-risk parents. The next research study was designed to evaluate the PPQ as a more specific measure of PTSD.

Quinnell and Hynan (at press) reported a convergent and discriminant validity study of the PPQ. A new sample of 83 mothers of premature infants, 51 mothers of healthy, full-term infants, and 8 mothers of full-term infants hospitalized in a NICU participated. Mothers were recruited from the same sources as the two previous validity studies. Mothers answered the PPQ and two other well-validated measures of PTSD: the IES (Horowitz et al., 1979) and the Penn Inventory (PI; Hammarberg, 1992). Mothers also answered a divergent measure, the Need for Cognition Scale (NCS; Cacioppo & Petty, 1982). The PPQ, IES, PI, and NCS have similar levels of internal consistency and test-retest reliablility. Mothers also provided information on the six perinatal stressor measures, demographics, and any psychotherapy for postpartum distress.

Mothers were instructed to answer the PPQ and IES with reference to their feelings during the 6 months after the birth of the child. Items on the PI represent the phenomenological expression of PTSD. Most of these items focus on present symptoms, so a modification of PI items to reflect a time frame of 6 months after a birth would have been problematic. We decided to use instructions on the PI directing participants to report on feelings "during the past few months, including today." Thus, the time frame for the PI reflected the recent past; the time frame for the PPQ and IES reflected the 6-month period following the birth. These different referents in time allowed us to examine a correlation of postnatal reports and residual symptoms.

Table 1 illustrates significant correlations among the convergent measures. An analysis of differences between dependent correlations showed that in all cases the magnitude of correlation among the convergent measures was significantly larger than the correlation among divergent measures—all ps < .01. The correlation between the PPQ and IES was also significantly larger than (a) the correlation between the PPQ and the PI and (b) the correlation between the IES and the PI.

Table 2 illustrates the mothers' scores on the PPQ, IES, PI, and NCS. Missing data concerning gestational age and the PCR reduced the number of subjects in these analyses. Mothers of premature infants and mothers of full-term, sick infants

Table 1: Intercorrelations among the Convergent and Divergent Measures

Scales	PPQ	IES	PI	NCS
PPQ	----	.78**	.50**	-.04
IES		----	.50**	-.08
PI			----	-.25*
NCS				----

Note: PPQ = Perinatal Posttraumatic Stress Disorder Questionnaire; IES = Impact of Events Scale; PI = Penn Inventory; NCS = Need for Cognition Scale.

*p < .05.

**p < .01.

did not differ on any of the four scores, so these two groups were combined to form the group of high-risk mothers. Mothers of high-risk infants had larger scores on both the PPQ and IES; $F(1,113)$ = 55.8 and 52.2, respectively; both ps < .001. The two groups of mothers did not differ on their scores on the PI—F = (1,113) = 2.9, p > .05—and the NCS.

A hierarchical multiple-regression was performed using the PPQ as the criterion. Socioeconomic status (SES) of the mothers was entered first as a control variable, accounting for 2% of the variance in the PPQ, $F(1,133)$ = 2.81, p < .10. Three additional control variables were then entered into the formula: (a) mother's age at the time of giving birth, (b) mother's age at the time of completing the questionnaire, and (c) their number of other children to whom the mother had given birth. These three control variables accounted for an additional 1.6% of variance in PPQ scores. The PCR was entered into the equation next, accounting for an additional 22.3% of the variance in PPQ scores, multiple R = .51, $F(5,129)$ = 9.05, p < .001. Of the remaining perinatal stressors (i.e., gesta-

Table 2: Scores for the Two Groups of Mothers on the Measures

Measure	Mothers	
	High-Risk Baby	Healthy-Term Baby
PPQ		
M	6.14	1.79
SD	3.50	1.86
IES		
M	19.01	6.79
SD	9.72	6.67
PI		
M	23.47	20.07
SD	10.04	9.27
NCS		
M	22.14	21.33
SD	24.80	21.76

Note: PPQ = Perinatal Posttraumatic Stress Disorder Questionnaire; IES = Impact of Events Scale; PI = Penn Inventory; NCS = Need for Cognition Scale.

tional age, birth weight, days hospitalized, and Apgar scores at 1 and 5 minutes), only gestational age accounted for significant additional variance, multiple $R = .54$, $F(6,128) = 8.83$, $p < .001$.

Only 3 of 51 mothers of healthy infants sought formal counseling or therapy for their childbirth experiences, whereas 46 of the 91 mothers of high-risk infants sought therapy. Follow-up analyses were conducted to determine the relationship between scores on the convergent and divergent measures and whether mothers sought therapy for childbirth experiences. Point biserial correlations were calculated with therapy (yes/no) as the nominal dimension. The correlation between the NCS and seeking therapy was not significant, $r = -.13$. Significant correlations were found between therapy seeking and the convergent measures: (a) PPQ, $r = ./1$; (b) IES, $r = .71$; and (c) PI, $r = .33$; all $ps < .001$.

Because we were concerned with the retrospective nature of the mothers' reports, we examined the relationship between mothers' scores on the convergent and divergent measures and the time elapsed since the child's birth. There were no significant correlations between the time elapsed since childbirth and scores on the PPQ, IES, PI, and NCS; $rs = -.01$, $-.08$, $-.07$, and $-.05$, respectively. The distribution of the number of years between the birth and questionnaire completion was skewed, $M = 7.09$, $SD = 7.22$, median $= 4$, mode $= 2$ years.

The results of the Quinnell and Hynan (at press) study show substantial support for the validity of the PPQ as a measure of PTSD. The PPQ correlates significantly with well-validated measures of PTSD, and the PPQ has discriminant validity. The construct validity of the PPQ was also supported by significant relationships of the PPQ with both the emotional consequences of the birth (seeking therapy for experiences related to childbirth and the NICU) and stressful antecedent perinatal events (e.g., the PCR and gestational age).

High-risk mothers and mothers of healthy babies differed in the frequency of responses on the PPQ and IES. These two groups of mothers did not differ in their responses to the PI. Also, the PPQ correlates more highly with the IES (.78) than the PI (.50). An interpretation of this pattern is problematic because the instruments are confounded with the time frame given in the instructions. On the PPQ and IES, mothers were asked to describe their feelings during the 6 months after giving birth, whereas on the PI, mothers were asked to report on the last few months. We propose that the counseling received by many highrisk mothers accounts for this pattern, rather than any differences in construct validity among the convergent measures.

We suspect that highrisk mothers with more symptoms of PTSD after giving birth sought counseling, which in turn decreased some symptoms. Counseling might account for the lack of a difference between highrisk and normal mothers on their answers to the PI, which reflected the recent past, not the 6 months after birth. This hypothesized decline in PTSD symptoms was not sufficient, however, to obscure a modest correlation between postnatal (i.e., PPQ and IES) and residual (PI) symptoms of PTSD observed in our data. We recognize that other explanations are possible. For example, counseling may have sensitized highrisk mothers to report more symptoms of PTSD after giving birth, but fewer symptoms after counseling had been completed.

Conditions for Use

Anyone may use the PPQ for research purposes. In clinical settings, the PPQ should be administered and interpreted by staff trained in the use of psychometric instruments. Although we believe that the data show encouraging support for the validity of the PPQ as a measure of PTSD symptoms, no single questionnaire should be used in forming a diagnosis. In addition, users of the PPQ may wish to administer additional validity scales to evaluate response bias.

Applications

In practical terms, we believe that the PPQ would be best administered to mothers (and fathers) when their babies are discharged from the NICU and when the parents return with their infants to follow-up clinics. Although it is premature to establish cutoff scores for the PPQ, endorsement of a large number of items could be used to channel parents into a more complete diagnostic evaluation. A perinatal follow-up clinic in Milwaukee has routinely administered the PPQ to mothers bringing in their infants for their 6-month physical evaluation. This clinic has added an additional item to the PPQ. This yes/no item asks parents whether they would like to talk to someone about any emotional distress they may have. A yes answer begins a referral process.

Benefits and Limitations

Our research suggests that both the PCR and the PPQ may be of value in family-centered perinatal settings. The PCR may be useful in identifying parents most at risk for PTSD because of the severity of their infant's medical complications. Interventions prior to the onset of PTSD may reduce the severity of parental psychological distress. If the PPQ is administered routinely in perinatal settings, parents with high scores can be referred to parent support groups and/or therapists.

The major limitation to our findings lies in the retrospective nature of the mothers' reports (Henry, Moffitt, Caspi, Langley, & Silva, 1994). In a few cases, mothers described births that had occurred more than 20 years before. Despite the retrospective nature of our data, our results are consistent with those of Affleck et al. (1991), who used a prospective design to collect parental data on the IES 6 and 18 months after the baby was discharged from the hospital. Also, we found no relationship between the amount of time elapsed since the birth and the mother's endorsement of items on the PPQ. We believe that subsequent research should use a prospective design and additional validity criteria. Specifically, we believe that a more stringent evaluation of the PPQ would involve additional divergent and convergent measures (especially a structured, diagnostic interview) administered within 6 months to 2 years after childbirth.

Chapter References

Affleck, G., Tennen, H., & Rowe, J. (1991). *Infants in crisis: How parents cope with newborn intensive care and its aftermath.* New York: Springer.

American Psychiatric Association. (1987). *Diagnostic and statistical manual of mental disorders* (3rd ed., rev.). Washington, DC: Author.

American Psychiatric Association. (1994). *Diagnostic and statistical manual of mental disorders* (4th ed.). Washington, DC: Author.

Anderson, J. C., & Gerbing, D. W. (1988). Structural equation modeling in practice: A review and recommended two-step approach. *Psychological Bulletin, 103,* 391–410.

Apgar, V. A., Holaday, D. A., James, L. S., Weisbrot, I. M., & Berrien, C. (1958). Evaluation of the newborn infant: Second report. *Journal of the American Medical Association, 168,* 1985–1988.

Bentler, P. M. (1992). *EQS Structural Equations Program Manual.* Los Angeles: BMDP Statistical Software.

Bentler, P. M. (1987). Comparative fit indexes in structural models. *Psychological Bulletin, 107,* 238–246.

Bentler, P. M., & Chou, C. (1987). Practical issues in structural modeling. *Sociological Methods and Research, 16,* 78–117.

Blumberg, N. L. (1980). Effects of neonatal risk, maternal attitude, and cognitive style on early postpartum adjustment. *Journal of Abnormal Psychology, 89,* 139–150.

Cacioppo, J. T., & Petty, R. E. (1982). The need for cognition. *Journal of Personality and Social Psychology, 42,* 116–131.

Davidson, J., & Foa, E. B. (1991). Diagnostic issues in posttraumatic stress disorder: Considerations for DSM-VI. *Journal of Abnormal Psychology, 100,* 346–355.

DeMier, R. L. (1994). *Predictors of posttraumatic stress disorder in mothers of high-risk infants.* Unpublished doctoral dissertation, University of Wisconsin–Milwaukee.

DeMier, R. L., & Hynan, M. T. (1994). Symptoms of posttraumatic stress disorder in mothers of high-risk infants [Abstract]. *Journal of Perinatology, 14,* 332.

DeMier, R. L., Hynan, M. T., Harris, H. B., & Manniello, R. L. (1996). Perinatal stressors as predictors of symptoms of posttraumatic stress in mothers of infants at highrisk. *Journal of Perinatology, 16,* 276–280.

DeMier, R. L., Hynan, M. T., Hatfield, R. F., Harris, H. B., Manniello, R. L., & Varner, M. W. (1997). *A measurement model of perinatal stressors: Identifying risk factors for posttraumatic stress in mothers of high-risk infants.* Unpublished manuscript.

Derogatis, L. R. (1983). *SCL-90: Administration, scoring and procc dure manual—II.* Baltimore, MD: Clinical Psychometric Research.

Gennaro, S. (1988). Postpartal anxiety and depression in mothers of term and preterm infants. *Nursing Research, 37,* 82–85.

Hammarberg, M. (1992). Penn Inventory for posttraumatic stress disorder: Psychometric properties. *Psychological Assessment: A Journal of Consulting and Clinical Psychology, 4,* 67–76.

Harrison, H., & Kositski, A. (1993). *The premature baby book.* New York: St. Martin's.

Henry, B., Moffitt, T. E., Caspi, A., Langley, J., & Silva, P. A. (1994). On the "remembrance of things past": A longitudinal evaluation of the retrospective method. *Psychological Assessment, 6,* 92–101.

Horowitz, M. J., Wilner, N. R., & Alvarez, W. (1979). Impact of event scale: A measure of subjective distress. *Psychosomatic Medicine, 13,* 139–145.

Hoyle, R. H., & Smith, G. T. (1994). Formulating clinical research hypotheses as structural equation models: A conceptual overview. *Journal of Consulting and Clinical Psychology, 62,* 429–440.

Hynan, M. T. (1987). *The pain of premature parents: A psychological guide for coping.* Lanham, MD: University Press of America.

Hynan, M. T. (1991). The perinatal stress composite: A validation study. *Bulletin of the Psychonomic Society, 29,* 1–3.

Lazarus, R. (1966). *Psychological stress and the coping process.* New York: McGraw-Hill.

Lazarus, R. (1981). The stress and coping paradigm. In C. Eisdorfer, D. Cohen, A. Kleinman, & P. Maxim (Eds.), *Models for clinical psychopathology* (pp. 177–214). New York: Spectrum.

Lobel, M. (1994). Conceptualizations, measurement, and effects of prenatal maternal stress on birth outcomes. *Journal of Behavioral Medicine, 17,* 225–272.

Lobel, M., & Dunkel-Schetter, C. (1990). Conceptualizing stress to study effects on health: Environmental, perceptual, and emotional components. *Anxiety Research, 3,* 213–230.

Lobel, M., Dunkel-Schetter, C., & Scrimshaw, S. C. M. (1992). The role of prenatal maternal stress in infant prematurity. *Health Psychology, 11,* 32–40.

Lubin, B. (1967). *Depression Adjective Checklist.* San Diego: Educational and Industrial Testing Service.

March, J. S. (1993). What constitutes a stressor? The "criterion A" issue. In J. Davidson & E. B. Foa (Eds.), *Post-traumatic stress disorder: DSM-IV and beyond* (pp. 37–54). Washington, DC: American Psychiatric Press.

Muliak, S. A., James, L. R., Van Alstine, J., Bennett, N., Lind, S., & Stillwell, C. D. (1989). Evaluation of goodness-of-fit indices for structural equation models. *Psychological Bulletin, 105,* 430–445.

Nance, S. (1982). *Premature babies: A handbook for parents.* New York: Arbor House.

Quinnell, F. A. & Hynan, M. T. (at press). Convergent and discriminant validity of the Perinatal PTSD Questionnaire (PPQ). *Journal of Traumatic Stress.*

Solomon, Z., Weisenberg, M., Schwarzwald, J., & Mikulincer, M. (1987). Posttraumatic stress disorder among frontline soldiers with combat stress reactions: The 1982 Israeli experience. *American Journal of Psychiatry, 144,* 448–454.

Spielberger, C., Gorsuch, R., & Luchine, R. (1970). *Manual for the State-Trait Anxiety Inventory.* Palo Alto, CA: Consulting Psychologists Press.

Thompson, R. J., Oehler, J. M., Catlett, A. T., & Johndrow, D. A. (1993). Maternal psychological adjustment to the birth of an infant weighing 1500 grams or less. *Infant Behavior and Development, 16,* 471–485.

The Personal Style Inventory

A Measure of Stress Resiliency

Charles L. Sheridan, University of Missouri–Kansas City*
Sally A. Radmacher, Missouri Western State College

■ Instrument Name

The Personal Style Inventory (PSI)
The Personal Style Inventory: A Measure of Stress Resiliency
The PSI

■ Developer

Charles L. Sheridan, Ph.D., The University of
Missouri–Kansas City

■ Contact Information

Dr. Charles L. Sheridan, University of Missouri–Kansas City,
5319 Holmes, Kansas City, MO 64110
Telephone: (816) 235-1069; e-mail: csheridan@cctr.umkc.edu
Sally A. Radmacher, Ph.D., Missouri Western State College,
4525 Downs Dr., St. Joseph, MO 64507
Telephone: (816) 271-4445;
e-mail: radmache@griffon.mwsc.edu.

Description and History of Instrument

The Personal Style Inventory (PSI) was designed to measure
stress resiliency. We define stress resiliency as a person's abil-

---

*The Personal Style Inventory (PSI) is copyrighted by Charles L. Sher-
idan.

221

ity to recover or "bounce back" from stressful events. The scale was designed to provide a broad-spectrum assessment of the range of personal factors that mediate reactions to stressful events. The items reflect the attitudes, coping styles, cognitive patterns, habits, and competencies that were identified from an extensive review of the relevant literature. Many items that involve personal qualities related to stress resistance were taken or derived from an earlier instrument, the Inventory of Stress Resistance Resources (ISRR; Sheridan & Smith, 1987). The ISRR deals with specific activities and circumstances that influence reactions to stress. Besides personal activities, the ISRR includes material, social, and what Antonovsky (1979) termed "macrosociocultural" circumstances. In addition to the items gleaned from the ISRR, new items were created for the PSI that encompass dimensions believed to influence stress reactions. For example, items were added to assess optimism, skill at communicating feelings about stress, and some characteristics that have been observed in "resilient" children (e.g., feeling special). Furthermore, some items were constructed on the basis of our own observations of people who seem to manage stress exceptionally well or very poorly. Examples of these items include the possession of self-calming skills and the tendency to amplify stressful stimuli.

Construction of the PSI was heavily influenced by the work of the late Aaron Antonovsky (1979), who held that internal and external generalized resistance resources contribute to the formation of a "sense of coherence" that permits an individual to resist stress. He theorized that sense of coherence (SOC) is the degree to which an individual finds life meaningful, manageable, and comprehensible. Antonovsky (1987) developed a scale to measure SOC called the Orientation to Life Inventory that many investigators, including ourselves, have used to collect data in support of his theory and the instrument. However, factor analyses provided no solid support for the three theoretical components of sense of coherence. Moreover, the literature on the mediating factors of stress reveals many other efficacious dimensions that are at least nominally different than SOC. For example, early longitudinal studies indicated that certain key styles of coping (suppression, anticipation, altruism, and humor) fostered health, whereas other styles (denial, fantasy, and repression) did not (Vaillant, 1977). More recently, dimensions and measures mediating health status have burgeoned, and, again, each is nominally different from the other. Lazarus and Folkman (1984), and other investigators who have been influenced by them, have examined the impact of modes of coping. Similarly, the concept of the "hardy personality" has stimulated a substantial body of research (Kobasa, 1979). Seligman (1991) has identified optimism as an important stress mediator, and Pennebaker, Colder, and Sharp (1990) have shown that discussing stressful events and expressing the accompanying emotions may minimize the stress reaction. These and many other researchers have identified significant, and seemingly nonoverlapping, factors that regulate the impact of stress. It is apparent that to fully assess stress resiliency, all of these factors should be combined into one instrument.

Conceptual Structure of the PSI

The PSI is based on the conceptualizations of resistance resources and sense of coherence that form the foundation of stress resistance according to Antonovsky (1979). The deviation from the concept of sense of coherence was based on the recognition that, in spite of Antonovsky's impressive effort to identify the core features of stress resistance, it was not obvious that the core he identified really encompassed all of the significant dimensions described by other researchers. The approach used in constructing the PSI was to include a full range of dimensions from other theorists and investigators that might or might not be independent of Antonovsky's core constructs and then to determine the structure of stress resistance empirically through factor analyses.

Factor Analyses

Factor analyses were conducted independently on two different data sets using a common protocol for the analyses and the labeling of factors. This procedure was based largely on the protocol advocated by Kline (1994). Kline's protocol involves running an initial principal components analysis to determine the appropriate number of factors. Rather than using an eigenvalue of 1 as a criterion for determining the number of factors, a Scree test is conducted, and then a final determination of the number of factors is made on the basis of items loading clearly on the factors (i.e., loading heavily on no more than one factor). For both data sets, three factors appeared appropriate based on the preliminary principal components analyses; therefore, subsequent factor analyses stipulated the three-factor solution. Various forms of factor analysis (e.g., oblimin vs. varimax) were then done on the two data sets, and all yield basically the same factors. Correlation coefficients between similar factors from the two sets of data ranged from .84 to .97, indicating that the same dimensions had been identified independently in the separate analyses. The resulting factors provided a basis for an empirically derived conceptual structure of the PSI.

- The first dimension of the PSI encompasses most of the familiar concepts found to be important in the stress resistance literature including, "hope," "optimism," "sense of coherence," "coping skills," "primitive versus mature defense," "meaningfulness," "challenge," "social competence," "structure and organization," and "self-efficacy." In essence, it appears to reflect negative versus positive attitudes and various competencies for resisting stress.
- The second dimension reflects perfectionistic sensitivity coupled with self-criticism, self-abnegation, and overinvolvement with others.
- The third dimension reflects a communication/expres-

siveness dimension previously linked to stress reactivity by such investigators as Pennebaker (1990) and Gross and Levenson (1993).

Social Desirability Scale Subscale

In addition to the items designed to assess stress resiliency, the PSI includes 10 items designed to assess the tendency to "fake good." Although these were newly constructed items, they were modeled after the Social Desirability Inventory (Crowne & Marlowe, 1960). The impetus for including these items was research conducted by Ingersoll (1990) and Cloud (1995), which indicated that the relationship between stress and stress reaction may be obscured by the tendency to "fake good." Specifically, these investigators independently found that the relationship between avowed stress and essential hypertension became clear only after the effects of social desirability were partialed out. A further rationale for including a "lie" scale was that assessments of stress are often done in contexts in which the people undergoing assessment may be motivated to seem more or less distressed—for example, workers who may see the assessment as a vehicle to complain about their working conditions or chronic pain patients who may want to avoid any indications of a psychological component to their problems.

Negative Affectivity Subscale

After the initial development of the PSI, the important role of negative affectivity (NA) or neuroticism in the stress-health relationship began to be emphasized in the literature. This interest developed primarily from the work of Watson and Pennebaker (1989) and Costa and McCrae (1987), who took the view that NA tends to lead to exaggerated reports of both stress and illness, which inflates the correlation between these two variables. However, some research has provided strong evidence that both stress and NA have an influence on health when the health measure is not subject to distortions in self-reporting (Cohen, Tyrrell, & Smith, 1993). Negative affectivity has been viewed as one of the early manifestations of breakdown when resources failed to neutralize stressors (Sheridan & Smith, 1987). This conceptualization of NA corresponds quite closely to that of Frankenhaeuser (1991).

With either of these perspectives, the role of NA was considered important to the understanding of the stress-health relationship. Because habits of nervous tension and worry correspond quite closely to the usual indications of NA and had been included in the PSI, it was decided to identify a subset of items in the PSI to function as an index of NA. Mulhern (1994) administered the PSI to a diverse group of 107 people along with two widely used measures of NA, the NEO-PI, Form S (Costa & McCrae, 1985), and the Negative Emotionality Scale (Tellegen, 1982). Based on Mulhern's data, 21 items were selected from the PSI to form a Negative Affectivity subscale (PSINA). The criteria for inclusion were (a) face validity (i.e., items had to reflect NA directly rather than indirectly), and (b) each item had to have a statistically significant correlation with the NEO. This selection procedure resulted in an r of .72 between the PSINA and the NEO and an r of .63 between PSINA and NEM. Given that the correlation between the NEM and NEO is .70, we concluded that PSINA is an adequate measure of NA.

Administration, Format, and Scoring

The PSI is a 65-item checklist inventory developed to measure the full range of personal factors influencing reactions to stressors. It is appropriate for use with adults with at least a seventh-grade reading level. Versions of the PSI have been adapted for use with secondary and middle-school children and are currently being evaluated. The inventory takes about 5 to 15 minutes to complete. Respondents check a yes box if the item applies to them and a no box if the item does not apply to them. The PSI can be and is used as a checklist-type of scale; however, the yes/no format prevents the problem that arises when only a few items are checked, leaving the researcher to wonder whether the items checked were the only ones that applied or if the respondent simply failed to complete the scale.

Each yes response is counted as one point except for the 29 reverse-keyed items. In those cases, a no response is counted as one point. A high score indicates a high degree of stress resiliency. (Early in the construction of the PSI, it was conceptualized as a measure of stress vulnerability/resiliency. As the psychometric analyses continued, it became apparent that the majority of the most robust items were reflecting resiliency rather than vulnerability. Therefore, many of the validation studies used a reverse-scoring method and have titles that reflect the earlier conceptualization.) A total PSI score is obtained by summing the number of points. In addition, the three subscales are scored by totaling points for the appropriate subset of PSI items. The three subscales are scored in the same manner and are described as follows:

- Positive Attitude is the first subscale and consists of 30 items that reflect positive attitudes and competencies. Examples are "I frequently take good care of, calm, and comfort myself," "I am likely to look at the bright side of troublesome situations," "I commonly see difficult situations as a challenge," "In general, my life experiences make sense to me," and "Often, when dealing with difficult situations, I do things that end up making things worse for me."
- The second subscale, Hypersensitivity/Self-Criticism, reflects a hypersensitivity to criticism from others and self-criticism. A sample of this subscale's 19 items follow: "When something bad happens to me, I get angry or critical with myself for having gotten into the situation," "I spend a lot of time painfully worrying about things that end up not happening at all," "I can't stand disapproval,

even when it comes from someone who isn't very important to me," "I feel that I am more anxious than most people about what other people think of me," and "I spend a lot of time inwardly criticizing myself (my appearance, my skills, what I've done, etc.)."

- The third subscale, Communications/Expressiveness, has eight items that reflect effective communication and self-expression. Examples of this subscale are "When under stress, I usually talk out my feelings with someone who is likely to understand and care," "When I am troubled and talk over my problems with others, I am likely to come away feeling better," and "I usually feel okay about saying how I feel."

Psychometric Characteristics

Reliability

Reliability is an index of test consistency (i.e., the extent to which a test score is stable and free from error). There are two types of reliability: temporal stability and internal consistency. Temporal stability is the degree to which the results of a measure are stable over time and is established through test-retest. This involves giving the measure to the same group of participants at two different times and correlating the two sets of scores. A test-retest correlation of .70 or above is considered acceptable. Internal consistency is the extent to which the items of the test are homogeneous. Internal consistency is usually established with a coefficient alpha of .70 or greater.

Several coefficient alphas have been reported that establish the internal consistency of the PSI. For example, an alpha of .95 was obtained from a sample of 87 employees of a mental health facility (Bigham, Sheridan, & Martin, 1994). An alpha of .90 in a heterogeneous convenience sample of 80 adults was reported (Martin & Sheridan, 1994). Harmless (1996) obtained an alpha of .90 from a sample of 256 college students.

Finally, in a heterogeneous sample of 758 participants (Sheridan, Radmacher, & Petren, 1997) an alpha of .91 was reported for the PSI. Internal consistencies were also established for the three PSI subscales using the sample of 758 just mentioned. The coefficient alphas for Positive Attitudes, Hypersensitivity/Self-Criticism, and Communications/Expressiveness were .86, .84, and .80, respectively.

Temporal stability was established for the full PSI with test-retest data obtained on 157 college students, which yielded an r of .89. The tests were separated by a period of 2 to 4 weeks.

Criterion-Related Validity

Criterion validity is the extent to which a test is effective in predicting some criterion that is an independent measure of the construct being measured (Anastasi, 1988). A substantial body of evidence has been gathered in support of the validity of the PSI and its subscales using two measures of health status as criterion variables. One measure is a generic health status scale that places heavy emphasis on major and chronic illnesses, although it also includes minor illnesses. This measure is probably best suited to older, less healthy samples. The second measure is a somatic symptom checklist that is carefully limited to somatic symptoms and has little of its variance attributable to distortions from negative affectivity (Mulhern, 1994; Sheridan, Mulhern, & Martin, at press).

Bigham et al. (1994) found the PSI correlated significantly with these measures of health status, with correlation coefficients ranging from .50 to .56, depending on the measure. They further found that the PSI made an additional contribution to the prediction of health status even after first forcing Cohen's Perceived Stress Scale (PSS; Cohen, Kamarck, & Mermelstein, 1983) into a multiple-regression equation (PSS: $B = .41, p < .001$; PSI: $B = .24, p < .05$). Because perceived stress is presumably due in part to recognition of environmental stressors and in part to secondary appraisals, this is a particularly demanding test of PSI predictive validity. Statistically significant relationships between all of the PSI subscales and the same health status measures were found, with correlation coefficients ranging from .31 ($p < .005$) to .59 ($p < .0001$). When the PSS (Cohen et al., 1983) was forced into a multiple-regression equation and then followed by the PSI subscales, the subscales made an additional contribution to the prediction of health status.

Using the same two health status measures, another study (Martin & Sheridan, 1994) also found that the PSI predicted overall health. The Hypersensitivity/Perfectionism factor was a significant predictor of health, again after the effects of the PSS had already been taken into account. Statistically significant correlations between health status and PSI were reported in a study of chronic fatigue syndrome (CFS) patients, non-CFS chronic patients, and nonpatient controls (Schmidt & Sheridan, 1994). The PSI was a significant predictor of the two health status measures and scores on the Fatigue Severity Scale (Krupp, LaRocca, Muir-Nash, & Steinberg, 1989). All probability values were less than .02. These data also showed that PSI scores were significantly elevated in both groups, chronic patients compared with the controls. This study is one that used the reversed scoring, which means that a high score indicates low resiliency (see the explanation in the "Administration, Format, and Scoring" section).

Several significant correlation coefficients were found between PSI subscales and blood lipid levels in a sample of 175 employees participating in a state college wellness screening program (Radmacher & Sheridan, 1995a). The subscales were Communications/Expressiveness and a subscale that resulted from an earlier factor analysis labeled Self-Nurturance that contains many of the items from the Positive Attitude subscale. Communications/Expressiveness was a statistically significant predictor of high-density lipoprotein (HDL) cholesterol even when age, sex, and avowed levels of physical activity were forced into the equation first. Self-Nurturance was a statistically significant predictor of the HDL/total cholesterol ratio, again with the other variables just mentioned being forced into the equation first. However, these findings were not replicated in the second phase of this ongoing study.

Construct Validity

Construct validity refers to the extent to which the test measures a theoretical construct or trait and involves the labels we give our tests (e.g., does an IQ test really measure intelligence, or does it measure exposure to the mainstream culture?). Construct validity is established in two steps: first by testing for a convergence across different measures of the same variable, then testing for a divergence between measures of related but conceptually distinct variables. A moderately high correlation with the convergent measure and a moderately low correlation with the divergent measure is preferred. The multiple-regression analyses forcing the PSS into the equations provide support for the discriminant validity of the PSI by indicating that it measures a dimension relevant to health yet distinct from perceived stress. Convergent validity has also been established in a study (Martin & Sheridan, 1994) that found a statistically significant correlation between the PSI and the Orientation to Life Inventory (OTLI), a measure of Sense of Coherence developed by Antonovsky (1987). In addition, the PSI was found also to correlate significantly with a measure of borderline personality organization (Oldham et al., 1985). Borderline is a personality style that is generally acknowledged to be associated with vulnerability to stress. In a study yet to be published (Ficken & Sheridan, 1997) a correlation was found with the Hope Scale (Snyder et al., 1991), $r = -.55, p = .005$. This study also confirmed that the PSI has a strong correlation with the OTLI, $r = -.69, p < .001$.

Applications

Currently the PSI is being used as a screening tool in a state college wellness program. A 54-item abridged version of the

PSI, along with QuickScan, a 27-item stressor checklist (Radmacher & Sheridan, 1995b), is contained in an extensive wellness questionnaire that is completed by employees who volunteer to participate in the state college wellness program mentioned earlier. Employees are given feedback from their responses to the PSI in the form of a Stress Profile that provides them with overall QuickScan and PSI scores, six subscale scores, and group norms. Although these subscales are loosely based on those derived from the factor analyses, they were primarily created conceptually to provide self-help information to employees. Confidentiality is strictly maintained through wellness identification numbers that are assigned by the director of nursing.

Stress Profile Description

The Stress Profile is presented on one sheet generated by a computer program developed by the college. It begins with the following paragraph:

> Your scores on the "QuickScan" and the "Personality Style Inventory" (PSI) and PSI subscales follow. An explanation of these measures and the meaning of your scores with some suggestions for coping with stress is provided in the attached summary entitled "Coping with Stress." Your scores on these scales should be used strictly as a tool to help you become more aware of your stressors and the resources you already have, or can develop, to help you manage stress better. Although these scales are based on an extensive body of literature and 20 years of research, they do not replace a thorough assessment by a professional. The high, average, and low scores are based on quartiles from the 1996 wellness questionnaire data.

Each employee's score on the QuickScan, the PSI, and the PSI subscales follow with a brief description of the concept each represents, its norm, and a reference to the appropriate section of the "Coping with Stress" summary. An example follows:

You scored 37 on the total PSI, a measure of stress resiliency. Stress resiliency refers to those attitudes and behaviors that contribute to your ability to recover from stressful events. A high score is 38, an average score 32, and a low score 25.

SEE COPING WITH STRESS TIP #2

"Tips" Handout

"Tips for Coping with Stress" is a six-page handout that contains brief suggestions for coping with stress and improving stress resiliency. It begins with the following explanation:

> Stress is a difficult construct to measure because it has so many dimensions, not the least of which is the individual's appraisal and perception of stressful events (stressors). As a result, stress can't be measured like blood pressure or cholesterol, but your responses on the QuickScan and Personal Style Inventory can help identify your stressors and the resources you have (or can develop) to help you manage them more effectively. There are times when self-help strategies may not be sufficient to help us cope with the stressful events in our lives and professional counseling may be required. The Employee Assistance Program is part of the MWSC Wellness Program and provides confidential assistance to qualified employees and their family members for a variety of problems, including marital, family, emotional, legal, and substance abuse. See the MWSC Policy Guide for more information.

This paragraph is followed by seven "Coping with Stress Tips" that are referred to in the Stress Profile. Each tip contains the items that were included in the subscale to which it was referenced. In addition, each tip provides (a) a more complete, but still brief, description of the concept being measured; (b) suggestions for improvement in the area; and (c) suggested readings.

We feel that this kind of broad-based, low-cost screening for stress resiliency is an effective use of this type of scale. As the evidence linking stress to health outcomes becomes more compelling, it seems appropriate to help people identify areas in which they can improve their ability to cope with stress. The wellness screenings will continue over the next several years and involve a relatively stable population of administrators, faculty, and support staff. This will give us a unique opportunity to determine whether there is a relationship between scores on the PSI and long-term health outcomes.

Benefits and Limitations

The PSI is a comprehensive measure of stress resiliency that emphasizes personal, potentially modifiable activities and covers the entire range of known factors that mediate stress responses. A particular advantage of the PSI is the identification of specific activities that moderate reactions to stressful stimuli. This information can be used to provide constructive feedback to respondents and to develop broad-based, cost-effective interventions.

The data reported here indicate that the PSI is a comprehensive as well as reliable and valid measure of stress resiliency. Although its construction was heavily influenced by the work of Antonovsky (1979, 1987), it also synthesizes dimensions from other leading researchers in the field of stress resiliency. Additionally, the PSI has a clear factor structure and therefore provides a well-delineated assessment of empirically derived dimensions relevant to stress resiliency. For research purposes, the inclusion of social desirability and negative affect subscales provide an efficient means to control for these possible confounding variables. The PSI has not yet been used in a clinical setting; however, we believe that it has the potential to help clients become aware of and identify their areas of stress resiliency. Because it is a quick and easy scale to administer, it is also useful for wellness screening programs.

Use of the PSI is limited to adults with at least a seventh-grade reading level. Versions of the PSI have been adapted for use with secondary and middle-school children and are currently being evaluated but not yet available.

Chapter References

Anastasi, A. (1988). *Psychological testing* (6th ed.). New York: Macmillan.

Antonovsky, A. (1979). *Health, stress, and coping.* San Francisco: Jossey-Bass.

Antonovsky, A. (1987). *Unravelling the mystery of health.* San Francisco: Jossey-Bass.

Bigham, S., Sheridan, C. L., & Martin, D. M. (1994). Validation of a comprehensive measure of stress vulnerability. In *First World Conference on Stress, No. 19. Program and Abstracts* (p. 40). Bethesda, MD: International Society for the Investigation of Stress.

Cloud, L. D. (1995). *Psychosocial life-style stressors and the African-American hypertensive.* Unpublished doctoral dissertation, University of Missouri-Kansas City.

Cohen, S., Kamarck, T., & Mermelstein, R. (1983). A global measure of perceived stress. *Journal of Health and Social Behavior, 24,* 385–396.

Cohen, S., Tyrrell, D. A., & Smith, A. P. (1993). Negative life events, perceived stress, negative affect, and susceptibility to the common cold. *Journal of Personality and Social Psychology, 64*(1), 131–140.

Costa, P. T., & McCrae, R. R. (1987). Hypochondriasis, neuroticism, and aging: Why are somatic complaints unfounded? *American Psychologist, 40,* 19–28.

Crowne, D., & Marlowe, D. (1960). A new scale of social desirability independent of psychopathology. *Journal of Consulting Psychology, 24,* 349–354.

Ficken, S., & Sheridan, C. L. (1997). [Relationship between self-reports of hope and stress resiliency.] Unpublished raw data.

Frankenhaeuser, M. (1991). The psychophysiology of workload, stress, and health: Comparison between the sexes. *Annals of Behavioral Medicine, 13,* 197–204.

Gross, J. J., & Levenson, R. W. (1993). Emotional suppression: Physiology, self-report, and expressive behavior. *Journal of Personality and Social Psychology, 64,* 970–986.

Harmless, M. J. (1996). *Stress revisited: Exploring the role of attachment in the etiology of stress vulnerability and perceived stress.* Unpublished doctoral dissertation, University of Missouri–Kansas City.

Ingersoll, W. (1990). *Differential grouping of psychological and physiological characteristics in essential hypertension.* Unpublished doctoral dissertation, University of Missouri–Kansas City.

Kline, P. (1994). *An easy guide to factor analysis.* London: Routledge.

Kobasa, S. C. (1979). Stressful life events, personality, and health: An inquiry into hardiness. *Journal of Personality and Social Psychology, 37,* 1–11.

Krupp, L. B., LaRocca, N. G., Muir-Nash, J., & Steinberg, A. D. (1989). The fatigue severity scale: Application to patients with multiple sclerosis and systematic lupus erythematosus. *Archives of Neurology, 46,* 1121–1123.

Lazarus, R. S., & Folkman, S. (1984). *Stress, appraisal and coping.* New York: Springer.

Martin, D. M., & Sheridan, C. L. (1994). Stress, health, and borderline personality organization. In First World Conference on Stress, No. 152. Program and Abstracts (p. 62). Bethesda, MD: International Society for the Investigation of Stress.

Mulhern, M. (1994). *The validation of the inventory of health status.* Unpublished doctoral dissertation, University of Missouri–Kansas City.

Oldham, J., Clarkin, J., Applebaum, A., Carr, A., Kernberg, P., Lotterman, A., & Haas, G. (1985). A self-report instrument for borderline personality organization. In T. H. McGlashan (Ed.), *The borderline: Current empirical research* (pp. 3–18). Washington, DC: American Psychiatric Press.

Pennebaker, J. W. (1990). *Opening up: The healing power in confiding in others.* New York: Morrow.

Pennebaker, J. W., Colder, M., & Sharp, L. K. (1990). Accelerating the coping process. *Journal of Personality and Social Psychology, 58,* 528–537.

Radmacher, S. A., & Sheridan, C. L. (1995a). Employee stress vulnerability: Relationship to glucose, cholesterol, and triglyceride levels. Paper presented at the Joint Conference of the American Psychological Association, National Institute for Occupational Safety & Health, U.S. Office of Personnel Management, and Health Administration, Washington, DC.

Radmacher, S. A., & Sheridan, C. L. (1995b). An investigation of the demand-control model of job strain. In S. L. Sauter & L. R. Murphy (Eds.), *Organizational risk factors for job stress* (pp. 127–138). Washington, DC: American Psychological Association.

Schmidt, S. A., & Sheridan, C. L. (1994). *Avowed fatigue and symptom range as a function of stress in chronic fatigue syndrome patients with reporting distortions controlled.* Paper presented at the Annual Scientific Conference of the American Association for Chronic Fatigue Syndrome, Fort Lauderdale, FL.

Seligman, M. E. P. (1991). *Learned optimism.* New York: Knopf.

Sheridan, C. L., Mulhern, M., & Martin, D. M. (at press). Validation of a brief self-report measure of organic health status independent of social desirability and negative affectivity. *Psychological Reports.*

Sheridan, C. L., Radmacher, S. A., & Petren, S. (1997). *Validation of a measure of stress resiliency.* Unpublished manuscript, University of Missouri–Kansas City.

Sheridan, C. L., & Smith, L. K. (1987). Toward a comprehensive scale of stress assessment: Norms, reliability, and validity. *International Journal of Psychosomatic, 34,* 48–54.

Snyder, C. R., Harris, C., Anderson, J. R., Holleran, S. A., Irving, L. M., Sigmon, S., Yoshinobu, L., Bibb, J., Lagelle, C., & Harney, P. (1991). Development and validation of an individual-differences measure of hope. *Journal of Personality and Social Psychology, 60,* 570–585.

Tellegen, A. (1982). *Brief manual for the differential personality questionnaire.* Unpublished manuscript, University of Minnesota, Minneapolis.

Vaillant, G. (1977). *Adaptation to life.* Boston: McGraw-Hill.

Watson, D., & Pennebaker, J. W. (1989). Health complaints, stress, distress: Exploring the central role of negative affectivity. *Psychological Review, 96,* 234–254.

The School Refusal Assessment Scale

Christopher A. Kearney and Cheryl A. Tillotson,
University of Nevada, Las Vegas

■ **Instrument name**

School Refusal Assessment Scale
SRAS
SRAS-C (child version)
SRAS-P (parent version)

■ **Developers**

Christopher A. Kearney, Department of Psychology,
University of Nevada, Las Vegas, and Wendy K. Silverman,
Department of Psychology, Florida International
University

■ **Contact Information**

Dr. Christopher A. Kearney, Department of Psychology,
University of Nevada, Las Vegas, 4505 Maryland Parkway,
Las Vegas, NV 89154-5030
Telephone: (702) 895-3305; fax: (702) 895-0195

Description and History of the Instrument

Before proceeding with a description of the School Refusal
Assessment Scale (SRAS) and its revision (currently in development), a definition of school refusal behavior is necessary.
In essence, school refusal behavior refers to child-motivated

refusal to attend school or difficulties remaining in classes for an entire day (Kearney & Silverman, 1996). This definition excludes cases where a parent deliberately keeps a child home or withdraws the child from school. More specifically, school refusal behavior refers to those youngsters aged 5 to 17 years who are:

- completely absent from school,
- attend school but leave during the course of the school day,
- go to school only after significant behavior problems in the morning, and/or
- display unusual distress about attending school that leads to pleas for future nonattendance.

School refusal behavior is a common problem faced by psychologists and educators. Approximately 5% of school-aged youngsters refuse school on a regular basis, although this rate is much higher in some urban areas. School refusal behavior is seen fairly equally in boys and girls, and the mean age of onset is 11 to 12 years. Children entering a new school building for the first time are especially prone to refuse school. The problem appears to be independent of familial socioeconomic status, child intelligence, or academic performance up to the point of initial school refusal behavior (see King, Ollendick, & Tonge, 1995).

A key aspect of school refusal behavior is its heterogeneity. Common internalizing problems include general and social anxiety, fear, depression, suicidal ideation, withdrawal, fatigue, and somatic complaints (especially headaches and stomachaches). School refusal behavior is often considered within the realm of childhood anxiety disorders because of its strong linkage to generalized anxiety disorder, separation anxiety disorder, and social and specific phobia (Kearney & Silverman, 1996). In addition, the problem is often quite stressful for youngsters, as described in more detail in later sections. Common externalizing problems include noncompliance, refusal to move, clinging, verbal and physical aggression, running away from home or school, and tantrums (Kearney, 1995). Short-term school refusal behavior has several consequences, including alienation from others, declining school performance, family conflict, and substantial disruption to the family's daily life routine. Long-term consequences of school refusal behavior may include alcohol use, criminal behavior, anxiety, depression, and occupational and marital problems (see Berg & Nursten, 1996).

Despite the seriousness of school refusal behavior, few devices are available to assess youngsters with this problem. Two reasons may explain why this is so. First, traditional methods have concentrated on internalizing symptoms such as fear and anxiety. Such a concentration was largely the result of early thinking in the area, which emphasized psychodynamically based concepts like "school phobia" and "separation anxiety" to explain school refusal behavior (e.g., Johnson, Falstein, Szurek, & Svendsen, 1941). Although these concepts help explain why a subset of children refuse school, they do not cover the entire population. For example, many youngsters display absenteeism not because of something fearful or otherwise aversive at school but rather because they wish to pursue something much more positive outside school (see Kearney, Eisen, & Silverman, 1995).

A second reason that few assessment methods have been designed for this population is the overwhelming set of behaviors shown by youngsters with school refusal behavior. Clinical researchers find it difficult to chart all of these behaviors accurately and often have to rely on broad-band measures of behavior such as the Child Behavior Checklist and the Teacher's Report Form (Achenbach, 1991a, 1991b). Although measures such as these are useful and psychometrically sound, evidence supports the idea that school refusal behavior is a separate factor representing a conglomeration of internalizing and externalizing behaviors (e.g., Lambert, Weisz, & Thesiger, 1989). In addition, school refusal behavior is not listed as a formal diagnostic condition in either the current *Diagnostic and Statistical Manual of Mental Disorders* (American Psychiatric Association, 1994) or the *International Classification of Diseases* (World Health Organization, 1992). As a result, psychologists and educators are faced with the need to evaluate many children who refuse school, and their myriad behaviors, without a specific protocol for doing so. The School Refusal Assessment Scale was designed to partially meet this need.

Underlying Assumptions and Objective

Because psychologists and educators are faced with the unenviable task of sifting through a variety of school refusal behaviors, we believe it may be better to focus on the limited number of reasons that youngsters miss school. These reasons, or functions, may represent the best way of classifying this population. The underlying assumption of the SRAS, therefore, is that youngsters with school refusal behavior may be organized according to their reason for missing school. In particular, the SRAS measures the relative influence of each of four functions for school refusal behavior. The objective of the SRAS is to help clinicians and educators identify the primary reason or function for a particular child's school refusal behavior. Specifically, we postulate that youngsters refuse school for one or more of the following reasons or functions:

- To avoid something at school that causes the child to feel general dread or negative affectivity (anxiety/depression). This refers to youngsters who often cannot say why they are upset about school but report an overall sense of malaise. These children are often trying to stay away from school because stimuli there cause them to feel upset and experience physiologically based symptoms such as nausea or trembling.
- To escape aversive social and/or evaluative situations at school. This includes youngsters who experience difficulties making or keeping friends and thus feel isolated

and also those who find evaluative situations unpleasant. Common situations that are avoided include tests, oral presentations, writing in front of others, recitals, athletic events, and peer interactions.

■ To get attention from significant others. This refers to youngsters who act out to stay home from school and to spend time with parents or others. In most cases, these children will act out in the morning. Some children, however, become disruptive at school so they will be sent home or call their parents several times a day from school.

■ To pursue positive tangible reinforcement outside school. This refers to youngsters, usually adolescents, who skip school because it is more fun to be out of school. In many cases, these youngsters leave school with friends to attend parties, shop, gamble, sleep, watch television, play sports, or travel.

The first two functional conditions refer to youngsters who are refusing school for negative reinforcement (i.e., to get away from something negative at school). The latter two functional conditions refer to youngsters who are refusing school for positive reinforcement (i.e., to pursue something positive outside of school). In our experience, youngsters tend to be referred for treatment more so if they refuse school for positive reinforcement. Also, about one-quarter of youngsters refuse school for two or more reasons or functions. For example, it is not uncommon to see a child initially refuse school to escape aversive social situations but then discover the amenities of staying home. Such children subsequently refuse school for such positive reinforcement as well.

The SRAS is a 16-item measure that assesses the degree to which four functions impact upon a child's school refusal behavior. Separate child (SRAS-C) and parent (SRAS-P) versions have been developed. Four items are devoted to each function, and each item is rated on a 7-point Likert-type scale ranging from never (0) to always (6) as follows:

- Items 1, 5, 9, and 13 comprise the first functional condition (avoidance of stimuli that provoke negative affectivity).
- Items 2, 6, 10, and 14 comprise the second functional condition (escape from aversive social/evaluative situations).
- Items 3, 7, 11, and 15 comprise the third functional condition (attention getting).
- Items 4, 8, 12, and 16 comprise the fourth functional condition (positive tangible reinforcement).

Examples of items from the SRAS-C include the following:

- 13. Do you feel scared about school when you think about it on Saturday and Sunday? (functional condition 1)
- 14. Do you often stay away from places where you would have to talk to someone? (functional condition 2)
- 15. Do you ever refuse to go to school in order to be with your parents? (functional condition 3)
- 16. Do you ever skip school because it's more fun to be out of school? (functional condition 4)

Administration and Scoring Procedures

When administering the School Refusal Assessment Scale, we ask the child and parents to complete the SRAS-C and SRAS-P, respectively. This is done separately and takes about 5 minutes. For young children or those just learning to read, we present the SRAS items verbally and allow them to answer on their own. Ideally, SRAS ratings should be obtained from the child, mother, and father if all are available.

Following the completion of each questionnaire, item means are derived for each function. On the original version of the SRAS-C and each SRAS-P, therefore, scores are added for:

- items 1, 5, 9, and 13 (first function);
- items 2, 6, 10, and 14 (second function);
- items 3, 7, 11, and 15 (third function); and
- items 4, 8, 12, and 16 (fourth function).

These four total scores are then each divided by 4 (or the number of items answered in each set). For example, if a child's total rating score across:

- the first item set was 10, then the item mean would be 2.50;
- the second item set was 13, then the item mean would be 3.25;
- the third item set was 22, then the item mean would be 5.50;
- the fourth item set was 5, then the item mean would be 1.25.

This is done separately for ratings from the child, mother, and father. After this is done, mean item scores are averaged across all of the SRAS versions administered. Assume, for example, that:

- the child's mean item scores from the SRAS-C were 2.50, 3.25, 5.50, and 1.25;
- the mother's mean item scores from the SRAS-P were 4.25, 4.50, 6.00, and 1.25;
- the father's mean item scores from the SRAS-P were 4.00, 4.50, 5.25, and 1.50.

In this case, therefore:

- the overall mean for the first function would be 3.58 (2.50 + 4.25 + 4.00/3);
- the overall mean for the second function would be 4.08 (3.25 + 4.50 + 4.50/3);

- the overall mean for the third function would be 5.58 (5.50 + 6.00 + 5.25/3);
- the overall mean for the fourth function would be 1.33 (1.25 + 1.25 + 1.50/3).

The highest-scoring function is considered to be the primary reason a particular child is refusing school. Scores within 0.25 points of one another are considered equivalent. In this case, therefore, the highest-scoring function is the third one, or attention seeking (5.58). However, these numbers also provide a profile of related influences. In this case, for example, the child may be refusing school to some extent for the first and second functions (i.e., avoidance of stimuli provoking negative affectivity and escape from aversive social/evaluative situations; 3.58 and 4.08). However, the relative influence of the fourth functional condition, positive tangible reinforcement, is low (1.33). Thus, clinicians are able to make hypotheses about the primary motivator of a child's school refusal behavior and organize potential treatment targets hierarchically.

Following this determination, we assign one or more of four treatment strategies specific to each functional condition as follows:

- For children who refuse school to avoid stimuli that provoke negative affectivity, we use a combination of relaxation training, breathing retraining, and gradual return (exposure) to the regular classroom setting.
- For children who refuse school to escape aversive social and/or evaluative situations, we use a combination of modeling, role-play, and cognitive therapy.
- For children who refuse school for attention, we use parent training in contingency management. For children who refuse school for positive tangible reinforcement, we use familial contracting, communication skills training, and peer refusal skills training.

■ For children who refuse school for two or more reasons, we use a combination of these treatment approaches.

In essence, the School Refusal Assessment Scale represents a new strategy for classifying, assessing, and assigning treatment for youngsters with school refusal behavior. Rather than trying to find one "magic bullet" treatment for all youngsters who refuse school, therapeutic strategies are assigned individually and prescriptively to enhance effectiveness.

Summary of Research Regarding Psychometrics

A full explication of the psychometric data for the SRAS may be found elsewhere (Kearney & Silverman, 1993). A summary as well as preliminary psychometric data for a revision of the SRAS are presented here. These data surround reliability, concurrent validity, and construct validity.

Reliability

The original version of the SRAS was tested on 42 clients referred to specialized clinics that addressed youngsters with primary school refusal behavior. Test-retest reliability over a 7 to 14-day period for the child and parent versions of the SRAS was examined in addition to parent interrater reliability at the time of initial assessment. Item reliability correlations were generally quite good across both versions of the SRAS. As a synopsis, reliability figures for each functional condition subscore (FCS) are presented here (see previous section for items assigned to each functional condition):

■ SRAS-C test-retest: .73 (FCS1), .87 (FCS2), .68 (FCS3), and .44 (FCS4)
■ SRAS-P test-retest: .65 (FCS1), .81 (FCS2), .85 (FCS3), and .81 (FCS4)

- SRAS-P interrater: .49 (FCS1), .69 (FCS2), .62 (FCS3), and .56 (FCS4)

All figures are significant at $p < .01$ except SRAS-C test-retest FCS4 ($p < .05$).

Concurrent Validity

With respect to concurrent validity, tests were conducted separately for the first two functional conditions (negatively reinforced school refusal behavior) and the second two functional conditions (positively reinforced school refusal behavior) of the SRAS-C and SRAS-P. In general, negatively reinforced school refusal behavior was expected to be associated with internalizing variables, whereas positively reinforced school refusal behavior was expected to be associated with externalizing variables.

With respect to negatively reinforced school refusal behavior, correlations were calculated between relevant SRAS-C scores and measures of internalizing behavior. Such measures included those related to fear, general anxiety, social anxiety, depression, and low self-esteem. All variables except fear were, as expected, significantly correlated with SRAS-C subscores relevant to avoidance of stimuli provoking negative affectivity (functional condition 1) and escape from aversive social/evaluative situations (functional condition 2). In addition, SRAS-P scores for the first two functional conditions were, as expected, significantly correlated with internalizing T-scores from the Child Behavior Checklist.

DSM diagnoses from child and parent reports were also examined as a measure of concurrent validity. For youngsters with primarily negatively reinforced school refusal behavior, 60.0% were diagnosed with a primary internalizing disorder, as expected. In fact, internalizing diagnoses derived from child reports accounted for 83.3% of all diagnoses given in this group. In addition, parents who rated their children with negatively reinforced school refusal behavior indicated that the youngsters also met criteria for primary internalizing disorders in 58.8% of cases. In fact, internalizing diagnoses derived from parent reports accounted for 77.1% of all diagnoses given in this group.

Concurrent validity figures were less clear-cut for positively reinforced school refusal behavior (attention getting and positive tangible reinforcement) but generally sound. As expected, SRAS scores for the third and fourth functional conditions were not significantly correlated with depression, self-esteem, or social anxiety. Some correlation was found between fear, anxiety, and attention-getting functional condition scores. In addition, externalizing T-scores from the Child Behavior Checklist were found to be significantly correlated with positively reinforced school refusal behavior, as expected.

With respect to diagnoses, youngsters self-rated with positively reinforced school refusal behavior were diagnosed with primary separation anxiety disorder or no mental disorder, as expected, in 85.7% of cases. These categories accounted for 72.0% of all those given in this group. Parents who rated their children with positively reinforced school refusal behavior indicated that the youngsters met criteria for primary separation anxiety disorder, no mental disorder, or externalizing diagnoses such as attention deficit, oppositional, and conduct disorder in 72.7% of cases. These categories accounted for 46.2% of all those given in this group. Overall, these findings were taken as supportive of the concurrent validity of the SRAS-C and SRAS-P.

Construct Validity

Preliminary work has been done regarding the construct validity of the SRAS using combined scores from the child and parent versions. As expected, the correlation between the two subscales of the negatively reinforced division of the SRAS (avoidance of stimuli that provoke negative affectivity and escape from aversive social/evaluative situations) is significant (.43, $p < .01$). In addition, the correlation between the two subscales of the positively reinforced division of the SRAS (attention getting and positive tangible reinforcement) is significant (.32, $p < .05$). As expected, however, a correlation between the first two functional conditions and the second two functional conditions is not significant. Finally, a preliminary factor analysis of combined SRAS ratings indicated three factors: a combined negative reinforcement factor, an attention factor, and a positive tangible reinforcement factor. These data support the construct validity of the SRAS, although additional work is needed.

Versions and Editions

A revision of the School Refusal Assessment Scale is currently being developed to more accurately pinpoint functional condition subtypes. For example, newer items regarding functional condition 1 (avoidance of stimuli that provoke negative affectivity) are more reflective of general negative affectivity and not specific fear. The structure of the revised scale is identical to the original version, but 24 items are listed. Preliminary data on the revised SRAS from 34 clients are briefly presented here (Socha, Carpenter, Roblek, Thurman, & Kearney, 1995).

With respect to SRAS-C (revised) test-retest reliability, all item scores were correlated significantly over a 7- to 14-day period (mean = .71; range = .58–.92). With respect to SRAS-P (revised) test-retest reliability, all but two item scores were correlated significantly over a 7- to 14-day period (excluding these two items: mean = .70; range = .51–.90). With respect to SRAS-P (revised) interrater reliability, 16 questions were correlated significantly (mean = .63; range = .35–.79).

For purposes of concurrent validity, SRAS (revised) functional condition scores were correlated with SRAS functional condition scores from the original scale. For example, SRAS (revised) scores from functional condition 1 correlated significantly with SRAS (original) scores from functional condition 1 (.61). Similarly calculated correlations for functional conditions 2 (.71), 3 (.77), and 4 (.61) were also reported. All correlations are significant at $p < .01$. These data provide preliminary support for the psychometric strength of the revised versions of the SRAS.

Conditions for Use

The School Refusal Assessment Scale is a versatile measure that can be used for many different types of clients with problematic absenteeism. However, we remind the reader that the SRAS was originally designed for use with youngsters with *primary* school refusal behavior. The scale may be useful for assessing youngsters who refuse school in addition to other behavior problems, but data are not available for this population, and so caution is urged. In addition, the SRAS is meant to be used as part of a larger assessment protocol that involves interviews, child self-report measures, parent/teacher checklists, behavioral observations, and other techniques such as intelligence tests deemed preferable for a certain case. Whereas the SRAS is a useful tool for measuring the relative strength of different functions of school refusal behavior, we recommend that other procedures be used to confirm SRAS ratings and provide additional information for treatment.

Interviews with families of children who refuse school will have to be broadly based and cover areas related to social functioning, academic status, drug use, family interactions, mood, parameters of the school refusal problem, related behaviors, and extenuating circumstances. More specific to school refusal, we recommend asking questions that supplement the SRAS and give the assessor more data on which to base a decision about function. The following represent examples of interview questions that mirror each of the four functional conditions described before:

- How often does the child refuse school because of nervousness or anxiety about something related to school (e.g., bus, teacher, classroom, gym)? What physical symptoms does the child show when going to school?
- How often does the child refuse school because of peer-related situations such as difficulty talking to other kids or making/keeping friends? How often does the child refuse school to avoid situations where he or she would have to perform in front of others?
- How often does the child refuse school because he or she wishes to be home with his or her parents? Would it be easier for the child to attend school if a parent went with him or her?
- How often does the child refuse school because it is more fun to be out of school? What does the child do when not in school during the weekday?

Care should be taken, of course, to note any inconsistencies between child/parent SRAS ratings and information obtained from the interview. If discrepancies exist, a therapist should discuss them immediately and at length with relevant family members. In some cases, a readministration of the SRAS is warranted.

We have also found it useful to have children, parents, and teachers complete a series of questionnaires to supplement information gained from the interview and the SRAS. The questionnaires we commonly use are described in more detail elsewhere (see Kearney, 1995) but include those related to general anxiety, social anxiety, fear, depression, self-esteem, daily stress, and acting-out behaviors. In addition, we ask our clients to rate, in daily logbooks, levels of child anxiety, depression, overall distress, noncompliance, disruption to the family routine, and school attendance.

Finally, we encourage therapists to conduct a behavioral observation of the family's routine in the morning and the child's school refusal behaviors. Protocols for doing so are available (see Kearney & Albano, at press). If a formal behavioral observation is not feasible, then a therapist should watch for key behaviors in session that may indicate why a child is refusing school. For example, a youngster who is generally tearful, passive, and withdrawn during assessment may be the type who refuses school to avoid school-related stimuli that provoke negative affectivity. A youngster who seems anxious about interacting with others in the clinic may be the type who refuses school to escape aversive social/evaluative situations. A youngster who has difficulty separating from a parent or throws a tantrum to avoid speaking alone with the therapist may be the type of child who refuses school for attention. Finally, a youngster who argues forcefully with his or her parents in the session may be the type of child who refuses school for positive tangible reinforcement.

All of the assessment approaches described here must be combined to reach conclusions about (a) a particular child's major school refusal behaviors, (b) why the child is refusing school, and (c) the best treatment approach. The SRAS gives an excellent thumbnail sketch of why a child is missing school and what the best treatment might be, but the heterogeneity and fluidity of school refusal behaviors mandate a comprehensive and ongoing assessment protocol.

Case Example

We present here a case example that illustrates the use of the SRAS. Actual names are not used. Graham was a 12-year-old male referred for acute school refusal behavior. Upon entering a new building for seventh grade, he experienced difficulties adjusting to a large set of new peers and a complex class schedule. During September, Graham missed approximately 10 days of school, a problem that worsened during October. By the initial assessment on November 2, Graham had missed a total of 25 days from school, including all of the past two weeks. Graham's parents, Mr. and Mrs. C, had tolerated their son's behavior and tried to encourage his school attendance, but to no avail.

In the assessment session, Graham reported that he felt "awful" at school but could not identify anything in particular that caused his distress. He did say that he felt overwhelmed by the new setting and that he was having a hard time making new friends. His primary symptoms were vague but included general and social anxiety, fatigue, somatic complaints (particularly stomach aches), and some oppositional behavior. Graham said that, when missing school, he would sleep, watch television, or ride his bicycle around the neighborhood. He acknowledged that school attendance was something he would eventually have to restart, and expressed some moderate desire to do so.

Graham's parents reported that their son had experienced some difficulties attending school at the end of the previous academic year. His behavior over the summer was normal, although he was repeatedly asking questions about the new school building during August. When Graham initially refused to attend school, his parents were supportive and generally tolerated the behavior by allowing him to remain home. After Graham refused school for much of September, Mr. and Mrs. C became more angry and tried to force their son to attend school. Following 2 weeks of physical struggles in the morning, Mr. and Mrs. C began to seek counseling. Their reports regarding Graham's recent behavior mirrored their son's, and they said they were at a loss to explain the recent events.

In addition to the interviews, the therapist asked Graham and his parents to complete a variety of questionnaires. These forms are described in more detail elsewhere (see Kearney, 1995) but included those related to fear, general and social anxiety, depression, self-esteem, daily stress, and overall internalizing and externalizing behaviors. These forms revealed a variety of problematic behaviors, especially those related to social anxiety. In addition, the therapist conducted a behavioral observation of the family's morning routine and Graham's attempt to attend school. Although Graham generally prepared for school without difficulty, he became anxious and combative in the car on the way to school. He refused to get out of the car to enter the school building, stating that he wanted to return home. Interestingly, Graham slouched in his seat so that none of the other youngsters would see him in the car. Upon returning home, Graham's anxiety level was reduced, and he engaged in several pleasurable activities.

In addition to these assessment procedures, the therapist administered the SRAS to Graham and each of his parents. Scores were produced for each functional condition:

- avoidance of stimuli that provoke negative affectivity,
- escape from aversive social/evaluative situations,
- attention getting, and
- positive tangible reinforcement.

On the SRAS-C, total scores for each functional condition were 18, 20, 4, and 12 (for mean item scores of 4.50, 5.00, 1.00, and 3.00). On the mother's SRAS-P, total scores for each functional condition were 21, 21, 8, and 12 (for mean item scores of 5.25, 5.25, 2.00, and 3.00). On the father's SRAS-P, total scores for each functional condition were 15, 19, 0, and 3 (for mean item scores of 3.75, 4.75, 0.00, and 0.75).

Mean item scores were then averaged across each of these SRAS versions. In this case, therefore:

- the overall mean for the first function was 4.50 (4.50 + 5.25 + 3.75/3);
- the overall mean for the second function was 5.00 (5.00 + 5.25 + 4.75/3);
- the overall mean for the third function was 1.00 (1.00 + 2.00 + 0.00/3);
- the overall mean for the fourth function was 2.25 (3.00 + 3.00 + 0.75/3).

In this case, Graham's school refusal behavior was determined to be primarily maintained by a desire to escape aversive social/evaluative situations (functional condition 2). However, a secondary influence was Graham's wish to avoid stimuli that provoked negative affectivity (functional condition 1); in Graham's case, this primarily involved physical feelings of nausea and lightheadedness. To some extent, Graham appeared to refuse school as well for positive tangible reinforcement such as watching television at home (functional condition 4). Attention getting, the third functional condition, did not appear to influence this particular case.

Treatment was prescribed based on this functional profile. The bulk of therapy concentrated on building Graham's social skills and rearranging his schedule so that he would have more contact with people he already knew. In addition, breathing exercises were conducted so that Graham could control his physical symptoms. A gradual program of reintroducing Graham to the school setting was established. In this case, Graham was initially required to attend three classes in the afternoon. Classes were gradually added over a 5-week period to complete the school day. Later in therapy, a reward system for full-time school attendance was set up to compensate Graham for his loss of positive tangible reinforcement at home during the day. Graham's level of overall functioning was determined to be good at posttreatment.

Benefits and Limitations

The primary benefit of the School Refusal Assessment Scale is that it provides clinicians and educators with a straightforward and useful clinical picture of a child's school refusal behavior. Because practitioners are often faced with a myriad of interwoven symptoms, the SRAS gives a thumbnail sketch of the primary maintaining factors that influence a particular case. In addition, profiles from the SRAS may be used to assign prescriptive treatment options. The SRAS is thus a sound vehicle for classifying, assessing, and assigning treatment for youngsters with primary school refusal behavior.

The main limitation of the School Refusal Assessment Scale is that the instrument remains in development. As a result, data are only available for youngsters with primary school refusal behavior and not those with general behavior problems. We therefore recommend that the SRAS be integrated with a comprehensive assessment protocol. In addition, the SRAS is intended for clinicial samples only; thus, no normative data exist. Future research will explore revisions of the scale, usefulness with other clinical samples, and treatment validity.

The SRAS remains the only measure specifically designed for youngsters with problematic absenteeism. Given the serious and potentially debilitating nature of school refusal behavior, the development of pertinent assessment devices for this population should be a high priority for researchers. We invite any questions or comments from readers regarding the SRAS.

Chapter References

Achenbach, T. M. (1991a). *Manual for the Child Behavior Checklist/4-18 and 1991 profile.* Burlington: University of Vermont Department of Psychiatry.

Achenbach, T. M. (1991b). *Manual for the Teacher's Report Form and 1991 profile.* Burlington: University of Vermont Department of Psychiatry.

American Psychiatric Association. (1994). *Diagnostic and statistical manual of mental disorders* (4th ed.). Washington, DC: Author.

Berg, I., & Nursten, J. (1996). *Unwillingly to school* (4th ed.). New York: American Psychiatric Press.

Johnson, A. M., Falstein, E. I., Szurek, S. A., & Svendsen, M. (1941). School phobia. *American Journal of Orthopsychiatry, 11,* 702–711.

Kearney, C. A. (1995). School refusal behavior. In A. R. Eisen, C. A. Kearney, & C. E. Schaefer (Eds.), *Clinical handbook of fear and anxiety disorders in children and adolescents* (pp. 19–52). Northvale, NJ: Aronson.

Kearney, C. A., & Albano, A. M. (at press). *Therapist's guide for school refusal behavior*. New York: Psychological Corporation.

Kearney, C. A., Eisen, A. R., & Silverman, W. K. (1995). The legend and myth of school phobia. *School Psychology Quarterly, 10,* 65–85.

Kearney, C. A., & Silverman, W. K. (1993). Measuring the function of school refusal behavior: The School Refusal Assessment Scale. *Journal of Clinical Child Psychology, 22,* 85–96.

Kearney, C. A., & Silverman, W. K. (1996). The evolution and reconciliation of taxonomic strategies for school refusal behavior. *Clinical Psychology: Science and Practice, 3,* 339–354.

King, N., Ollendick, T., & Tonge, B. (1995). *School refusal: Assessment and treatment*. Boston: Allyn & Bacon.

Lambert, M. C., Weisz, J. R., & Thesiger, C. (1989). Principal components analyses of behavior problems in Jamaican clinic-referred children: Teacher reports for ages 6–17. *Journal of Abnormal Child Psychology, 17,* 553–562.

Socha, K. E., Carpenter, K., Roblek, T., Thurman, J., & Kearney, C. A. (1995, March). *Kids who miss school: The School Refusal Assessment Scale-Revised*. Paper presented at the meeting of the Western Psychological Association, Los Angeles.

World Health Organization. (1992). *International Classification of Diseases* (10th ed.). Geneva: Author.

The Self-Reliance Inventory

An Approach to Interdependence and Secure Social Attachments

J. Lee Whittington, Texas Wesleyan University
Janice R. W. Joplin, Southern Illinois University
Debra L. Nelson, Oklahoma State University
Jonathan D. Quick, World Health Organization
James Campbell Quick, University of Texas at Arlington

■ Instrument Names

The Self-Reliance Inventory: An Approach to
Interdependence and Secure Social Attachments
The SRI
The Self-Reliance Inventory (SRI, English)
The Self-Reliance Inventory II (SRI-II, English)
Self-Reliance Inventar (SRI-G, German)
Inventario de Auto-Suficiencia (IAS, Spanish)

■ Contact Information

The SRI and IAS are available from James Campbell Quick,
Box 19467, The University of Texas at Arlington,
Arlington, TX 76019-0467.
Telephone: (817) 272-3869; e-mail: jquick@uta.edu
The SRI-II is available from Janice R. W. Joplin, Department
of Management, Southern Illinois University, Edwardsville,
IL, 62026.
Telephone: (618) 692-2731; e-mail: jjoplin@siue.edu
The SRI-G is available from Joachim Stöber, Freie Universität
Berlin, Institut für Psychologie—WE 7, FB 12, FU Berlin,
Habelschwerdter Allee 45, D-14195 Berlin, FRG
Telephone: 49-30-838-5633;
e-mail: jstoeber@zedat.fuberlin.de

Description and History of the Instrument

The Self-Reliance Inventory (SRI) was developed as a self-report measure of a person's interpersonal attachment orientation. The first version of the instrument focused on a bipolar distinction among interdependent and counterdependent behavior (Quick, Nelson, & Quick, 1987, 1990). The original scale was revised into two subscales (Quick, Joplin, Nelson, & Quick, 1992):

- Interdependence/C measures a person's orientation to interdependent or counterdependent behavior.
- Interdependence/O measures a person's orientation to interdependent or overdependent behavior.

The two-subscale version of the SRI consists of 20 items and uses a 6-point Likert scale response format (0 = strongly disagree, 5 = strongly agree). A low score on both subscales indicates a higher degree of self-reliance and interdependence.

In an effort to refine the measurement of self-reliance, work was begun on a second Self-Reliance Inventory (SRI-II) in 1992. Confirmatory factor analyses of data collected using the second version revealed three factors that are closely aligned with the conceptual basis of self-reliance: interdependence, counterdependence, and overdependence (Joplin, Nelson, & Quick, 1996). Scale responses for the SRI-II are identical to the 6-point format used on the original SRI.

The Self-Reliance Inventory was translated into Spanish by Deborah Pérez Mojica, under the direction of Dr. Rubén Vélez García, at the Centro Caribeño de Estudios Postgraduados, Instituto Psicológico de Puerto Rico. The translation was based on the original 20-item SRI and resulted in the Spanish-language *Inventario de Auto-Suficiencia* (IAS). No validity or reliability data are available on the IAS from Spanish-speaking or bilingual samples.

The Self-Reliance Inventory was translated into German by Dr. Joachim Stöber at Freie Universität Berlin, Institut für

Psychologie. The translation was based on the original 20-item SRI and resulted in the German-language *Self-Reliance Inventar* (SRI-G). Dr. Stöber subsequently used the SRI-G in validity research specifically related to the Worry In Management (WIM) scale.

Underlying Assumptions, Premises, and Objectives

The concept of self-reliance is rooted in the ethological approach to personality and attachment pioneered by Ainsworth and Bowlby (1991). Attachment was originally developed by Ainsworth and colleagues to explain the nature of the relationship that develops between a child and an attachment figure during early childhood. Attachment figures serve two functions for children. First, the attachment figure provides protection and support. Second, the attachment figure is the individual the child seeks and turns to spontaneously when confronted with distress. Ainsworth, Blehar, Waters, and Walls (1978) identified three dominant patterns of attachment in children:

- secure,
- avoidant, and
- anxious-ambivalent.

Because the attachment patterns developed in early childhood may become dominant ways of relating to others, the consequences of these patterns may be manifest throughout the life cycle. Several researchers (Hazan & Shaver, 1987; Kobak & Hazen, 1991; Kobak & Sceery, 1988; Weiss, 1982) have suggested that these patterns influence a person's seeking and forming of relationships well into the adult years. In fact, these attachment patterns may be central to an individual's effectiveness and satisfaction in work activities (Hazan & Shaver, 1990).

As applied to adults, attachment theory suggests that individuals orient themselves to others in one of three patterns.

These orientations are based on underlying beliefs, established in childhood, about the availability and responsiveness of potential social resources. These underlying beliefs thus influence the individual's perceptions of others, as well as the decisions made about interactions and relationships with those others.

The patterns of attachment identified by Ainsworth et al. (1978) form the basis for the patterns measured by the SRI (Nelson, Quick, & Joplin, 1991; Quick et al., 1987). Originally conceptualized along the two distinct dimensions of counterdependence and overdependence, (Quick, Nelson, & Quick, 1991), three patterns emerged in a study of behavioral responses to anxiety (Quick et al., 1992). However, items contained in the third factor in this study were descriptive of circumscribed work behaviors and were conceptually closer to counterdependence than to self-reliance or interdependence.

One of the primary objectives of the SRI-II instrument was, along with improving psychometric qualities, to construct items that would directly tap into interdependence. One issue that emerged in the use of the original version of the SRI was that of cultural biases in the self-reliance label. Bowlby (1988), a British researcher, used the term *self-reliance* to describe interdependent support systems. In the United States, *self-reliance* is often used to imply independence and more frequently borders on our conception of counterdependence. Thus, when we began construction of the SRI-II, we asked graduate and undergraduate students in our management classes at two universities to write descriptions of the terms *interdependence, counterdependence*, and *overdependence* and to give examples of behaviors that would illustrate each term. From these descriptions and behaviors, we constructed a pilot instrument of 52 items. Using confirmatory factor analyses, three factors emerged in the SRI-II. The interdependent factor measures secure, or self-reliant, patterns of attachment; the avoidant pattern is measured as counterdependence; and the anxious-ambivalent pattern is measured as overdependence. Each of these three orientations may be seen as a dominant way of relating to others.

Self-reliance thus reflects a pattern of forming and maintaining attachments that are essential to health. Because self-reliant individuals reach out to others appropriately and yet are comfortable working alone, their behavior may appear paradoxical. Self-reliant adults function autonomously or interdependently as situations require. In contrast, counterdependence and overdependence reflect patterns that are unhealthy alternatives to self-reliance. Counterdependence leads to separation in relationships with others, while overdependence leads to preoccupied attempts to achieve security through relationships.

Definitions of Primary Dimensions

Individuals whose dominant attachment style is interdependence seek to form relationships characterized by reciprocity and flexibility. This orientation is based on the individual's secure knowledge that others will be available for support in stressful situations. Furthermore, interdependent individuals see themselves as a source of support for others in their time of need. Interdependent individuals develop broad support systems consisting of several quality relationships. This support network may span several life arenas (Quick, Paulus, Whittington, Larey, & Nelson, 1996) and thus act as a buffer against distress (Linville, 1987). The interdependent orientation has been described elsewhere as self-reliance (Bowlby, 1982, 1988; Quick, Joplin, Nelson, Mangelsdorff, & Fiedler, 1996).

Counterdependence encompasses behaviors that rely on too little support. As such, it is rooted in the belief that no one will be available in distressful situations. Thus, counterdependent individuals are driven to be their own best support system, often believing that no one can do a job as well as they can. These "rugged individualists" often spurn supportive overtures and withdraw into themselves in stressful situations. Frequent refusal to accept support ensures that others will not, in fact, be available for future support, thus reinforcing the initial belief in the general lack of available social support.

Overdependence is also based on a general belief that others may not be available when needed, but the behavioral response differs from that of counterdependence. Overdependence is manifested by the seeking out and relying on more support than necessary or appropriate for the situation. Anxious and disorganized in the face of stressful situations, overdependent individuals cling to others in any way possible. This often leads to the relinquishment of personal responsibility and an overreliance on others for task accomplishment. The lack of reciprocity that characterizes overdependence may eventually drive available sources of support away, further fueling the overdependent individual's fear of lack of support.

Related Constructs

Empirical results to date suggest that self-reliance is related to both the tendency to worry and self-esteem. In a study of 138 German, Austrian, and Swiss managers, Stöber and Seidenstücker (1996) found that counterdependence is related to general worrying. This suggests that managers who have few, if any, close personal or professional relationships are more likely to experience pathological worry symptoms such as anxiety and insomnia. Overdependence is related to both general worrying and job-related worrying, but more so the latter. Managers who develop inappropriate relationships worry more about organizational processes such as performance appreciation. The insecure attachment subscale also was related to job-related worrying, but not general worrying. These results indicate that no matter which insecure relational strategy a manager adopts, managers with low levels of self-reliance are likely to display higher levels of worry and all the associated negative effects.

Self-reliance also may be associated with self-esteem and burnout. An early study (Quick, Joplin, et al., 1996) reported counterdependence was related to low self-esteem and high burnout and that these relationships intensified as subjects experienced problems. Without implying causality, these results suggest that counterdependent individuals may be at greater risk regarding their personal well-being and ability to function normally. These results may also suggest that counterdependent individuals have not developed adequate coping skills or may be lacking a healthy social support network.

In addition to the empirically supported relationships between self-reliance and worry, and self-reliance and self-esteem, we believe there are other related constructs. The interpersonal patterns measured by the Self-Reliance Inventory are similar to the three styles of relating to others developed by Horney (1945). Horney believed that neurosis was rooted in what she called basic anxiety. Basic anxiety refers to the feeling a child has of being isolated and helpless in a potentially hostile world. From the perspective of Bowlby (1982, 1988), basic anxiety seems to stem from the lack of secure attachments. Horney believed that people develop a variety of coping strategies for dealing with feelings of isolation and hopelessness. These strategies function to minimize the anxiety of dealing with others. The first strategy involves "moving toward people." This is a self-effacing strategy in which the individual demonstrates dependency on others. Extreme forms of this style parallel the overdependent style of the SRI. The second strategy involves "moving away from people." This style is characterized by lack of commitment to relationships or total withdrawal from relationships. By becoming aloof, individuals using this style seek to avoid interpersonal pain. This style parallels the counterdependent style measured by the SRI. The third interpersonal strategy identified by Horney is "moving against people." This style is the manifestation of a power and mastery orientation. Horney believed that healthy people integrated these three styles into a balanced strategy for dealing with others. However, neurotic individuals, because of their heightened sense of anxiety, use only one strategy, while denying or repressing the other two. In fact, the neurotic becomes rigidly locked into a dominant interpersonal style. We believe that self-reliant individuals display the healthy pattern of balance among the three styles. Future self-reliance research should examine these relationships.

Administration, Scoring, and Norms

SRI, SRI-G, and IAS. Scoring for the original SRI instrument is to sum items as follows:

- Counterdependence = 2 + 6 + 13 + 14 + 17 + 20 + (20 − [4 + 5 + 9 + 18])
- Overdependence = 3 + 7 + 12 + 16 + 19 + 20

Scoring of the SRI-G and IAS follows the same pattern using the same 20 items.

Norms have not been established, but means for our civilian and military samples are as follows:

	Civilian (N = 310)	Military— Basic Trainees (N = 96)	Military— Officer Trainees (N = 126)
Counterdependence	16.81	17.36	13.78
Overdependence	15.43	15.25	13.56

Means for basic military trainees are based on scores of trainees in regular squadrons as the trainees had been classified by the military system. Means for military officer trainees are those from our second data collection point, approximately 4 weeks into training.

SRI-II. Scoring of items in the second Self-Reliance Inventory (SRI-II) is calculated as follows:

- Interdependence = (2 + 6 + 10 + 12 + 14 + 16) / 6
- Counterdependence = (1 + 3 + 5 + 7 + 9 + 11 + 13) / 7
- Overdependence = (4 + 8 + 15) / 3

Means for the civilian sample (N = 297) using this measure are as follows:

Interdependence	3.91
Counterdependence	1.27
Overdependence	1.81

Summary of Research

Reliability

Cronbach's coefficient alpha for our study of civilians (Quick, Joplin, Nelson, & Quick, 1992) were .69 for counterdependence and .58 for overdependence, both at acceptable levels for developmental scale work according to Nunnally (1979), who treated .50 as the marginally acceptable level in developmental and exploratory research circumstances. In the same article, test-retest reliabilities were reported to be .80 for counterdependence and .67 for overdependence. The military samples showed similar internal consistency calculations, and test-retest reliabilities were not calculated for those samples. Cronbach's alpha coefficients for the SRI-II subscale measures obtained from a sample of 297 students (Joplin, Nelson, & Quick, 1996) were .70 for counterdependence, .71 for interdependence, and .72 for overdependence. The internal consistency and test-retest reliabilities are shown in Table 1.

Internal Relationships among Measures and Confirmation of Dimensional Structure

As shown in Table 1, the three subscales of the SRI are significantly but not highly correlated. Specifically, counterdependent-2 is significantly correlated with overdependent-2 (r = .53) and autonomy at work (r = .53). Overdependent-2

Table 1: Test-Retest Reliabilities for Self-Reliance Subscales ($n = 44$)

	1	2	3	4	5	6
Time 1						
1. Counterdependence	1.00					
2. Overdependent-2	.532	1.00				
3. Autonomyatwork	.534	.336	1.00			
Time 2						
4. Counterdependent-2	_.799_	.390	.407	1.00		
5. Overdependent-2	.520	_.666_	.426	.367	1.00	
6. Autonomyatwork	.457	.233	_.729_	.542	.230	1.00

is significantly correlated with autonomy at work ($r = .34$). To further examine the relationships among the self-reliance subscales, an exploratory factor analysis using principal components was conducted. A three-factor solution based on a varimax rotation is shown in Table 2. Factor loadings greater than .30 were considered significant and are italicized in the table. Factor I was labeled Counterdependent-2 and is composed of 10 items. Factor II was labeled overdependence-2 and is composed of six items. Four items compose Factor III, which appears to measure autonomous behavior in the work environment. Taken together, the results of the correlation and exploratory factor analysis suggest that the SRI is providing a measure of three separate aspects of an individual's attachment behavior.

A confirmatory factor analysis of the SRI-II using LISREL VIII was conducted on data obtained from a sample of 297 students (Joplin et al., 1996). This analysis revealed that Fornell and Larcker's (1981) measure of the average variance each latent variable accounted for in its indicator was .58 for counterdependence, .42 for interdependence, and .53 for overdependence. The means of the squared standardized item load-ings for each factor (.35 for counterdependence, .29 for interdependence, and .43 for overdependence) were higher than the squared intercorrelations of the factors, thus sup-porting substantial discriminant validity (Fornell & Larcker, 1981). The overall fit was quite good as measured by several fit indices: Bentler's (1990) comparative fit index (CFI = .90), Bollen's (1989) incremental fit index (IFI = .90), Joreskog and Sorbom's (1993) goodness-of-fit index (GFI = .92), and Tucker and Lewis's (1973) fit index (NNFI = .88).

Profiles across Age Groups

The development and validation of the SRI instruments to date has been based on student and military samples. Thus, the results to date have some range restriction, with most of the subjects being under 34 years of age. Specifically, in the military sample (Quick et al., 1992), 12% of the subjects were under 20 years, 66% were in their 20s, 14% were in their 30s, 7% were in their 40s, and 1% were in their 50s. The student sample showed a similar distribution: 5.6% under 20, 77.3% in their 20s, 13% in their 30s, and 4.1% in their 40s. Age and education may contribute to the development of interdepen-dent behavior (Joplin, Quick, Nelson, & Turner, 1995).

Case Examples

Early studies conducted to examine the relationships among adult attachment patterns, health outcomes, and social sup-port involved military trainees. More recently, these relation-ships have been examined in comparable nonmilitary, young adult working populations. In a study involving basic military trainees (Quick, Joplin, et al., 1996) differences were examined in self-reliance between two successful groups of trainees and a third group of trainees experiencing a variety of behavioral, psychological, and medical problems with training. The re-

Table 2: Factor Analysis of the 20-Item Self-Reliance Inventory ($n = 310$)

	Factor I	Factor II	Factor III
Counterdependent-2			
2	0.43630	0.29607	0.10069
4	-0.53794	0.16159	0.07477
5	-0.46345	-0.03090	-0.23860
6	0.51973	0.13371	0.26987
9	-0.53301	0.13917	0.11857
13	0.61475	-0.02146	0.30793
14	0.39460	0.23764	0.15853
17	0.37884	0.02847	0.35374
18	-0.57702	-0.02145	0.13073
20	0.39092	0.43639	-0.05345
Overdependent-2			
3	0.22874	0.57122	0.14133
7	-0.15130	0.57497	0.25457
12	-0.04685	0.66086	0.13278
16	0.11363	0.56558	0.04603
19	-0.12064	0.45013	-0.0110
Autonomous behavior			
1	0.37615	0.10852	0.64727
11	-0.05036	-0.17507	0.73052
15	-0.11623	0.17367	0.55930
8	0.23455	-0.21214	0.06727
10	0.21582	0.03570	0.27015

sults of that study suggest that self-reliance measures can discriminate among groups expected to report different levels of self-reliance. Further analysis of data from this study suggested strong relationships among self-reliance, self-esteem, and burnout in both regular and problem trainees. Specifically, counterdependence was found to be related to low self-esteem and high burnout. These relationships were intensified for those individuals who experienced problems in training. Without implying causality, it appears that individuals who have counterdependent styles, low self-esteem, and high burnout levels may be at greater risk with regard to their personal well-being and their ability to function normally in a training situation.

A second study (Quick, Joplin, et al., 1996) using military subjects assessed the predictive validity of the self-reliance measures. This study found that graduates of basic military training school were significantly more self-reliant at the beginning of training than those who did not graduate. The nongraduating counterparts were significantly more overdependent and experienced problems associated with overdependence. Because the self-reliance inventory was administered before training began, it can be inferred that the training process did not induce the overdependence.

This conclusion is also supported by the results of a longitudinal study of military officer trainees (Joplin et al., 1995). In a study involving 297 students enrolled at two universities where the majority of students are employed full-time, the relationships among attachment orientations, social support, and health were examined with nonmilitary subjects. The results of this study underscore the relationships between attachment orientations and health. Specifically, interdependence was negatively related to perceived social dysfunction. This indicates that interdependent (self-reliant) attachment behaviors are more frequently exhibited by healthy individuals. Conversely, both counterdependence and overdependence were positively related to five perceived symptoms of distress: psychological, physiological, somatic, anxiety/

insomnia, and social dysfunction. These results indicate an adverse impact associated with counterdependence and over-dependence, which is consistent with previous attachment theory research.

In this study, counterdependent individuals perceived significantly less social support from the three potential sources of social support measured (supervisory, coworkers, family and friends). This suggests that counterdependent individuals may either enact relationships in ways that are not supportive or fail to enact any supportive relationships. In contrast, over-dependent individuals reported more support from coworkers, as well as family and friends.

Conclusion

The Self-Reliance Inventory provides a tangible method for applying attachment theory to several aspects of the organizational and personal life of adults. Research to date has found significant relationships between self-reliance and executive success (Quick, Nelson, & Quick, 1992), self-reliance and newcomer adjustment (Nelson & Quick, 1991), self-reliance and worry (Stöber & Seidenstücker, 1996) self-reliance and self-esteem (Quick, Paulus, et al., 1996), and self-reliance and felt security (Quick, Joplin, Nelson, & Quick, 1991). These results suggest that the SRI is an important tool for evaluating the attachment strategies of individuals for the purpose of predicting potential success or dysfunction and for developing appropriate intervention strategies for relationally based problems.

Chapter References

Ainsworth, M., Blehar, M., Waters, E., & Walls, S. (1978). *Patterns of attachment: A psychological analysis of the strange situation.* Hillsdale, NJ: Erlbaum.

Ainsworth, M., & Bowlby, J. (1991). An ethological approach to personality. *American Psychologist, 46,* 333–341.

Bentler, P. (1990). Comparative fit indices in structural models. *Psychological Bulletin, 107,* 238–246.

Bollen, K. (1989). A new incremental fit index for general structural equation models. *Sociological Methods and Research, 17,* 303–316.

Bowlby, J. (1982). *Attachment* (2nd ed.). New York: Basic Books.

Bowlby, J. (1988). *A secure base.* New York: Basic Books.

Fornell, C., & Larcker, D. (1981). Evaluating structural equation models with unobservable variables and measurement error. *Journal of Marketing Research, 18,* 39–50.

Hazan, C., & Shaver, P. (1987). Romantic love conceptualized as an attachment process. *Journal of Personality and Social Psychology, 52,* 511–524.

Hazan, C., & Shaver, P. (1990). Love and work: An attachment-theoretical perspective. *Journal of Personality and Social Psychology, 59,* 270–280.

Horney, K. (1945). Our inner conflicts, a constructive theory of neurosis. New York: Norton.

Joplin, J., Nelson, D., & Quick, J. (1996). *Attachment behavior and health: Relationships at work and home.* Unpublished manuscript.

Joplin, J., Quick, J., Nelson, D., & Turner, J. (1995). Interdependence and personal well-being in a training environment. In L. Murphy, J. Hurrell, S. Sauter, & G. Keita (Eds.), *Job stress interventions* (pp. 309–322). Washington, DC: American Psychological Association.

Joreskog, K., & Sorbom, D. (1993). *LISREL VIII: Analysis of linear structural relationships by maximum likelihood, instrument variables and least squares methods* (8th ed.). Morresville, IN: Scientific Software.

Kobak, R., & Hazan, C. (1991). Accommodating working models in marital relationships: The role of attachment security and communication. *Journal of Personality and Social Psychology, 60,* 861–869.

Kobak, R., & Sceery, A. (1988). Attachment in late adolescence: Working models, affect regulation, and representation of self and others. *Child Development, 59,* 135–146.

Linville, P. W. (1987). Self-complexity as a cognitive buffer against stress-related illness and depression. *Journal of Personality and Social Psychology, 52,* 663–676.

Nelson, D. L., & Quick, J. C. (1991). Social support and newcomer adjustment in organizations: Attachment theory at work? *Journal of Organizational Behavior, 12,* 543–554.

Nelson, D., Quick, J., & Joplin, J. (1991). Psychological contracting and newcomer socialization: An attachment theory foundation. *Journal of Social Behavior and Personality (Special Stress Issue), 6,* 55–72.

Nunnally, J. C. (1979). *Psychometric theory.* New York: McGraw-Hill.

Quick, J. C., Joplin, J., Nelson, D., Quick, J. D. (1991). *Self-reliance for stress and combat.* Paper presented at the 8th Combat Stress Conference, U.S. Army Health Services Command, Fort Sam Houston.

Quick, J. C., Joplin, J., Nelson, D., Mangelsdorff, A., & Fiedler, E. (1996). Self-reliance and military service training outcomes. *Military Psychology, 8*(4), 279–293.

Quick, J. C., Joplin, J., Nelson, D., & Quick, J. D. (1992). Behavioral responses to anxiety: Self-reliance, counterdependence, and over-dependence. *Anxiety, Stress, and Coping, 5,* 41–54.

Quick, J. C., Nelson, D., & Quick, J. D. (1987). Successful executives: How independent? *Academy of Management Executive, 1*(2), 139–146.

Quick, J. C., Nelson, D., & Quick, J. D. (1990). *Stress and challenge at the top: The paradox of the successful executive.* Chichester, England: Wiley.

Quick, J. C., Nelson, D., & Quick, J. D. (1991). The self-reliance inventory. In J. W. Pfeiffer (Ed.), *The 1991 annual: Developing human resources* (pp. 149–161). San Diego: University Associates.

Quick, J. C., Paulus, P. B., Whittington, J. L., Larey, T. S., & Nelson, D. L. (1996). Management development, well-being, and health. In M. J. Schabracq, J. A. M. Winnubst, & C. L. Cooper (Eds.), *Handbook of work and health psychology* (pp. 369–388). Chichester: Wiley.

Quick, J. D., Nelson, D., Matuszek, P., Whittington, J., & Quick, J. C. (1995). Social support, secure attachments and health. In C. L. Cooper (Ed.), *Handbook of stress, medicine and health* (pp. 269–287). Boca Raton, FL: CRC Press.

Stöber, J., & Seidenstücker, B. (1996). Worry in managers: An inventory of job-related worries and correlates with job involvement and self-reliance. Unpublished manuscript.

Tucker, L., & Lewis, C. (1973). The reliability coefficient for maximum likelihood factor analysis. *Psychometrika, 38,* 1–10.

Weiss, R. (1982). Attachment behavior in adult life. In C. Parkes & J. Stevenson-Hindes (Eds.), *The place of attachment in human behavior* (pp. 171–184). New York: Basic Books.

The Stress Response Scale

A Measure of Children's Behavioral Adjustment

Louis A. Chandler, University of Pittsburgh

■ Instrument Names

Stress Response Scale

SRS

■ Developer

Louis A. Chandler, Ph.D., Psychoeducational Clinic,
University of Pittsburgh

■ Contact Information

Dr. Louis A. Chandler, Department of Psychology
in Education, 5C Forbes Quadrangle, University
of Pittsburgh, Pittsburgh, PA 15261
Telephone: (412) 624-1262; fax: (412) 624-7231; e-mail:
chandler@fs1.sched.pitt.edu

The SRS is distributed exclusively by Psychological
Assessment Resources, Inc. For availablity, ordering, and
distribution information, contact PAR directly:
Psychological Assessment Resources, Inc., P.O. Box 998,
Odessa, FL 33556; telephone: (800) 331-8378

A software program for scoring the SRS by means of a
personal computer is also available. Information on
computer scoring of the SRS is available from Dr. Mark
Shermis, IUPUI Testing Center, 620 Union Dr. (#G003),
Indianapolis, IN 46202-5168; telephone: (317) 278-2288;
e-mail: MShermis@eval.iupui.edu

Description and History of the Instrument

The Stress Response Scale is a 40-item behavior rating scale with items rated by frequency of occurrence on a 6-point Likert-type scale ranging from 0 ("never") to 5 ("always"). It is generally used with elementary school-aged children (i.e., those between 5 and 14 years of age), although experimental norms are available that extend the age range to 18 years (Shermis, Ruden, & Chandler, 1992). The SRS is normally completed by an adult familiar with the child's behavior, usually a teacher or parent. Items are written in such a way as to not be specific to either home or school.

The SRS is based on a model of the response styles often adopted by children under stress (Chandler, 1983). In addition to its Total score, which may be seen as an overall measure of behavioral adjustment, the SRS yields five subtest scores consistent with the behavioral response style predicted by the model: Dependent, Acting-out, Overactive, Passive-Aggressive, and Repressed. The results may be profiled to depict the child's characteristic stress response.

The Stress Response Scale was developed for use in clinics, schools, and community agencies as one measure of children's emotional adjustment. It was originally conceived to fill the need for a useful conceptual approach for studying and assessing children referred to the University of Pittsburgh's Psychoeducational Clinic. The clinic was established in 1982, and very early on we discovered that we were seeing a subtle but increasingly apparent shift in the nature of problems children presented when being seen for treatment. Our services had been built along a traditional model used for children, oriented to meet the needs of those seen as high-risk children: emotionally disturbed, troubled youth; the mentally handicapped; and, more recently, children with specific learning disabilities. We used standard assessment instruments to identify those problems.

But beginning in the mid-1980s we saw a new phenomenon begin to unfold. A different type of child was showing up in increasing numbers among those being referred to school psychologists, guidance counselors, and mental health workers in our child guidance clinics. These were children who did not neatly fit any of our traditional categories of "at-risk" youth, yet they were clearly having a difficult time meeting the demands of learning and growing up in today's society.

The most obvious manifestations were seen in school functioning. Increasingly we saw children who had limited attention spans and difficulty concentrating. They seemed unable to marshall their resources for the focused and sustained effort required for learning. Such school functioning problems were often manifested in reading, in which case the child was likely to be seen as having a "reading problem," or they first showed up in math, leading to special tutoring in that area. These children were likely to be diagnosed as learning disabled or, increasingly as the decade went on, as children with attention deficits disorders.

Because of the obvious educational manifestations, these children were likely to end up in special education programs, where they swelled the ranks of burgeoning remedial programs. Yet, in spite of all the educational efforts, the school performance of such children remained, at best, marginal. With barely passing grades, they were likely to be minimally involved in the school experience. As they proceeded through school, essentially untouched by the educational process, they were more likely to drop out spiritually, if not physically. Given a reported widespread grade inflation in the schools, these children were likely to be passed on, and eventually to graduate, although their low achievement test scores showed they were barely literate and often poorly equipped to deal with life as literate citizens—as their low achievement test scores showed (Office of Educational Research and Improvement, 1994).

These were the children who are experimenting with drugs and sex at increasingly earlier ages, and in such large numbers that alarmed school officials called it a national epidemic (*Newsweek*, 1994). They were running away from home, and they were committing suicide in record numbers. They tended to be both the perpetuators and victims of violence in the schools. Since more "average" children were showing such behavior that was regarded as a sign of a troubled child only 20 years ago, it became obvious some new paradigm was necessary to understand those children being referred for treatment. It would be a paradigm more sensitive to the context in which development and schooling took place. What seemed to be called for was a wider psychosocial perspective, one that was sensitive to the rapid pace of social change and how that change affected the lives of children.

In examining the cases we saw for a relevant common denominator, we observed that such troubled children often showed a "driven" quality, most evident in their behavior. They had a great deal of difficulty coping and adopted behavior patterns that were often counterproductive, further exacerbating their situation. This driven quality led us to adopt a view of these children as children under stress.

Once this conceptual overview had been adopted, we examined the literature on psychosocial stress to see what factors might have been identified as relevant to children's life-stress experience. The effects of stress on children's lives have been well documented (Compas, 1987). In his excellent review of the extensive literature on stressful life events of children, Compas has described the linkages between such events and a wide range of somatic, psychological, and behavioral outcomes. He shows that stress has been linked to school functioning and academic achievement, to behavior disorders and short-term emotional adjustment reactions, and to long-term personality disorders, as well as being found to be associated with a wide range of somatic symptoms.

Stress is a complex physiological and psychosocial phenomena. For our purposes, stress may be defined as a state of emotional tension arising from unmet needs and/or environmental demands that involve the threat of harm or loss. From this perspective, stress may be seen as affecting children's development and general well-being in terms of health, family, social relations, and school functioning. The effects of stress are most often apparent in children's behavior when, for example, in attempting to meet stress demands, children adopt various behavioral responses. If these responses are socially desirable and effective, they may be labeled "coping responses"; if such efforts are self-defeating and/or socially undesirable, they may be labeled as "behavior disorders" or "emotional adjustment reactions" (Chandler, 1982, 1985; Chandler, Shermis, & Marsh, 1985).

To systematically study childhood stress, a theoretical paradigm is useful because it suggests relationships among the elements of the stress experience and encourages the assessment of stress outcomes. A paradigm indicates the type of data to collect, guides the study of the relevant variables, and suggests ways to validate the stress experience. It would also have clear implications for clinical assessment. Figure 1 presents a possible paradigm for childhood stress.

This paradigm provides a perspective by interpreting a child's life-stress experience within a psychosocial interactive framework (Endler, 1980; Endler & Magnusson, 1976; Lazarus & Folkman, 1984; Magnusson, 1982). It suggests that those who wish to study childhood stress should concern themselves with (a) identifying stressors in the child's history and current situation; (b) exploring the moderators of those

Figure 1: An Interactive Paradigm of a Child's Experience with Stress

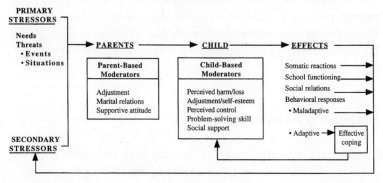

stressors (e.g., the child's perception of harm or loss involved in those situations); and (c) assessing stress outcomes,—that is, the impact on the child's health, school and social functioning, as well as his or her behavioral adjustment (Chandler & Shermis, 1990). While other measures were designed to examine the other aspects of the stress experience, the SRS was developed specifically to address the last component,—that is, the behavioral response to stress. These are the behavioral indicators of maladjustment that frequently cause school functioning problems.

Our objective was to couple the theoretical model underlying the assessment measure with a rating scale format so as to take advantage of the advances in rating scale development. With few notable exceptions at that time, rating scales had mostly been developed for use in research contexts, and few attempts were made to show their clinical relevance. The use of these scales with children seems particularly appropriate because, unlike those techniques typically used with adults (e.g., self-reports, interviews), rating scales are not dependent on more mature levels of reasoning, language development, or even client cooperation. Because such scales focus on observable characteristics, they bring potentially greater objectivity to clinical reporting. Finally, the reliability of many of the more popular scales has been consistently demonstrated.

Although rating scales have been widely accepted in research in child development and psychopathology, they have not enjoyed the same popularity among practitioners. One reason may be a validity issue, in that many of the scales in use seem to have questionable clinical relevance. The Stress Response Scale was designed to provide clinically relevant information.

Underlying Assumptions

The behavior a child adopts in response to stress may be viewed on a continuum from adaptive, effective coping behaviors to extreme maladaptive efforts to meet stressful demands. To assess children's behavioral responses to stress, it was decided to develop a behavior rating scale—the Stress Response Scale (Chandler 1983, 1984).

Designing the SRS necessitated a model of the stress response to provide the conceptual framework for construction of the instrument. The response to stress may be understood within the broader context of the organism's response to the environment. Within this context, the response to stress is simply a response to one specific type of stimulus—that is, one that has been characterized as a stressor. Therefore, we looked to personality theory to provide a model of how, in general, the person responds to the world and adopted from the work of various personality theorists two dimensions of personality: activity-passivity and introversion-extroversion. These were placed in a circumflex model. This model was put forth as a way of predicting how children might theoretically respond to stress (see Figure 2).

Next, we tried to predict the type of behavioral response pattern that might be seen if children were responding according to the model. From a review of the literature and from our own clinical experience, we initially proposed eight patterns of possible stress responses (as seen along the inner edge of the circle in Figure 3). However, as we developed the model it became apparent that it was more reasonable to subsume the eight patterns into just four: Impulsive, Dependent, Passive-Aggressive, and Repressed.

The next step was to test the validity of the hypothesized categories. For this we turned to the clinical reports of children seen for psychological services and asked a number of experienced clinicians to classify the sample of reports using the classification scheme. Once there was some evidence of construct validity and the initial reliability of the classification scheme proved to be satisfactory, we reviewed clinical reports to extract 10 behavioral descriptors that corresponded to each of the four categories. These descriptors were then randomly

Figure 2: Two Dimensions of Personality

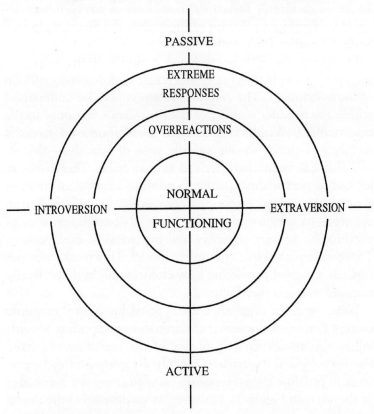

assigned to item positions in a Likert-type behavior rating scale.

A series of developmental studies were then conducted to gather data using the SRS with various populations of children. SRS data were factor analyzed to establish factorial validity with both referred and nonreferred populations of children; the results consistently showed a five-factor solution, consonant with the model (Shermis & Chandler, 1985). The following subscale scores were established by factor analysis:

- *Impulsive (Acting-out)*: Acting-out children are often described as demanding, selfish, and defiant with frequent

Figure 3: Four Common Response Patterns to Stress

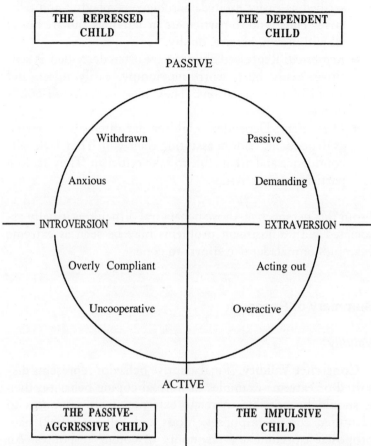

temper outbursts. They are prone to fighting and picking on other children. They are impulsive, uncooperative, and stubborn, and they have difficulty accepting criticism. They are sometimes mischievous, willful, and detached.

- *Passive-Aggressive*: Passive-Aggressive children are often described as underachievers who procrastinate, have a poor attitude toward school, tend not to complete assignments, and show declining grades. They also tend to be uncooperative and stubborn.

- *Impulsive (Overactive)*: Overactive children are often described as easily excited, mischievous, playful, and talkative. They tend to participate in activities and are not at all withdrawn, passive, or shy.
- *Repressed*: Repressed children are often described as sensitive, easily hurt, worrying, jumpy, easily upset, and afraid of new situations. They tend to lack self-confidence.
- *Dependent*: Dependent children are often characterized as dependent, seldom asserting their will. They lack self-confidence and are unable to take criticism. They seldom participate in activities.

From this perspective, those behavioral difficulties usually associated with adjustment problems may be seen as extreme examples of maladaptive efforts to cope.

Summary of Research

Validity

Construct Validity. If maladaptive behavior represents distorted or extreme examples of normal coping behavior, then it should be possible to relate extreme stress responses to identified coping responses. Moos and Billings (1982) have proposed a preliminary taxonomy of coping responses. An examination of the behavioral response patterns predicted by the stress response model, and selected coping responses from those proposed by Moos and Billings, finds some stress response patterns that show some similarities to coping responses such as Resigned Acceptance (Dependent), Emotional Discharge (Impulsive), Developing Alternate Rewards (Passive-Aggressive), and Cognitive Avoidance (Repressed).

Further evidence of the validity of this perspective comes from the work of Klerman (1979), who sees adult depressive disorders as vain attempts on the part of the individual to adapt. Clinical depressions are, from his perspective, maladaptive outcomes of partially successful efforts at adaptation. In a similar way, it is likely that children's emotional adjustment problems may be seen as maladaptive responses to stress. These extreme responses call attention to themselves and interfere with the child's effective functioning at home, at school, and in social relations.

Still another approach to construct validity comes from the work of personality theorists who view coping styles as traits of personality that are relatively stable across time and situations (Coyne & Lazarus, 1980; Haan, 1977; White, 1974; Witkin & Goodenough, 1977). The well-known studies of Thomas and Chess (Thomas & Chess, 1977; Thomas, Chess & Birch, 1968) provide additional evidence of the persistence of response styles and examples of their use in establishing personality typologies.

Reed (1993) examined the relationships between parent behavior ratings of their children's stress response patterns and their ratings of their children's temperament using the Revised Dimensions of Temperament Survey. He found that higher activity levels were associated with more active stress responses, whereas higher temperamental withdrawal was associated with more passive stress response patterns.

If behavioral responses to stress form characteristic patterns that are relatively stable, evidence might be found for similar patterns manifested by children in different cultures. Similar patterns have been found using the SRS with children in Venezuela (Gibson & DiPaula, 1989), Egypt (Chandler, El-Samadony, Shermis, & El-Khatib, 1991), and Poland (Chandler & Maurer, 1996). The SRS has been translated into Spanish, French, German, Polish, Hebrew, Arabic, and Indonesian/ Malaysian.

To examine behavioral responses to stress within the context of children's life stress experiences, a series of studies were conducted that focused on stressful life events and those variables that might act as moderators between stressors and stress outcomes (Johnson, 1989; Johnson & Chandler, 1987;

Million, 1987). These studies have found a consistent moderate relationship between the number of stressful life events experienced and the total score of the SRS with a sample of 53 clinic-referred children ($r = .38$), a sample of 364 randomly selected schoolchildren ($r = .47$), and a sample of 43 clinic-referred children ($r = .39$). Further evidence confirming this relationship was found in a study using SRS scores as one element of a proposed paradigm for children's life-stress experience (Chandler, 1988). An examination of the interrelationships within that paradigm, using the scores of a sample of 60 clinic-referred children, found the relationship between behavioral adjustment and the number of stressful life events to be similar to that found in previous studies ($r = .35$). These findings are consistent with the literature on stressful life events that reports the typical relationship between stressful events and psychological disturbance to be between .30 and .40 (Thoits, 1983).

A second series of studies looked at the stress experiences of children in terms of the relationship between children's behavioral adjustment, as measured on the SRS, and such mediating variables as the influence of a significant male in their lives (Winikoff, 1986), the quality of intimate relationships between significant adults (Curlee, 1986), and the number of depressive symptoms reported by single mothers (Bartolomucci, 1986). In all cases significant moderate relationships were found in the predicted directions.

In examining still another aspect of construct validity, Hoover (1987) investigated the relationships among constructs theoretically related to childhood stress using the teacher ratings of a sample of fifth-grade students ($n = 99$). He found that children who showed a repressed stress response style tended to have poorer self-concepts and more problems with self-control, with the absolute value of coefficients among the constructs in the .67 to .71 range. Similarly, another study (Vercruysse & Chandler, 1992) found a significant, although modest, relationship between certain styles of coping and behavioral adjustment, as well as a moderate relationship between self-concept and behavioral adjustment as measured on the SRS ($r = .36$).

Finally, several studies were conducted using the SRS with children in various situations that might be seen as potentially stressful, including special education (Robinson & Chandler, 1985; Rodriguez, 1994), dental treatment (Riva & Chandler, 1989), family relocations (Vercruysse & Chandler, 1992), remedial classes (Atherley, 1990), and with children referred because of emotional adjustment difficulties (Chandler et al., 1985; Rocchio, 1986).

Content Validity. If the predicted behavioral patterns are commonly found among children, and especially among children showing emotional adjustment difficulties, then it should be possible to identify similar patterns in the literature on childhood psychopathology. Although the labels sometimes differ, similar patterns have been identified in the literature (Clarizio & McCoy, 1978; Quay, 1979). In addition, similar syndromes have also been found through empirical studies that identified clusters of behavior using statistical techniques (Edelbrock, 1979). Finally, evidence of the predicted behavior patterns was found in the psychological reports of children referred for clinical study (Chandler, 1979). From the literature, and from the psychological reports of children, characteristics for each type were collated, and composite descriptions developed. Descriptors from each composite description were then randomly assigned to item positions on a rating scale format.

Further evidence for the existence of the predicted behavior patterns came from a study that employed a cluster analysis technique to identify the patterns found most frequently among a population of school-aged children (Chandler and Shermis, 1985). Several patterns were found that clustered within various sex/age subgroups, further confirming that these patterns are commonly found with children and that developmental and sexual identity considerations may influence behavioral responses.

To determine more specifically how age affects the behavioral response patterns children tend to adopt, Batterman (1989) examined the relationship between age and children's behavioral response style with a sample of referred children ($n = 93$). She found that the Overactive response style is generally associated with younger children, whereas the Passive-Aggressive response style is more typically found with older children. Correlations of stress response styles with age confirmed this relationship (Acting-out, $r = .08$, n.s.; Passive-Aggressive, $r = .42$, $p < .001$; Overactive, $r = .22$, $p < .05$; Repressed, $r = .08$, n.s.; Dependent, $r = .13$, n.s.).

Factorial Validity. A series of developmental studies were conducted with early versions of the rating scale. An initial factor analytic-study with a sample of clinic-referred children ($n = 120$) found a five-factor solution consonant with the types predicted by the model, which accounted for 62% of the variance (Chandler, 1979). Replication with a modified version of the scale and a larger group of clinic-referred children ($n = 200$) also found a five-factor solution accounting for 70% of the variance (Piso, 1981). One important finding was that a similar factor structure existed with a group of non-referred children ($n = 376$), lending additional support to the notion that emotional adjustment reactions may be seen as extreme patterns of normal coping behavior (Chandler, 1982, 1983).

A factor-analytic study of the current version of the scale with nonreferred children ($n = 167$) once again yielded the five-factor solution, accounting for 64% of the variance (Chandler & Lundahl, 1983). Thirty-four of the 40 items were included in the analysis, and the cluster sizes ranged from 6 to 12 items each. Three of the clusters seemed consistent with the predicted categories of the model. These were labeled as Passive-Aggressive, Dependent, and Repressed. The two remaining clusters seemed to reflect a division of the fourth predicted type, the Impulsive, into two subtypes: Impulsive (Overactive) and Impulsive (Acting-out). Replication with a larger sample ($n = 962$) has confirmed the five-factor solution (Shermis & Chandler, 1985).

Concurrent Validity. Concurrent validity was tested by comparing the data derived from the SRS with that derived from other instruments designed to assess children's behavioral and emotional status. Hughes (1986) compared SRS scores with those from the Walker Problem Behavior Identification Checklist (WPIBC), a behavior rating scale designed to identify children with behavior problems. Using a sample of 30 schoolchildren in grades K through 6 who had been referred for psychological evaluation, Hughes showed that the total scores on both instruments were positively related ($r = .84$). There was also evidence of overlap between the SRS Acting-out subscale and the WPIBC Acting-out ($r = .76$) and Distractibility ($r = .78$) subscales.

Johnson (1989) examined the relationship between scores derived from Koppitz's list of emotional indicators as applied to children's human figure drawings (HFD) and the SRS scores derived from teacher ratings of the children's behavior. Results pointed to a significant moderate relationship between HFD scores and the SRS Total T scores ($r = .54$), and a similar relationship between HFD scores and the SRS Acting-out subscale scores ($r = .58$). A weaker relationship, although also significant, was found between HFD scores and the SRS Passive-Aggressive subscale score ($r = .41$).

In another study of the relationship between children's behavior and their expressive productions, Rosenberg (1987), using a sample of 56 clinic-referred children, performed a content analysis of children's stories as told on the Children's Apperception Test to examine the protocols for evidence of frequent concerns with various needs and threats. She then compared the results with the children's SRS scores as derived from parent ratings. The findings showed that children who show Passive-Aggressive behavioral patterns have significantly more concerns with aggression and punishment than those who show other behavioral patterns.

Discriminant Validity. The discriminant validity of the Stress Response Scale has been tested by a series of studies examining the ability of scores on the scale to discriminate among various clinical groups and subgroups, and their peers (Chandler, 1979). Findings have consistently shown that referred children are rated significantly higher than nonreferred children (Piso, 1981) and children in the general population of schoolchildren (Chandler, 1983; Dasuki, 1986; Kemmerer, 1984). Children assigned to special education classes for the emotionally disturbed are also given significantly higher ratings than their peers (Krotec, 1982; Tartaglione, 1991).

Further support for the discriminant validity of the scale was provided by a study that examined the relative frequency of the various profile types in both clinic-referred and randomly selected populations (Chandler & Shermis, 1986). The results showed that within the clinic-referred group, subgroups labeled as Acting-out and Repressed were identified frequently. A subsequent study of the distribution of response patterns among various groups of children compared the scores of samples of children who had been referred to a university's psychoeducational clinic and those who had been referred to a psychiatric clinic, against the scores of the randomly selected normative sample (Chandler, 1987).

Once discriminative validity had been well established, a series of studies were conducted to examine possible clinical implications of the various subgroups identified by their scores on the SRS. Rocchio (1986) identified two clinical subgroups of children established on the basis of their SRS profile patterns (30 Acting-out; 30 Repressed). These children were compared with each other and with a group of 60 nonreferred children to determine whether the groups differed in terms of health, school, and family/social functioning as assessed by parent interviews. Significant differences were found among the groups. The Repressed group had more health problems than either the Acting-out or the nonreferred group; and the Acting-out group had significantly more reported school functioning and family/social problems than either of the other two groups.

Criterion-Related Validity. If the scale is to prove useful in assessing children's emotional adjustment, it should be judged against its ability to predict mental health and educational outcomes. Within the clinical setting, one of the more common outcomes involves differential diagnosis among the psychiatric categories assigned to children. The descriptions that define the diagnostic categories in the American Psychiatric Association's (1980) *Diagnostic and Statistical Manual of Mental Disorders* seem to have some correspondence to SRS response patterns: Conduct Disorder (Acting-out), Oppositional Disorder (Passive-Aggressive), Attention Deficit Disorder (Overactive), and Anxiety Disorder (Repressed).

Using these matched comparisons, the ability of the SRS was tested to predict psychiatric group membership in a clinical setting (Chandler et al., 1985). When the SRS subscale scores were compared against the diagnoses assigned to a sample of clinic-referred children (*n* = 60), they were found to reduce the error in predicting psychiatric group membership. The ratings of both parents and teachers were useful; however, those of teachers proved to be superior in this context. This study suggests that the SRS may prove useful as one element in a diagnostic assessment.

Subsequently, the scale's criterion-related validity was tested in terms of educational outcomes in a school setting. A study was conducted to determine whether SRS scores could be useful in predicting from among a group of children referred for psychological evaluation, those who subsequently would be recommended for special educational placement, and from among those recommended for special education, those who would be referred for a program for children with emotional disturbance (S&ED) (Robinson & Chandler, 1985). The results showed that the Acting-out subscore may be the best predictor of special education placement, while children with a combination that includes a high Acting-out score along with low Repressed and Dependent scores, are more likely to be specifically referred for S&ED placement. These findings suggest that the SRS may prove to be a useful aid in psychoeducational decision making.

Reliability

Initial reliability was found to be good with children in regular education classes ($n = 45$) using teachers as raters, and a test-retest interval of 2 weeks (80.7 mean percent of agreement across all items). A reliability study with the current version of the scale shows good results ($r = .86$) with a similar population ($n = 25$) in a test-retest procedure using a 1-month interval. Test-retest coefficients for the five subscales were Acting-out, $r = .79$; Passive-Aggressive, $r = .90$; Overactive, $r = .85$; Repressed, $r = .78$; and Dependent, $r = .87$.

A subsequent study was conducted using the ratings of teachers of 68 elementary school-aged children (age range 7 to 11 years) in a test-retest procedure with a 4-week interval (Mramor, 1986). The following coefficients were found: Total Score, $r = .87$; Acting-out, $r = .83$; Passive-Aggressive, $r = .83$; Overactive, $r = .72$; Repressed, $r = .80$; and Dependent, $r = .73$.

Coefficient alpha, a measure of internal consistency, was found to be .94 with the normative population. A subsequent study (Bartolumucci, 1986), using the ratings of 100 mothers of (nonreferred) children, showed a similar level of internal consistency (alpha coefficient, $r = .89$).

One important psychometric property of any rating scale is interrater agreement. In the case of the SRS, the agreement between parents and teachers is especially important. Marsh (1984), who studied 60 children who had been referred for clinical study, found an agreement level of $r = .21$ between parent and teacher ratings. This slight positive relationship is consistent with that reported in the literature (Goyette, Connors, & Ulrich, 1978; Quay, 1979).

To further study interrater reliability, the agreement between parent and teacher ratings on the SRS was examined using a sample of 45 referred school children between the ages of 5 and 12 years (Lantz-Hecker & Chandler, 1988). Pearson product-moment correlations were calculated between parent's and teacher's SRS scores. Moderate agreement was found on the Total SRS T-scores (r = .50). In terms of subscale scores, a strong relationship was found between rating groups on the Passive-Aggressive subscale (r = .72); a moderate relationship on the Acting-out (r = .54), Repressed (r = .51), and Dependent (r = .45) subscales; and a weak relationship on the Overactive (r = .24) subscale.

To better understand the nature of that agreement, Lantz-Hecker (1988) performed a series of t-tests on the group means of the two rating groups. The results showed that there were no significant differences between parent and teacher ratings on the SRS scores on that sample of referred children. Finally, an examination of the absolute differences between parent and teacher Total T-scores showed that nearly 80% of the scores differed by 10 or fewer points, with a mean difference between parent and teacher ratings of 7.02 (SD = 4.92).

Hoover (1987), using a sample of 99 randomly selected children, found substantially lower correlations between teacher and parent ratings than those found in the Lantz-Hecker (1988) study. However, he reported a similar pattern of relationships with better agreement, in general, on the ratings of boys than on girls in his sample. These results suggest that interrater agreement may be higher for boys and for those children whose behavior is seen as problematic.

Conditions for Use

The Stress Response Scale was developed for use in clinics, schools, and community agencies as one measure of children's emotional adjustment. It may help decision making, in both screening and making a differential diagnosis. The scale was designed for use with children referred for possible emotional adjustment problems or behavior disorders. Children whose problems are primarily the result of mental retardation or psychoneurological learning disabilities are not considered to be an appropriate population for clinical use of the scale.

Likewise, children with severe emotional disturbance are not typically seen as appropriate subjects for this measure. The SRS is generally used with elementary school–aged children (i.e., those between 5 and 14 years of age), although experimental norms are available that extend the age range to 18 years. It is normally completed by an adult familiar with the child's behavior as part of the clinical assessment.

Case Example

The case presented here illustrates how the Stress Response Scale results may be incorporated within the context of a more comprehensive life-stress assessment.

Rachel was a 12-year-old who lived with both parents. Early developmental history included pregnancy and birth complications, but there were no other unusual childhood health problems. She was referred for psychological assessment by her parents, who expressed their concerns about her school performance. In particular, they reported that she was not performing up to her potential and that she had become more irresponsible and disrespectful at home.

Rachel's early school history was relatively uneventful, and she received all A grades through the end of the fifth grade. During the past year, however, Rachel's grades steadily declined, and her parents and teachers believed she was not working up to her potential. Rachel often seemed to be careless with school or home assignments, and she sometimes failed to turn in work that had been completed. According to her parents' report, Rachel needed considerable monitoring and prompting to complete homework assignments.

Socially, Rachel was relatively active, involved with many extracurricular activities. She tended to interact well with peers and was generally an affectionate child at home. At the time, however, Rachel had been demonstrating problematic behaviors involving oppositional behavior toward adult authority figures. When difficulties arose, Rachel frequently blamed others and often complained that adults were "unfair."

Life Stress Assessment

A survey of Rachel's life history indicated that she had experienced nine potentially stressful life events and situations: beginning school, changing schools, learning problems, speech problems, poor grades, change in peer acceptance, hospitalization of a parent, increased arguments with parents, and increased incidence of lying and dishonesty. This number of potentially stressful experiences means that, when compared with a sample of other 12-year-olds, Rachel placed at the 71st percentile, or the high range, of risk on this factor.

The Thematic Apperception Test was administered to identify those experiences that might be perceived as potentially stressful for Rachel. A need-threat analysis of the results indicated that, for Rachel, the most important experiences were those events and situations where the need for achievement or the threat of failure was involved. Content analysis suggested that Rachel's concerns about achievement were tied to her perceptions of parental expectations.

A review of Rachel's background and current situation suggested that stress effects were particularly evident in the school functioning and, to a lesser extent, in the family relations domains. Rachel tended to cope with stress by adopting a passive-aggressive response style. This response style is characterized by passive resistance, evident in Rachel's low level of motivation, underachievement, and carelessness. In addition, Rachel was employing more active oppositional behavior including stubborn and defiant behaviors and temper outbursts. While this response is often an ineffective and counterproductive means of coping, it was one that Rachel was likely to adopt in a situation perceived as stressful. Parent ratings placed her behavior at the level of a severe emotional adjustment reaction when compared with other 12-year-olds. The life-stress assessment, therefore, suggested that Rachel was responding to the perceived stress of parental expectations, which she saw as unrealistic, by adopting a passive and resistant response pattern.

Summary

Rachel was a 12-year-old functioning within the high average to superior range of intelligence, with the potential for academic success at her age/grade level. She was seen for psychological assessment because she had been demonstrating problematic behavior in school and at home.

Rachel seemed to have many of the concerns of a young adolescent, especially those relating to adult authority. She had been demonstrating both passive and active oppositional behaviors that were affecting her home and school functioning. The developing conflict around Rachel's achievement was not likely to be resolved in the absence of a planned behavioral intervention.

Benefits and Limitations

Six major benefits are as follows:

- Unlike many behavior rating scales, the SRS is theory based. It provides for interpretation of results in the context of the child's life-stress experience.
- Using SRS information within the context of a child's life-stress assessment helps facilitate communication with parents and teachers. Stress is an experience familiar to the general public, and most people can easily understand that children may have difficulty in responding to stress, real or perceived.
- The SRS is a relatively brief form (one page; 40 items), and teachers and parents show little resistance to completing it.
- It provides a look at behavior to complement other

methods of assessment often used with children, such as projective techniques, standardized tests, and interviews, each of which might offer its own unique perspective and contribute to a comprehensive assessment.

■ The SRS Profile allows the child to be compared with other children who have shown a similar stress response pattern, thus aiding in grouping, prediction, and clinical decision making.

■ Intervention can be directly linked with assessment in that behavior management strategies that have been used effectively with children showing similar stress response patterns can be applied in the case under study (Chandler, 1992).

Major limitations are as follows:

■ The SRS is a theory-based instrument, and if the hypothesized model is not accepted, then the extent to which the results represent stress responses may be called into question.

■ The SRS yields information on only one perspective on the child, and it should never be used in isolation in making clinical decisions.

■ Some find the instrument tedious to score, and the use of the computer-assisted scoring is highly recommended for both accuracy and efficiency.

Chapter References

American Psychiatric Association. (1980). *Diagnostic and Statistical Manual* (3rd ed.). Washington, DC: American Psychiatric Association.

Atherley, E. A. (1990). *The relationship between coping responses and related variables in a group of high-risk adolescents.* Unpublished doctoral dissertation, University of Pittsburgh, Pittsburgh, PA.

Bartolomucci, E. (1986). *The effects of depressive symptoms on the quality of parenting and intimate relationships in single black women.* Unpublished master's project, University of Pittsburgh, Pittsburgh, PA.

Batterman, J. L. (1989). *The relationship between children's age and their stress response style.* Unpublished research project, University of Pittsburgh, Pittsburgh, PA.

Chandler, L. A. (1979). *A classification scheme for behavior disorders.* Unpublished manuscript, University of Pittsburgh, Pittsburgh, PA.

Chandler, L. A. (1982). *Children under stress: Understanding emotional adjustment reactions.* Springfield, IL: Thomas.

Chandler, L. A. (1983). The Stress Response Scale: An instrument for use in assessing emotional adjustment reactions. *School Psychology Review, 12*(3), 260–265.

Chandler, L. A. (1984). Behavioral responses of children to stress. In J. H. Humphrey (Ed.), *Stress in childhood.* New York: AMS Press.

Chandler, L. A. (1985). *Assessing stress in children.* New York: Praeger.

Chandler, L. A. (1988). *A stress paradigm for the assessment of children's emotional status: An interim report.* Paper presented at the annual convention of the American Psychological Association, Atlanta, GA.

Chandler, L. A., El-Samadony, E. I., Shermis, M. D., & El-Khatib, A.T. (1991). Behavioral responses of children to stress. *School Psychology International, 12*, 197–209.

Chandler, L. A., & Lundahl, W. T. (1983). Empirical classification of emotional adjustment reactions. *American Journal of Orthopsychiatry, 5*(3), 460–467.

Chandler, L. A., & Maurer, A. M. (1996). Behavioural responses of children to stress: A Polish-American cross-cultural study. *International Journal of Behavioral Development, 19*(3), 639–650.

Chandler, L. A., & Shermis, M. D. (1985). Assessing behavioral responses to stress. *Educational and Psychological Measurement, 45*, 825–844.

Chandler, L. A., & Shermis, M. D. (1986). Behavioral responses to stress: Profile patterns of children. *Journal of Clinical Child Psychology, 15*(4), 317–323.

Chandler, L. A., & Shermis, M. D. (1990). A paradigm for the study of childhood stress. In J. H. Humphrey (Ed.), *Human stress: Current selected research (Vol. 4,* pp. 111–124). New York: AMS Press.

Chandler, L. A., Shermis, M. D., & Marsh, J. (1985). The use of the Stress Response Scale in diagnostic assessment. *Journal of Psychoeducational Assessment, 3,* 15–29.

Clarizio, H. F., & McCoy, G. F. (1978). Behavior disorders of children. New York: Crowell.

Compas, B. E. (1987). Coping with stress during childhood and adolescence. *Psychological Bulletin, 101*(3), 391–403.

Coyne, J. C., & Lazarus, R. S. (1980). Cognitive style, stress perception, and coping. In I. L. Kutash et al. (Eds.), *Handbook on stress and anxiety* (pp. 144–158). San Francisco: Jossey-Bass.

Curlee, J. (1986). *Effects of intimate relationships on child adjustment in a sample of black inner-city women.* Unpublished master's project, University of Pittsburgh, Pittsburgh, PA.

Dasuki, M. A. (1986). *A comparison of Stress Response Scale scores among various groups of children.* Unpublished master's thesis, University of Pittsburgh, Pittsburgh, PA.

Edelbrock, C. (1979). Empirical classification of children's behavior disorders: Progress based on parent and teacher ratings. *School Psychology Review, 8,* 355–369.

Endler, N. S. (1980). Person-situation interaction and anxiety. In I. L. Kutash et al., (Eds.,) *Handbook on stress and anxiety* (pp. 249–266). San Francisco: Jossey-Bass.

Endler, N. S., & Magnusson, D. (1976). Toward an interactional psychology of personality. *Psychological Bulletin, 83,* 947–956.

Gibson, J. T., & DiPaula, M. (1989, May). Providing increased tactile contact in Venezuelan preschools: Touching and children's behavior. *Poster presentation,* American Psychological Association, Washington, DC.

Goyette, C. H., Connors, C. K., & Ulrich, R. F. (1978). Normative data on the Revised Connor's Parent and Teacher Rating Scale. *Journal of Abnormal Child Psychology, 6,* 221–236.

Haan, N. (1977). *Coping and defending: Processes of self-environment organization.* New York: Academic Press.

Hoover, J. (1987). *Using a multitrait-multimethod matrix to examine childhood stress.* Unpublished doctoral dissertation, University of Pittsburgh, Pittsburgh, PA.

Hughes, C. A. (1986). *Cross validation of children's behavior categories using behavior rating scales.* Paper presented at the annual convention of the National Association of School Psychologists, Hollywood, FL.

Johnson, G. (1989, July). Emotional indicators in the human figure drawings of hearing-impaired children: A small sample validation study. *American Annals of the Deaf*, 205–208.

Johnson, V. J. (1989). The contributions of children's histories, perceptions, and prior coping effectiveness to their behavioral responses to stress. Unpublished manuscript, University of Pittsburgh, Pittsburgh, PA.

Johnson, V. J., & Chandler, L. A. (1987). *Assessing the impact of stressful life events on children.* Paper presented at the annual convention of the National Association of School Psychologists, New Orleans, LA.

Kemmerer, A. (1984). *A comparison of the Stress Assessment System data of clinic-referred and non-referred children.* Unpublished master's project, University of Pittsburgh, Pittsburgh, PA.

Klerman, G. L. (1979). Stress, adaption, and affective disorders. In J. E. Barrett (Ed.), *Stress and mental disorder* (pp. 151–160). New York: Raven.

Krotec, S. C. (1982). *A comparison of behavior, personality, and academic variables of learning disabled, emotionally disturbed, and normal adolescents.* Unpublished doctoral dissertation, University of Pittsburgh, Pittsburgh, PA.

Lantz-Hecker, D. L. (1988). *Variables which relate to agreement between parent's and teacher's ratings of children's behavior.* Unpublished doctoral dissertation, University of Pittsburgh, Pittsburgh, PA.

Lantz-Hecker, D. L., & Chandler, L. A. (1988). *Parent and teacher agreement on behavior rating scales.* Paper presented at the annual convention of the National Association of School Psychologists, Chicago.

Lazarus, R. S., & Folkman, S. (1984). *Stress, appraisal, and coping.* New York: Springer.

Magnusson, D. (1982). Situational determinants of stress: An interactional perspective. In Goldberger & S. Breznitz (Eds.), *Handbook of stress: Theoretical and clinical aspects* (pp. 231–244). New York: Free Press.

Marsh, J. (1984). *An investigation of the validity and use of the Stress Response Scale.* Unpublished master's project, University of Pittsburgh, Pittsburgh, PA.

Million, M. E. (1987). Stressful life events, behavioral adjustment, and socioeconomic status as predictors of academic achievement. Unpublished doctoral dissertation, University of Pittsburgh.

Moos, R. H., & Billings, A. G. (1982). Conceptualizing and measuring coping responses and processes. In L. Goldberger & S. Brenitz (Eds.), *Handbook of stress: Theoretical and clinical aspects* (pp. 212–230). New York: Free Press.

Mramor, N. (1986). *Stress management for children through education and television.* Unpublished manuscript, Saybrook Institute, San Francisco.

Newsweek. (January 10, 1994). Pages 43–44.

Office of Educational Research and Improvement. (1994). *What do student grades mean: Differences across schools.* Washington, DC: U.S. Department of Education.

Piso, C. N. (1981). *A revision, factor analysis, and concurrent validity study of a children's behavior scale.* Unpublished doctoral dissertation, University of Pittsburgh, Pittsburgh, PA.

Quay, H. C. (1979). Classification. In H. C. Quay & J. S. Werry (Eds.), *Psychopathological disorders of childhood* (2nd ed., pp. 1–42). New York: Wiley.

Reed, R. A. (1993). A study of the relationship between childhood temperament and childhood stress response using theory-based behavior rating scales. Unpublished doctoral dissertation, University of Pittsburgh, Pittsburgh, PA.

Riva, M. T., & Chandler, L. A. (1989, August). *Developmental aspects of coping responses in children.* Paper presented at the annual convention of the American Psychological Association, New Orleans, LA.

Robinson, M. A., & Chandler, L. A. (1985, April). *Predicting school psychologists' recommendations from ratings on the Stress Response Scale.* Paper presented at the annual convention of the National Association of School Psychologists, Las Vegas, NV.

Rocchio, J. D. (1986). *Stress response patterns and associated characteristics of children referred for psychological services.* Unpublished doctoral dissertation, University of Pittsburgh, Pittsburgh, PA.

Rodriguez, T. K. (1994). *Student level of competency as related to the restrictiveness of their special education placement.* Unpublished doctoral dissertation, University of Pittsburgh, Pittsburgh, PA.

Rosenberg, L. (1987). *The association of children's thematic productions and their behavior.* Unpublished master's project, University of Pittsburgh, Pittsburgh, PA.

Shermis, M. D., & Chandler, L. A. (1985). *A confirmatory factor analysis of the Stress Response Scale.* Unpublished manuscript, University of Pittsburgh, Pittsburgh, PA.

Shermis, M. D., Ruden, D., & Chandler, L. A. (1992). An extension of the norms for the Stress Response Scale for Children. *Journal of Psychoeducational Assessment, 10,* 65–75.

Tartaglione, D. A. (1991). *The use of stress-related information with children referred for psychological services.* Unpublished doctoral dissertation, University of Pittsburgh, Pittsburgh, PA.

Thoits, P. A. (1983). Dimensions of life events that influence psychological distress: An evaluation and synthesis of the literature. In H. B. Kaplan (Ed.), *Psychosocial stress: Trends in theory and research* (pp. 33–87). New York: Academic Press.

Thomas, A., & Chess, S. (1977). *Temperament and development.* New York: Brunner/Mazel.

Thomas, A., Chess, S., & Birch, J. (1968). *Temperament and behavior disorders.* New York: New York University Press.

Vercruysse, N., & Chandler, L. A. (1992). Coping stragegies used by adolescents in dealing with family relocation overseas. *Journal of Adolescence, 15,* 67–82.

White, R. (1974). Strategies of adaption: An attempt at systematic description. In G. Coelho, D. Hamburg, & J. Adams (Eds.), *Coping and adaptation.* New York: Basic Books.

Winikoff, M. (1986). *Behavioral adjustment and quality of significant adult male/child relationship: A preliminary study of low income, school-aged black children.* Unpublished master's project, University of Pittsburgh, Pittsburgh, PA.

Witkin, H. A., & Goodenough, D. R. (1977). Field dependence and interpersonal behavior. *Psychological Bulletin, 34,* 661–689.

The Stress Response Scale for Adolescents

Gerald R. Adams, University of Guelph

■ Instrument Names

The Stress Response Scale for Adolescents
SRSA

■ Developers

Steven Curtis, Ph.D., and Gerald R. Adams, Ph.D., University
of Guelph

■ Contact Information

Gerald R. Adams, Department of Family Studies, University
of Guelph, Guelph, Ontario NIG 2W1 Canada
Telephone: (519) 824-4120; e-mail: gadams@uoguelph.ca

Description and History of the Instrument

Although specialists on adolescence have suggested specific developmental, social, physical, and environmental stresses on adolescent behavior, few reliable or valid measures of stress reactions have been constructed for use in a practice setting with adolescents. In discussions about stress among teenagers, considerable attention has been given to two forms of stressors. Normative stressors have been suggested (e.g., Cohen, Burt, & Bjorck, 1987; Hamburg, 1974; Konopka, 1980) that include, among others, hormonal changes affecting physical growth and emotions, changes in family and peer relationships, and environmental transitions due to changes in school structures, school organization, or new educational experiences. Nonnormative stressors have often been defined and identified in the form of social and emotional adjustment, developmental delay, and adolescent psychopathology. To remedy the shortage of measurement, a series of investigations have been undertaken (Curtis & Adams, 1991), with refinements and adaptations developed. The final outcome is a stress response scale for use with early through late adolescent populations.

The Stress-Response Scale for Adolescents prototype (Curtis, 1989) was designed to be a self-perceived stress response measure for ages 14 to 20. The original scale began with 62 items that were completed on a 5-point scale ranging from "not at all" to "extremely so." In a series of studies reported elsewhere (Curtis & Adams, 1991), the instrument was reduced to 32 items with separate scales for males and females. In further work, the scale has been reduced to 10 easy-to-read, quick-to-score items that can be commonly used for males and females. The items in this scale are based on large random samples of a known population. Reliability and validity are based either on purposeful group comparisons or experimental methodologies.

Underlying Assumptions and Concepts

Several definitions and conceptual models of stress underpin the development of the SRSA. Four common definitions of stress, for instance, focus on stimulus, response, interactional, and informational components (Feuerstein, Labbu, & Kuczmierczyk, 1986). These may be summarized as follows:

- The *stimulus* definition identifies stress in terms of the stimulus characteristics for the individual. The stimuli that are disruptive are called stressors, and the response is called the strain. Prior research focusing on the study of stressful situations or life events can be categorized as stimulus-focused perspectives (e.g., Csikszentmihalyi & Larson, 1984; Holmes & Rahe, 1967).

■ The *response* model of stress focuses on the response to a stressor. As Selye (1980) indicates, stress is "the non-specific response of the body to any demand" (p. 127). Therefore, the stress response is a psychological or physiological, pleasant (eustress) or unpleasant (distress) reaction to the stressor. In the Selye model, stress responses progress through various states of general adaptation. This includes a stage of alarm reaction leading to body adaptations to the stressor but a concurrent reduction in resistance to other stressors, then exhaustion and maladjustment, and finally decline, disease, and trauma.

■ In the *interactional* model of stress, the person is viewed as having an influence on the impact of a stressor through self-regulation mechanisms (Feuerstein et al., 1986). For example, perceptions of stressors, through a process of cognitive appraisals, can moderate the impact of stress (see Coyne & Lazarus, 1980). In this model, stress occurs when the person perceives a difference between the demands of the stressor and the ability to cope with it. Individual characteristics of the person are thought to lead to variations in cognitive appraisals, resulting in feedback loops that modify the impact of a stressor through self-regulation mechanisms.

■ *Informational-processing* definitions consider both the stressor and response and the individual's interpretation of the stimuli as stressful. For example, Hamilton (1980) proposed such a model of stress, indicating that stress means people are faced with demands on their behavior that they find difficult to meet. These demands require the use of physiological energy, rapid processing of stimuli, and a search for responses that yield a subjective state of calmness. When appropriate processes, operations, or outcomes are only partially available, the person is thought to be under stress.

All of these definitions of stress are useful. However, relatively little attention has been given to a model of stress for adolescents that includes a developmental perspective. Sometime ago, Petersen and Spiga (1982) described a *biopsychosocial developmental* model in which both normative developmental events and unpredictable life events serve as stressors. Furthermore, they suggested that stress responses are thought to have behavioral, affective, and physiological components. As a foundation to building on this model, an appropriate stress response scale was validated for use by practitioners to assess the influence of biological, social, and contextual stressor influences.

Operationalizations

Several basic conceptualizations have been formulated in the development of this measure, as follows:

- The term *stress* is replaced by the term *stress process*. The stress process is the continual transaction between the person and environment in which demands are placed on the individual requiring adaptation.
- *Adaptation* is the change in behavior that has survival value to handle current or impending environmental demands.

The stress process is divided into the stressor, mediation mechanisms, and stress response:

- *Stressors*, which can be internal or external, are those events in which the individual experiences discomfort and must make changes to adapt.
- *Mediation mechanisms* include such things as cognitive appraisal, coping skills, personality characteristics, individual vulnerabilities, and information evaluations to perceived threat. All of these mediation mechanisms influence how a person responds to a stressor and account

for variations between individuals in their stress responses to similar stressors.

■ *Stress responses* are simply the reactions to stressors. Stress responses have cognitive/emotional, physiological, and behavioral components. It is important to note that anxiety is a natural emotional component of a stress response. A stress response includes physiological reactions to stressors such as an increasing heart rate, a decrease in blood flow to the extremities, and a rise in blood pressure. It also includes subjective feelings of fear, depression, mind racing, mental confusion, and mood changes, among other cognitive/emotional components. Behavioral components can include such things as overt aggression, crying, restlessness, impulsive behaviors, or withdrawal. Psychological manifestations of the behavioral component can come in the form of defensive mechanisms. Finally, it is essential to restate that exposure to repeated stressors, which are recognized as threatening and overdemanding of one's energy and for which the impact has not been reduced, will result in psychological, behavioral, or physiological pathology.

Psychometric Characteristics

Four original psychometric studies were completed (Curtis & Adams, 1991). I have completed two additional unpublished studies. These six studies are summarized here to describe the psychometric foundation for this measure.

Study 1

Initially, 34 items were prepared that described physiological, behavioral, and cognitive/emotional components of stress. Items were developed in short "I" statements, and a 5-point Likert-type scale was used as follows: 1 = not at all; 2 = somewhat so; 3 = moderately so; 4 = quite a bit; 5 = extremely so. Instructions on how to complete the scale included a statement of whether and to what degree the respondent was currently experiencing (last 5 days) the circumstance stated in each item. Subjects also completed the Life Events Checklist (Johnson & McCutcheon, 1980), the State-Trait Anxiety Inventory (Spielberger, 1973), a brief version of the Marlowe-Crowne Social Desirability Scale (Strahan & Gerbasi, 1972), and measures of psychopathology and superior adjustment (Offer, Ostrov, & Howard, 1981).

One hundred forty-two adolescent high school and college-aged youths (14–21 years; 76 males, 66 females) completed all instrumentation. All subjects were middle-class, of white European ancestry, and had two parents in their home.

A standard principal components factor analysis using varimax rotation resulted in a single factor accounting for 46% of the variance. This factor included 19 items. Coefficient alpha for the 19 items was .95. The Stress Response Scale for Adolescents (SRSA) correlated .69 with state and .66 with trait anxiety ($ps < .01$). As expected, anxiety was associated with the stress response. However, when this association was extracted from the remaining associations using partial correlations, the stress response scores not only were predictive of greater self-reported psychopathology and adjustment problems but were also predicted by more frequent stressful life events. There was no association between the stress response score and social desirability. Finally, a test of normality revealed a normal distribution of scores. And when raw scale scores were converted to T-scores, subjects with scores greater than 60, when contrasted with those equal to or less than 60, were found on average to manifest greater psychopathology, less adjustment, and more state and trait anxiety and to have more life event stressors.

Study 2

Role enactment methodology (see Adams & Schvaneveldt, 1985) was used in this study. Students (12 males, 25 females;

mean age = 17.5 years) were provided with a low-stress or a high-stress script and asked to complete the SRSA items in a manner that reflected how they would feel in that context. A significant t-test ($p < .05$) revealed that subjects perceived themselves as being more stressed in the high-stress versus low-stress role enactment condition.

Study 3

Again, using role enactment methodology, subjects (23 male, 33 female high school students; mean age = 17.6 years) read a script depicting a scene that was stressful or nonstressful and completed the SRSA. Next, they were asked to read an opposite script and complete the SRSA again. Significant t-tests ($ps < .05$) were observed for both forms of reversal. That is, a high-stress condition resulted in higher SRSA scores, with the low-stress condition resulting in a lower stress score.

Study 4

In a large introductory class, 110 university students completed the SRSA and on a 5-point scale were questioned to what degree they viewed themselves as having test anxiety. During the midterm examination, subjects completed the SRSA items again. Subjects scoring low ("not at all") versus high ("extremely so") on the text anxiety item were compared on their SRSA scores. Ten males and 12 females scored low on test anxiety, and 11 males and 14 females scored high. An analysis of variance (ANOVA), using a 2 (high vs. low text anxiety) × 2 (male vs. female) factorial, revealed a significant main effect but no interaction. That is, high-anxiety subjects scored higher in their SRSA scores than did the low-anxiety comparison group.

A correlation was computed between the two tests of the SRSA measure. The test-retest reliability of the measure was moderate ($r = .64$, $p < .05$). Internal consistency was alpha = .84 and .82, for each of the two points of measurement.

Study 5

Research (Steinberg, 1987; Steinberg & Hill, 1978) suggests that when a comparison is made between prepubertal, early pubertal, and postpubertal adolescents, the family relationship patterns reflect little conflict for prepubertal adolescent families, considerable conflict for early pubertal families, and a return to less conflict for postpubertal families. A similar pattern in stress responses as measured by the SRSA should be expected, given that conflict is generally viewed as stressful.

In an unpublished investigation, 20 boys and 20 girls were compared, for each of the three pubertal statuses on perceived family conflict and stress. A 2 (boys vs. girls) × 3 (pre, early, and postpubertal) factorial ANOVA was computed for both stress and perceived conflict. Conflict was assessed using the Family Environment subscale measure of conflict in the family. A significant main effect for pubertal status was observed for both conflict and stress ($ps < .01$). Individual comparisons revealed the same pattern for both measures. Prepubertal children reported little stress or conflict, early pubertal adolescents reported the highest level of conflict and stress, and the postpubertal youths scored almost identically to the prepubertal children. Internal reliability, as measured by Cronbach's alpha, averaged to .83.

Study 6

The final investigation included a comparison of four groups of teenagers between the ages of 13 and 18 years (50 boys and 50 girls of mixed ethnic heritage for each group, overall 67% white, 14% black, 8% Asian, 2% Native American, with the remaining 9% undeclared). The first group, thought to be the least-stress group, consisted of students who were getting average to above-average grades, were regular school attenders, came from two-parent households, and were from homes with incomes above average for their community. The second group consisted of adolescents who were defined by school personnel as having chronic school absenteeism but obtaining passing grades. The third group consisted of youth who were school dropouts or facing suspension from school for one semester or more. Finally, the fourth group consisted of school drop outs who were facing legal charges of various types. Each of these groups, moving from first to fourth, was thought to have cumulatively greater stressors.

All adolescents completed the SRSA. The 400 respondents' scores were entered into a principal components factor analysis using varimax rotation. A single significant factor emerged that exceeded an eigenvalue of 1.0. This factor included the 10 items (alpha = .91) that comprise the recommended version of the SRSA. These items are found in Table 1.

The sum of these items were compared for group differences using an ANOVA and a 2 (boys vs. girls) × 4 (successful school attenders, successful school nonattenders, dropouts

Table 1: Items for the Stress Response Scale for Adolescents

I feel overwhelmed.

I have tight muscles.

I am worried.

I have frequent accidents.

I get confused.

I am having trouble relating to people.

I am frustrated.

I feel stressed.

I find my mind goes blank.

I feel nervous.

---

or suspended, dropouts pending legal charges) factorial. Only a significant main effect ($p < .05$) for groups was observed (see Table 2 for means and standard deviations). The successful school attenders were the least stressed. The nonattenders and suspended groups were significantly more stressed than the school attenders. And the dropouts pending legal charges were the most stressed of the four groups.

Summary

The psychometric foundation of the SRSA is based on the conceptualization that a stress process involves a stress response to stressors that is mediated by contextual conditions or individual characteristics of the person. The instrument was revised and trimmed through a series of factor analyses to arrive at 10 highly internally consistent items. The items have been found to be predicted by life event stressors, even when state and trait anxiety are controlled for through partial correlation techniques. Likewise, high SRSA scores have been found to be related to poor adjustment. In none of the investigations did social desirability play a role in respondents' self-reports. No significant gender differences were observed in

Table 2: Means and Standard Deviations for Four Comparison Groups

Group	Mean	Standard Deviation
Successful school attender	17.2	4.2
Successful nonschool attender	26.5	6.0
Dropouts/suspended	31.9	5.6
Dropouts facing legal action	39.7	4.7

Note: Scale ranges from a low of 10 and a high of 50 based on the 10 items in Table 1.

the construction of the measure. Further, role enactment studies indicate that the levels of stress in social conditions predict theoretically appropriate stress response levels. Furthermore, in a field study students with high test anxiety were observed to manifest higher SRSA scores. A comparative study of pubertal status among adolescents demonstrated that the SRSA detects higher stress for adolescents in more conflicted homes based on entry into puberty. And comparisons between adolescents in different levels of stressful school and legal conditions can be differentiated by corresponding levels of stress responses as measured by the SRSA. These last two studies indicate that the SRSA can be used to assess stress responses based on a biopsychosocial developmental model (as suggested in Petersen & Spiga, 1982).

Applications

The Stress Response Scale for Adolescents is a self-report assessment of stress. It is a brief measure that can be used with children as young as 10 years of age and extended for use with early, middle, and late adolescents. It is most recommended for students in the high school and early college-age years. The items are simple self-statements and are based on limited reading skills. The instrument should only be used as a simple screening device of a child's or adolescent's current stress response (most recent 5 days). While it is a measure of individual differences, it can be used to detect changes in a child's state of stress. Higher scores suggest greater stressors in a child's or adolescent's life. Likewise, the Stress Response Scale is a measure of the combination of behavioral, emotional, cognitive, and physiological components of stress. It should be noted that the measure has a strong component of anxiety. However, it goes beyond anxiety as a measure of the stress response. Finally, the instrument can be used to detect stress in both normative and nonnormative contexts associated with adolescent development.

At this time no cutoffs are suggested for use in detecting an at-risk adolescent or in categorizing an adolescent as being at low, moderate, or high stress. Evidence in Table 2 suggests that youth with scores at or above 30 points are likely to be experiencing enough risk that interventions may be called for to reduce the stress process.

Chapter References

Adams, G. R., & Schvaneveldt, J. D. (1985). *Understanding research methods.* New York: Longman.

Cohen, L. H., Burt, C. E., & Bjorck, J. P. (1987). Life stress and adjustment: effects of life events experienced by young adolescents and their parents. *Developmental Psychology, 23,* 583–592.

Coyne, L. C., & Lazarus, R. S. (1980). Cognitive style, stress perception, and coping. In I. L. Kutash, & L. B. Schlesinger (Eds.), *Handbook of stress and anxiety: Contemporary knowledge, theory, and treatment* (pp. 144–158). San Francisco: Jossey-Bass.

Csikszentmihalyi, M., & Larson, R. (1984). *Being adolescent: Conflict and growth in the teenage years.* New York: Basic Books.

Curtis, S. (1989). *The development of the stress-response scale for adolescents.* Unpublished manuscript, Department of Psychology, Utah State University, Logan, UT.

Curtis, S., & Adams, G. R. (1991). The development of a stress response scale for adolescents. *Journal of Adolescent Research, 6,* 454–469.

Feuerstein, M., Labbu, E. E., & Kuczmierczyk, A. R. (1986). *Health psychology: A psychobiological perspective.* New York: Plenum.

Hamburg, D. A. (1974). Early adolescence: A specific and stressful stage of the life cycle. In G. V. Coelho, D. A. Hamburg, & J. E. Adams (Eds.), *Coping and adaptation* (pp. 101–124). New York: Basic Books.

Hamilton, V. (1980). An information processing analysis of environmental stress and life crisis. In I. G. Sarason & C. D. Spielberger (Eds.), *Stress and anxiety* (vol. 7, pp. 13–30). Washington, DC: Hemisphere.

Holmes, T. H., & Rahe, R. H. (1967). The social readjustment rating scale. *Journal of Psychosomatic Research, 11,* 213–218.

Johnson, J. H., & McCutcheon, S. (1980). Assessing life stress in older children and adolescents: Preliminary findings with the life events checklist. In I. G. Sarason & C. D. Spielberger (Eds.), *Stress and anxiety* (vol. 7, pp. 111–125). Washington, DC: Hemisphere.

Konopka G. (1980). Stresses and strains in adolescents and young adults. In L. A. Bond & J. C. Rosen (Eds.), *Competence and coping during adulthood* (pp. 178–194). Hanover, NH: University Press of New England.

Offer, D., Ostrov, E., & Howard, K. (1981). *The adolescent: A psychological self-portrait*. New York: Basic Books.

Petersen, A. C., & Spiga, R. (1982). Adolescent and stress. In L. Goldberger & S. Breznitz (Eds.), *Handbook of stress: Theoretical and clinical aspects* (pp. 515–528). New York: Free Press.

Selye, H. (1980). The stress concept today. In I. L. Kutash & L. B. Schlesinger (Eds.), *Handbook on stress and anxiety: Contemporary knowledge, theory, and treatment* (pp. 127–143). San Francisco: Jossey-Bass.

Spielberger, C. (1973). *Preliminary test manual for the State-Trait Anxiety Inventory for Children*. Palo Alto, CA: Consulting Psychologists Press.

Steinberg, L. D. (1981). Transformation in family relations at puberty. *Developmental Psychology, 17,* 833–840.

Steinberg, L. D., & Hill, J. P. (1978). Patterns of family interaction as a function of age, the onset of puberty, and formal thinking. *Developmental Psychology, 14,* 683–684.

Strahan, R., & Gerbasi, K. C. (1972). Short, homogeneous version of the Marlowe-Crowne Social Desirability Scale. *Journal of Clinical Psychology, 28,* 191–193.

Student-Life Stress Inventory

Bernadette M. Gadzella, Texas A & M
University–Commerce

- ## Instrument Name

Student-Life Stress Inventory*

- ## Developer

Bernadette M. Gadzella, Texas A & M
University–Commerce†[2]

- ## Contact Information

Dr. Bernadette M. Gadzella, Department of Psychology and
Special Education, Texas A & M University–Commerce,
East Texas Station, Commerce, TX 75429
Telephone: (903) 886-5588 or (903) 886-6862

Description and History of the Instrument

Stress is a complex concept, difficult to define. There are different kinds of stress, and most people experience some kind
of stress. Over the years, theorists and researchers have tried
to define stress and study it in various ways (Gadzella, 1994b).
Holmes and Rahe (1967) refer to stress as a *stimulus* event, a
relationship between one's stressful life events and physical
illness. Their theory is that changes in personal relationships,
work, and so forth (which could be welcomed events), can

---

*Registered under Bernadette M. Gadzella, Ph.D.
†Formerly known as East Texas State University, Commerce, TX 75429.

also be stressful. They developed the Social Readjustment Rating Scale in which readjustments due to changes in major life events were assigned numerical values. Critics argued that the scale did not measure changes exclusively and that it was difficult to interpret its findings (Weiten, Lloyd, & Lashley, 1990). Other researchers (Sarason, Johnson, & Siegel, 1978) have attempted to correct many of the problems criticized in the earlier scale. Horowitz and Wilner (1980) have studied stressful life events with their Life Events Questionnaire.

Selye (1976) views stress as a *response* (physiological arousal) elicited by some events (stimuli). He formulated a theory about stress reactions known as the General Adaptation Syndrome. In his model, stress responses go through three stages: alarm, resistance, and exhaustion. The alarm reaction occurs when an organism recognizes a threat. If the threat continues, a physiological arousal arises. It can then level off as the organism becomes accustomed to the threat. If the stress continues, the body's resources for fighting it may be depleted, and then the organism enters the exhaustive stage. Selye believes a relationship exits between a person's stress and illness.

Other researchers (Lazarus & Folkman, 1984) describe stress as a specific *stimulus-response transaction*. In this model, the stress one experiences is not in the event (situation) or in a person but in the *transaction* between the event and the person, depending on how the person appraises the situation and adapts to it (Goleman, 1979; Weiten et al., 1990). Lazarus and Folkman's focus is on the cognitive interpretations (appraisals) of the stressful situation. One appraisal is about the initial evaluation of the stressful event and the other about whether the individual has the resources and effective strategies to deal with the stress (Martin & Osborne, 1993).

The work done by these previous theorists and researchers helped me understand how stress can be defined, and influenced the development of my Student-Life Stress Inventory. Most of the research mentioned focuses on specific groups of people. The Student-Life Stress Inventory (Gadzella, 1991) is an instrument that focuses on understanding and assisting students to identify and evaluate their experiences both on and off campus. That is, it is meant to study students' global experiences rather than only those experiences related to their course work.

Stress can be viewed as a positive or negative experience. Evaluation of one's overall perception of stress may be mild, moderate, or severe. In the Student-Life Stress Inventory, stressors are considered to be events or conditions (stimuli) that demand adjustments beyond the normal trials of daily living. These stressors may cause various reactions or responses (physiological, emotional, and/or behavioral), which may or may not be difficult to cope with. The reactions to stressors can also be viewed as appraisals (cognitive interpretation) in which stressors are evaluated as relevant or irrelevant. The appraisals determine whether one can recognize the stressors and has the strategies to cope with them effectively (Gadzella, 1994b).

My interest and development of the Student-Life Stress Inventory began with undergraduate students who were enrolled in my psychology classes, which included the study of stress. Students were given the opportunity, as class assignments, to meet in small groups and list their stressors and the reactions to the stressors they experienced. They submitted their ideas in statements, and each student rated each of the statements. These statements were evaluated by all groups. The next semester, several other groups of students were given similar assignments on stress. They listed their stressors and reactions to stressors under the headings on stress suggested in the texts that were used by Coleman, Morris, & Glaros (1987) and Morris (1990). These headings became the model for the inventory. It included types of stressors (frustrations, conflicts, pressures, changes, and self-imposed) and reactions to stressors (physiological, emotional, behavioral, and cognitive).

During the following semesters, other groups of students evaluated and rated the statements. The data were analyzed by different (gender and class status) groups and provided to each of the classes. These data were only used as feedback for their class assignment and were not saved for future use. However, I felt that an instrument should be developed and used in my future classes that cover stress.

The Instrument

The items were set up in a questionnaire and copyrighted as the Student-Life Stress Inventory (Gadzella, 1991). An answer sheet was designed so that responses to the inventory could be collected systematically and analyzed. This inventory is a self-reporting instrument that consists of two types of responses. First, subjects report whether they perceive their overall stress as mild, moderate, or severe. Then, they rank each of the 51 items in the inventory using a 5-point Likert scale in which 1 = never, 2 = seldom, 3 = occasionally, 4 = often, and 5 = most of the time. The 51 items appear under nine categories (five stressors and four reactions to stressors). Each item is ranked separately.

Stressors

Following is a summary of examples under the Stressors category:

- *Frustrations* (7 items) deal with delays in reaching goals, experiencing daily hassles, lacking resources, failing to reach goals, being socially unacceptable, having dating frustrations, and perceiving denied opportunities.
- *Conflicts* (3 items) are things producing two or more desirable alternatives, things producing two or more undesirable alternatives, and things producing both desirable and undesirable alternatives.
- *Pressures* (4 items) are stress due to competition, deadlines, overload, and interpersonal relationships.
- *Changes* (3 items) are stress due to unpleasant changes,

too many occurring rapidly and those that disrupt a person from attaining life goals.

■ *Self-imposed* (6 items) are stress due to competing, seeking personal attention, worrying, procrastinating, assuming perfection, and experiencing test anxiety.

Reactions to Stressors

Following is a summary of examples under Reactions to Stressors.

■ *Physiological* (14 items): experiencing sweat, stuttering, trembling (biting fingernails), rapid movements, exhaustion, irritable bowels, asthma, backaches, hives, headaches, arthritis, viruses, weight loss, or weight gain.

■ *Emotional* (4 items): experiencing fear and anxiety, anger, guilt, grief, and depression.

■ *Behavioral* (8 items): having cried, abused others, abused self, smoked excessively, been irritable toward others, attempted suicide, used defense mechanisms, or separated oneself from others.

■ *Cognitive appraisal* (2 items): analyzed stressful situations and determined whether strategies used were effective.

A portion of the Student-Life Stress Inventory and its answer sheet are shown as illustrations of the instrument.

Scoring the inventory is done by summing the ratings of each item and recording the values for each of the first eight categories. In the last category (Cognitive), the ratings of the two items are first reversed, then summed and recorded. To obtain the total stress score, the values of the nine categories are summated.

The objectives in developing the inventory were to get students actively involved in evaluating their stressors and reactions to stressors. Over the years, scores were systematically collected and analyzed by total groups, gender, age, marital

Student-Life Stress Inventory
Bernadette M. Gadzella, Ph. D., 1991 Copyright
East Texas State University

Student-Life Stress Inventory
Bernadette M. Gadzella, Ph. D., 1991 Copyright
East Texas State University

This inventory contains statements dealing with student-life stress. Read it carefully and respond to each statement as it has related or is relating to you as a students. Use the 5-point scale which indicates the level of your experiences with:

| 1 = never, 2 = seldom, 3 = occasionally, 4 = often, 5 = most of the time |

Record your responses on the accompanying answer sheet.

I. Stressors:

A. As a student:

1. I have experienced frustrations due to delays in reaching my goal.
2. I have experienced daily hassles which affected me in reaching my goals.
3. I have experienced lack of sources (money for auto, books, etc.).
4. I have experienced failures in accomplishing the goals that I set.
5. I have not been accepted socially (became a social outcast).
6. I have experienced dating frustrations.
7. I feel I was denied opportunities in spite of my qualifications.

B. I have experienced conflicts which were:

8. Produced by two or more desirable alternatives.
9. Produced by two or more undesirable alternatives.
10. Produced when a goal had both positive and negative alternatives.

status, and stress levels (mild, moderate, and severe). Data were provided as feedback information for students to make their comparisons with different groups (gender, class status, etc.). The data were also used for various research studies that were presented in conferences and published as articles in journals.

Summary of Research

Validity

Studies were conducted to determine whether the inventory measures what it sets out to measure (i.e., students who per-

Answer Sheet to Student-Life Stress Inventory
Copyright 1991
Bernadette M. Gadzella, Ph.D.
East Texas State University

Answer Sheet to Student-Life Stress Inventory
Copyright 1991
Bernadette M. Gadzella, Ph. D.
East Texas State University

Name _____ Course _____	
Marital Status: Married _____ Single _____ Single Parent _____	
Number and Age of Children; None _____ Children _____	
Commuting: No ___ Single ___ If Yes, round-trip mileage _____	
Average hours studying per week: _____	
Average hours working (employed) _____	

Rate your overall level of stress
Mild _____ Moderate _____ Severe _____

Respond to each statement in the Student-Life Stress Inventory by
recording the level of your experience on the 5-point scale with
1 = never, 2 = seldom, 3 = occasionally, 4 = often, 5 = most of the time

	1	2	3	4	5			1	2	3	4	5
A. 1.	_	_	_	_	_	F.	27.	_	_	_	_	_
2.	_	_	_	_	_		28.	_	_	_	_	_
3.	_	_	_	_	_		29.	_	_	_	_	_
4.	_	_	_	_	_		30.	_	_	_	_	_
5.	_	_	_	_	_		31.	_	_	_	_	_
6.	_	_	_	_	_		32.	_	_	_	_	_
7.	_	_	_	_	_		33.	_	_	_	_	_
							34.	_	_	_	_	_
B. 8.	_	_	_	_	_		35.	_	_	_	_	_
9.	_	_	_	_	_		36.	_	_	_	_	_
10.	_	_	_	_	_		37.	_	_	_	_	_

ceive their stress as mild, moderate, or severe) and whether
student responses differed to the 51 items on the inventory
and, specifically, to the nine categories in the inventory and
the total score. Several studies in which the three groups of
subjects reported their overall perceptions of stress (mild,
moderate, or severe) were compared on their scores with each
of the nine categories as well as the total stress score. With 530

subjects (Gadzella, Fullwood, & Tomcala, 1992), 87 subjects (Gadzella & Guthrie, 1993), and 290 subjects (Gadzella, 1994b), research results have established that there were significant differences among the three groups (mild, moderate, and severe) on all nine categories and total stress scores. In each case (except the Cognitive appraisal), the group reporting mild stress had lower mean scores than the groups that reported moderate and severe stress, respectively. And the group that reported having moderate stress had lower mean scores than the group that reported having severe stress. In the Cognitive appraisal, the severe group had the lowest mean score and the mild group the highest mean score. A sample of these data is shown in Table 1 (Gadzella & Guthrie, 1993).

In a recent study (Gadzella & Masten, 1997), scores on the stress inventory were correlated with scores on two instruments (Inventory of Learning Processes [ILP] and the Internality, Powerful Others, and Chance [IPC] Locus of Control). The ILP (Schmeck, Ribich, & Ramanaiah, 1977) is a self-reporting learning-style questionnaire with four scales. The Deep Processing scale (18 items) assesses the extent to which subjects evaluate, analyze, organize, compare, and contrast information. The Elaborative Processing scale (14 items) assesses evaluative strategies, how information is translated into one's own terms or personalized. The Fact Retention scale (7 items) assesses how facts are retained in memory. The Methodical Study scale (23 items) assesses study skills and the use-of-drill and practice approaches. The results of the correlations between the stress inventory scores and the ILP scores showed (a) significant *positive* correlations between Elaborative Processing (ILP scale) and Cognitive appraisal (reactions to stress) and (b) significant *negative* correlations between Deep Processing (ILP scale) and Frustrations (stress scale) and between the Methodical Study (ILP scale) and the Conflicts and Self-Imposed (stress scales) and Emotional (reaction to stress), respectively. Stated differently, the Elaborative Processing scale and Cognitive appraisal scale are similar in that they are evaluative scales, whereas the Deep Processing

Table 1: Differences among the Three Stress Level Groups (Mild, $n = 22$; Moderate, $n = 43$); Severe, $n = 22$) on the Nine Categories of the Stress Inventory

Category	Subtest	Group	Mean	SD	F-ratio
I. Stressors	Frustration	Mild	15.23	3.34	17.62*
		Moderate	18.77	3.68	
		Severe	21.36	3.05	
	Conflict	Mild	6.59	2.09	16.15*
		Moderate	8.40	2.03	
		Severe	9.95	1.70	
	Pressure	Mild	12.77	3.74	16.18*
		Moderate	14.91	2.29	
		Severe	17.77	3.15	
	Change	Mild	6.27	2.14	5.02*
		Moderate	7.60	2.24	
		Severe	11.64	2.82	
	Self-Imposed	Mild	20.09	3.94	8.57*
		Moderate	22.19	3.78	
		Severe	24.50	2.43	
II. Reactions to Stress	Physiological	Mild	21.59	4.32	73.39*
		Moderate	32.37	6.49	
		Severe	44.95	7.83	
	Emotional	Mild	9.27	2.85	49.80*
		Moderate	12.81	2.76	
		Severe	44.95	7.83	
	Behavioral	Mild	14.82	3.00	27.48*
		Moderate	18.30	4.55	
		Severe	4.23	2.07	
	Cognitive	Mild	5.45	2.20	4.46*
		Moderate	5.84	2.00	
		Severe	4.23	2.07	
III. Totals		Mild	109.59	9.14	201.12*
		Moderate	141.09	10.06	
		Severe	177.59	14.87	

Note: From Gadzella and Guthrie (1993).

*$p < .05$.

scale measures the opposite to that measured by the Frustrations scale. Measures on the Methodical Study scale would also be the opposite to measures obtained from the Conflicts, Self-Imposed, and Emotional scales.

The other instrument used (Gadzella & Masten, 1997) was the Internality, Powerful Others, and Chance (IPC) Locus of Control inventory (Levenson, 1981). It has three scales measuring to whom individuals attribute their successes and failures. The Internality scale score attributes successes and failures to one's own understandings and responsibilities. The Powerful Others scale score attributes successes and failures to the influence of powerful people (significant others). The Chance scale score indicates whether successes and failures are a result of taking chances and having luck.

The results of the analyses between the IPC Locus of Control scores and stress scores showed (a) significant *positive* correlations between the Powerful Others scale (IPC Locus of Control) and the Frustrations and Changes (stress scales) scores, respectively, and (b) significant *positive* correlations between the Chance (IPC Locus of Control scale) score and the Frustrations, Conflicts and Changes (types of stressors), Physiological (reactions to stressors), and Total Stress scores, respectively. Stated simply, individuals who are influenced by others and take chances in their endeavors experience certain kinds of stressors and reactions to stressors.

In another study (Gadzella, 1994a), the three groups of subjects who perceived their stress to be mild, moderate, and severe were compared on their IPC Locus of Control scores. Significant differences were found in two different groups of subjects. The mild and moderate stress groups had significantly lower mean scores on Powerful Others scale than the severe stress group. On the Chance Locus of Control scale, data showed significant differences among all stress level groups, with the mild and moderate stress groups reporting lower scores than the severe stress group.

Reliability

Various studies have been conducted to determine whether the stress inventory measures consistently what it sets out to measure. Cronbach's alphas and Pearson product-moment correlations were used to analyze responses made to the Student-Life Stress Inventory by 95 subjects (Gadzella, 1991; Gadzella, Fullwood, & Ginther, 1991). Cronbach's alphas were computed for the total group on the nine categories of the stress inventory (see Table 2). The internal consistency values ranged from .52 (Frustrations) to .85 (Changes).

Using the two responses to the stress inventory made by

Table 2: Internal Consistency (Alpha) on the First Response to the Student-Life Stress Inventory by Sections for the Total Group

Category	Subtest	Alpha
I. Stressors		
	Frustration	.52*
	Conflict	.64*
	Pressure	.73*
	Change	.85*
	Self-Imposed	.63*
II. Reactions to Stressors		
	Physiological	.73*
	Emotional	.81*
	Behavioral	.71*
	Cognitive	.77*

Note: From Gadzella, Fullwood and Ginther (1991).

*$p < .05$.

the subjects within 12 days, Pearson product-moment correlations were computed for the total group (95 subjects), gender, and stress level (mild, moderate, and severe) groups for the nine categories. Tables from one study (Gadzella et al., 1991) are provided as illustrations (see Tables 3 and 4). The significant correlations ranged from .50 to .89.

In another study (Gadzella & Guthrie, 1993), Pearson product-moment correlations were computed with two responses to the Student-Life Stress Inventory (obtained within 3 weeks) for 87 subjects. Correlations for the total group were .78; for men, .92; and for women, .72.

Table 3: Correlations between Two Responses on the Student-Life Stress Inventory by Sections for the Total and Gender Groups

		Group		
Category	Subtest	Total (n = 95)	Men (n = 38)	Women (n = 57)
I. Stressors				
	Frustration	.72*	.69*	.75*
	Conflict	.59*	.67*	.54*
	Pressure	.73*	.79*	.70*
	Change	.67*	.80*	.55*
	Self-Imposed	.75*	.71*	.76*
II. Reactions to Stressors				
	Physiological	.75*	.54*	.78*
	Emotional	.76*	.68*	.80*
	Behavioral	.72*	.62*	.77*
	Cognitive	.57*	.67*	.50*

Note: From Gadzella, Fullwood and Ginther (1991).

*p < .05.

Table 4: Correlations between Two Responses on the Student-Life Stress inventory by Sections for Three Stress Level Groups

Category	Subtest	Mild (n = 17)	Moderate (n = 64)	Severe (n = 14)
I. Stressors				
	Frustration	.76*	.69*	.30
	Conflict	.68*	.54*	.55*
	Pressure	.84*	.63*	.53*
	Change	.60*	.63*	.30
	Self-Imposed	.68*	.72*	.83*
II. Reactions to Stressors				
	Physiological	.68*	.64*	.68*
	Emotional	.89*	.69*	.53*
	Behavioral	.72*	.67*	.79*
	Cognitive	.64*	.53*	.49*

Note: From Gadzella, Fullwood and Ginther (1991).

*$p < .05$.

Differences between Genders

Several studies reported differences between men and women on their stress scores. For example, differences were found for the 190 men and 340 women in one (Gadzella, Fullwood, & Tomcala, 1992). Findings showed that women reported significantly higher scores on Pressures and Self-Imposed (stressors) and Physiological, Emotional, and Behavioral (reactions to stress). In another study (Gadzella & Guthrie, 1993) with 87 subjects (23 men and 64 women), women reported significantly higher scores on Pressures and Changes (stressors), Physiological and Emotional (reactions to stressors), and the Total Stress score. In another (Gadzella, 1994b) with 290 subjects (106 men and 184 women), women reported significantly higher scores on Pressures and Changes (stressors), Physiological, Emotional, and Behavioral (reactions to stressors), and the Total Stress, whereas men reported significantly higher scores on Cognitive appraisal (reaction to stressors). Generally, it would appear that women report higher scores (more stress and reactions to stress) than men.

Differences in Age Groups

A study (Gadzella & Fullwood, 1992) was conducted with 528 students whose ages ranged from 16 to 57 years on their responses to the stress inventory. The students' responses were analyzed by four age groups: Group 1 (16–18 years, n = 104), Group 2 (19–21 years, n = 174), Group 3 (22–30 years, n = 129 years), and Group 4 (31–57 years, n = 121). Results of the analyses showed that Group 1 reported significantly higher scores than the other three groups on Self-Imposed (stressors). In reactions to stressors, there were three significant differences. In Physiological (reactions to stressors), data showed significant differences between Groups 1 and 2 and Groups 3 and 4. In each case, Groups 3 and 4 reported higher scores than Groups 1 and 2. On Emotional (reactions to stressors), Groups 1 and 3 had significantly higher scores than Group 4. On Cognitive appraisal (reaction to stressors), Groups 3 and 4 had significantly higher scores than Group 1; that is, the older students (ages 22–57 years) evaluated their stressors and used more effective strategies than the younger students). Analyses were also made between gender and the four age groups; significant differences were found in each of the stressors and reactions to stressors between the genders and among the four age groups in this study (Gadzella & Fullwood, 1992).

Differences between Marital Statuses

In a 1992 study (Gadzella et al.), differences for 530 students' stress scores were analyzed by marital status groups: single (308), married (190), and divorced/separated (32). Results showed that the singles group reported the highest scores on Self-Imposed (stressors), the married group reported the highest scores on Cognitive appraisal (stressors), and the divorced/separated group reported the highest scores on Frustrations (stressors) and Physiological (reactions to stressors).

Patterns of Relationships among Types of Stressors

A study (Gadzella, Ginther, & Fullwood, 1993) was conducted with 95 subjects who responded to the stress inventory. Intercorrelations were computed for stressors and reaction to stressors for gender and stress level (mild, moderate, and severe) groups. Results were presented in tables and figures, some of which are provided in Figures 1 and 2 and Tables 5, 6, and 7).

Data for intercorrelations between the stressors for the stress level (mild, moderate, and severe) groups are presented in Table 5. Interesting patterns are seen in the intercorrelations between the Self-Imposed and Conflict responses for the three groups. For instance, similar intercorrelations are seen between Self-Imposed and Conflict responses among the mild ($r = .28$), moderate ($r = .01$), and severe ($r = .22$) groups. In comparison, differences are noted in intercorrelations between Change and Frustration responses among the mild ($r = .64$), moderate ($r = .16$), and severe ($r = .49$) groups.

Intercorrelations between stressors for men and women are presented in Table 6. It is interesting to note, for instance, that intercorrelations (as shown in Table 6 between Pressure and Frustration responses for men [$r = .50$] and women [$r = .50$] and between Self-Imposed and Conflict responses for men

Figure 1: Stressors: Male and Female Groups (from Gadzella, Ginther, and Fullwood, 1993)

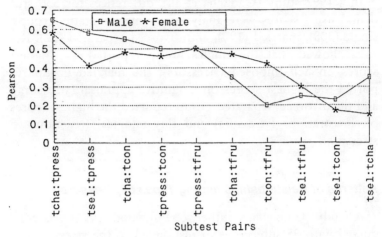

Figure 2: Stressors: Mild, Moderate, Severe Groups (from Gadzella, Ginther, and Fullwood, 1993)

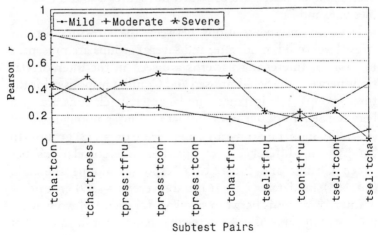

Table 5: Intercorrelations between Stressors for Mild ($n =$ 17), Moderate ($n = 64$), and Severe ($n = 14$) Stress Level Groups

Stressor	Group	TFRU	TCON	TPRESS	TCHA	TSEL
				Stressor		
TFRU	Mild	—				
	Moderate	—				
	Severe	—				
TCON	Mild	.37	—			
	Moderate	.21	—			
	Severe	.16	—			
TPRESS	Mild	.70*	64*	—		
	Moderate	.26*	.24*	—		
	Severe	.44	.61*	—		
TCHA	Mild	.64*	.81*	.75*	—	
	Moderate	.16	.34*	.49*	—	
	Severe	.49	.43	.32	—	
TSEL	Mild	.53*	.28	.63*	.43	—
	Moderate	.09	.01	.25	.08	—
	Severe	.23	.22	.51	.01	—

Note: TFRU = total frustration, TCON = total conflict, TPRESS = total pressure, TCHA = total change, and TSEL = total self-imposed. From Gadzella, Ginther and Fullwood (1993).

*$p < .05$.

[$r = .25$] and women [$r = .30$] were similar. On the other hand, intercorrelations between Conflict and Frustration responses for men [$r = .20$] and women [$r = .42$] were quite different.

In the intercorrelations to the reactions to stressors for the three stress level groups (Table 7), similarities are noted between the Emotional and Physiological responses among the mild ($r = .56$), moderate ($r = .55$), and severe ($r = .72$) groups, whereas differences between intercorrelations on the Cognitive and Behavioral responses are noted among the mild

Table 6: Intercorrelations between the Stressors for Men ($n = 38$) and Women ($n = 57$)

		Stressor				
Stressor	Group	TFRU	TCON	TPRESS	TCHA	TSEL
TFRU	Men	---				
	Women	---				
TCON	Men	.20*	---			
	Women	.42*	---			
TPRESS	Men	.50*	.50*	---		
	Women	.50*	.46*	---		
TCHA	Men	.35*	.55*	.65*	---	
	Women	.47*	.48*	.58*	---	
TSEL	Men	.25	.23	.58*	.35*	---
	Women	.30*	.17	.41*	.15	---

Note: TFRU = total frustration, TCON = total conflict, TPRESS = total pressure, TCHA = total change, and TSEL = total self-imposed. From Gadzella, Ginther and Fullwood (1993).

*$p < .05$.

($r = .14$), moderate ($r = .34$), and severe ($r = .18$) groups. These intercorrelational patterns among the stressors and reactions to stressor responses for the gender and stress level groups show that some of the subjects' responses overlapped (were similar) and other responses were quite different.

In the intercorrelations to reactions to stressors for men and women (Table 8), there is a great deal of similarity between the Behavioral and Emotional responses for men ($r = .60$) and women ($r = .61$) and differences in intercorrelations between Cognitive and Behavioral responses for men ($r = .44$) and women ($r = .10$).

Applications

A number of students have used and are using this inventory in work on honors (Boston, 1996) and master's (Berdahl,

Table 7: Intercorrelations between the Reactions to
Stressors for Mild (n = 17), Moderate (n = 64), and Severe
(n = 14) Stress Level Groups

Reactions to Stressor	Group	Reactions to Stressor			
		TPHY	TEMO	TBEH	TCOG
TPHY	Mild	—			
	Moderate	—			
	Severe	—			
TEMO	Mild	.56*	—		
	Moderate	.55*	—		
	Severe	.72*	—		
TBEH	Mild	.37	.77*	—	
	Moderate	.30*	.49*	—	
	Severe	.60*	.50*	—	
TCOG	Mild	.18	.08	.14	—
	Moderate	.01	.17	.34*	—
	Severe	.20	.15	.18	—

Note: TPHY = total physiological, TEMO = total emotional, TBEH = total behavioral, and TCOG = total cognitive. From Gadzella, Ginther and Fullwood (1993).

*p < .05.

1996) theses. Data are also being collected and analyzed with other variables in comparing group characteristics and predicting learning styles and academic performances. In a recent study (Gadzella, Ginther, Masten, & Guthrie, 1997) on prediction of deep and shallow processors of information (for 77 students), the total stress score was used, with four other measures (on learning styles and critical thinking), to predict students who were high processors versus those who were low processors. Using analyses of variance and discriminate function analysis, it was reported that the total stress score was one of the significant factors in determining high (deep) and low (shallow) processors. The low processors reported significantly higher stress scores when compared with the high processors.

Table 8: Intercorrelations between the Reactions to
Stressors for Men (*n* = 38) and Women (*n* = 57)

| Reactions to Stressor | Group | Reactions to Stressor | | | |
		TPHY	TEMO	TBEH	TCOG
TPHY	Men	---			
	Women	---			
TEMO	Men	.71*	---		
	Women	.60*	---		
TBEH	Men	.38*	.60*	---	
	Women	.55*	.61*	---	
TCOG	Men	.22	.42*	.44*	---
	Women	.10	.05	.10	---

Note: TPHY = total physiological, TEMO = total emotional, TBEH = total behavioral, and TCOG = total cognitive. From Gadzella, Ginther and Fullwood (1993).

*$p < .05$.

Benefits and Limitations

The use of the stress inventory has a number of benefits. Students who participate in the studies get actively involved in analyzing their own stressors and how they react to them. Data are collected and analyzed by groups (which serve as norms), and students can make their own comparisons. The results of studies reveal characteristics of student groups and indicate how stress affects their thinking and behaviors.

The limitations of an instrument like the Student-Life Stress Inventory should also be noted. First, stress is a complex concept to study, even when it is defined operationally. Stressors and reaction to stressors overlap. Second, in ranking a specific stressor high and a related stressor low, the result will be an average ranking for that category. Also, reactions to stressors may change over short or long periods of time as the individual learns to accept them and to use effective strategies. Therefore, multiple responses made to the inventory over long periods of time may result in different responses.

Chapter References

Berdahl, B. (1996). *Effects of stressors on learning performance in psychology students.* Unpublished master's thesis, Chico State College, Chico, CA.

Boston, J. B. (1996). *Stress and coping mechanisms in the university.* Honors thesis, Tulane University, New Orleans, LA.

Coleman, J. C., Morris, C. G., & Glaros, A. G. (1987). *Contemporary psychology and effective behavior* (6th ed.). Glenview, IL: Scott, Foreman.

Gadzella, B. M. (1991). *Student-Life Stress Inventory and answer sheet to Student-Life Stress Inventory.* Unpublished manuscript. Texas A & M University-Commerce, Commerce.

Gadzella, B. M. (1994a). Locus of control differences among stress groups. *Perceptual and Motor Skills, 79,* 1619–1624.

Gadzella, B. M. (1994b). Student-Life Stress Inventory: Identification of and reactions to stressors. *Psychological Reports, 74,* 395–402.

Gadzella, B. M., & Fullwood, H. L. (1992, March). Differences among university student age groups on their perceptions of stress. In *Proceedings of the Texas Academy of Science, 95th Annual Meeting* (pp. 176–180). Wichita Falls, TX: Midwestern State University.

Gadzella, B. M., Fullwood, H. L., & Ginther, D. W. (1991, January). *Student-Life Stress Inventory.* Paper presented at the Texas Psychological Convention, San Antonio, TX (ERIC 340 345).

Gadzella, B. M., Fullwood, H. L., & Tomcala, M. (1992, April). *Students' stressors and reactions to stressors.* Paper presented at the Southwestern Psychological Association Conference, Austin, TX (ERIC 345 172).

Gadzella, B. M., Ginther, D. W., & Fullwood, H. L. (1993, April). *Patterns of relationships among types of stressors.* Paper presented at the Southwestern Psychological Association Conference, Corpus Christi, TX.

Gadzella, B. M., Ginther, D. W., Masten, W. G., & Guthrie, D. (1997). Predicting students as deep and shallow processors of information. *Perceptual and Motor Skills, 84,* 875–881.

Gadzella, B. M., & Guthrie, D. L. (1993, March). Analysis of a stress inventory. In *Proceedings of the Texas Academy of Science, 96th Annual Meeting.* (pp. 301–308). Denton: University of North Texas.

Gadzella, B. M., & Masten, W. (1997, April). *Relationships between a stress inventory and two other instruments.* Paper presented at the Southwestern Psychological Association Conference, Fort Worth, TX.

Goleman, D. (1979). Interview with Richard S. Lazarus: Positive denial: The case for not facing reality. *Psychology Today, 13*(6), 44–60.

Holmes, T. H., & Rahe, R. H. (1967). The Social Readjustment Rating Scale. *Journal of Psychosomatic Research, 11,* 213–218.

Horowitz, M. J., & Wilner, N. (1980). Life events, stress, and coping. In L. W. Poon (Ed.), *Aging in the 1980s* (pp. 363–374). Washington, DC: American Psychological Association.

Lazarus, R. S., & Folkman, S. (1984). *Stress, appraisal and coping.* New York: Springer.

Levenson, H. (1981). Differentiating among internality, powerful others, and chance. In H. Lefcourt (Ed.), *Research with locus of control: Vol. 1. Assessment method* (pp. 15–63). New York: Academic Press.

Martin, G. L., & Osborne, J. G. (1993). *Psychology, adjustment and everyday living* (2nd ed.). Upper Saddle River, NJ: Prentice Hall.

Morris, C. G. (1990). *Psychology: An introduction* (7th ed.). Upper Saddle River, NJ: Prentice Hall.

Sarason, J. G., Johnson, J. H., & Siegel, J. M. (1978). Assessing the impact of life changes: Development of the Life Experiences Survey. *Journal of Consulting and Clinical Psychology, 46,* 432–446.

Schmeck, R. R., Ribich, F. D., & Ramanaiah, N. (1977). Development of a self report inventory for assessing individual differences in learning processes. *Applied Psychological Measurement, 1,* 413–431.

Selye, H. (1976). *The stress of life* (2nd ed.). New York: McGraw-Hill.

Weiten, W., Lloyd, M. A., & Lashley, R. L. (1990). *Psychology applied to modern life: Adjustment in the 90s* (3rd ed.). Pacific Grove, CA: Brooks Cole.

The Ways of Religious Coping Scale

Pamela Davis Martin, Pennington Biomedical Research Center, Louisiana State University
Sheryl L. Catz, Center for AIDS Intervention Research, Medical College of Wisconsin
Edwin Boudreaux, Department of Emergency Medicine, Earl K. Long Medical Center
Phillip J. Brantley, Pennington Biomedical Research Center, Louisiana State University

■ Instrument Names

Ways of Religious Coping Scale
WORCS

■ Developers

Edwin Boudreaux, Sheryl Catz, Laurie Ryan, Marta Amaral-Melendez, Louisiana State University, and Phillip J. Brantley, Louisiana State University Medical Center

■ Contact Information

Edwin D. Boudreaux, Department of Emergency Medicine, Earl K. Long Medical Center, 5825 Airline Highway, Baton Rouge, LA 70805

Description and History of the Instrument

Background

Research has long demonstrated that exposure to intense, frequent, or chronic stress is associated with numerous adverse effects on physical and psychological health (Cannon, 1929; Everly & Rosenfeld, 1981; Rabkin & Struening, 1976; Selye, 1956). However, not all people who experience stress develop adverse reactions. Consequently, inquiry into how and why people respond differently to stress is extremely valuable. Previous research has found that the way people manage stressful situations may determine, in part, the degree to which they are negatively impacted (Lazarus & Folkman, 1984). A greater understanding of the specific coping strategies that help minimize stress-related disorders is needed.

A variety of coping strategies have been identified as possible health moderators (Folkman & Lazarus, 1988; Lazarus & Folkman, 1984). Increasing evidence suggests religious coping may be a widely used strategy. In a Gallup (1985) poll, 72% of those surveyed agreed with the statement "my whole approach to life is based on my religion." Also, a large proportion of a church-attending sample (78%) reported that religion was involved in understanding or handling serious negative events (Pargament, Ensing, Falgout, Olsen, Reilly, Van Haitsma, & Warren, 1990), while 75% of a community sample reported using faith to cope with stressful events (Mc-Crae, 1984), further supporting the conclusion that religious coping is a commonly used strategy. Despite a wealth of data on religion and its impact on people's lives (Levin & Vanderpool, 1991), it has historically been ignored by many psychologists, prompting Larson and Larson (1992) to call it the "forgotten factor in physical and mental health." However, this situation appears to be changing, as religion is gaining increasing acknowledgment by psychologists as a fruitful and important area of study (American Psychological Association, 1994; Larson & Larson, 1992; Rowan, 1996).

Similarly, the impact of religion on physical health has been increasingly recognized. For many medical patients, the difficulties of facing a potentially life-threatening illness are often met with an increased reliance on religious beliefs. Religiosity has been associated with reduced distress, increased social support, and improved health outcomes among a wide range of medical populations (Larson & Larson, 1992). For instance, a number of published studies with cancer patients have found that various aspects of religiousness were negatively associated with anxiety, anger, distress, fear of death, sleep disturbance, social isolation, nurse ratings of distress, and reports of pain, while being positively associated with the patients' self-esteem, happiness ratings, and adjustment to illness (Acklin, Brown, & Mauger, 1983; Gibbs & Achterberg-Lawlis, 1978; Jenkins & Pargament, 1988; Kaczorowski, 1989; Yates, Chalmer, St. James, Follansbee, & McKegney, 1981).

Development

The development of the WORCS was prompted by the first author's attempts to find an appropriate instrument to further explore the relation between religious coping and physical and psychological symptoms in low socioeconomic status medical patients. Although Levin and Vanderpool (1991) suggested religion has been studied extensively, the psychometrics of religious coping remains in its infancy. The majority of research investigating religion is based on a few simple questions assessing religious affiliation, degree of religiosity, and religious service attendance (e.g., Anson, Carmel, & Bonneh, 1990; Schafer & King, 1990). In light of the growing interest in religion and its role in psychology (American Psychological Association, 1994; Larson & Larson, 1992; Rowan, 1996), reliable and valid measures of the religious coping construct are needed.

At the time the WORCS was developed, the Religious Coping Activities Scale (RCAS; Hathaway & Pargament, 1990; Pargament et al., 1990) was one of the few instruments that had been adequately subjected to psychometric scrutiny. The RCAS contained six short subscales: Spiritually Based Coping, Good Deeds, Discontent, Religious Support, Plead, and Religious Avoidance. Unfortunately, the RCAS had both measurement and conceptual limitations. First, the items were worded in incomplete sentences, and the reading level was appropriate for respondents with relatively high education levels. Second, the items did not appear to assess the domain comprehensively. For example, even though prayer is a common aspect of most religions and is conceivably an important and widely used act of religious coping, the RCAS did not have an item directly assessing prayer. A third flaw was the brevity of many of the RCAS's scales. Four of the six scales consisted of only three or fewer items, contributing to low subscale reliabilities and, consequently, questionable validity. Finally, a clear definition for "stressful" was not provided in the RCAS's ambiguous instructions. In conclusion, a scale that remedied the aforementioned problems was thought to be necessary to advance the study of religious coping.

The WORCS was specifically developed to address problems with previous measures of religious coping. An additional aim of scale development was to assess the domains of internal, primarily cognitive, coping strategies and external, primarily behavioral, religious coping strategies. Thus, the WORCS was designed to be an instrument with the sensitivity to investigate whether internal and external religious coping behaviors could be differentiated in terms of their ability to mediate the relation between stress and psychological/physical health.

Scale Description

The Ways of Religious Coping Scale is a 40-item self-report measure designed to assess the degree to which subjects engage in religious behaviors to cope with stressful situations (Boudreaux, Catz, Ryan, Amaral-Melendez, & Brantley, 1995). WORCS items are rated on a 5-point Likert scale from 0 ("not used at all/does not apply") to 4 ("used always"). The religious behaviors included in the scale range from passive, internally focused processes such as prayer, to active, externally focused processes such as participating in a church support group. The WORCS yields a total score and two factor-analytically derived subscale scores: Internal/Private and External/Social. The Internal score is the sum of religious behaviors that are private and not directly observable. The External score is the sum of religious behaviors that are observable and socially oriented.

Underlying Assumptions, Premises, and Objectives

The development of the WORCS was based on the transactional theory of stress and modeled after the Ways of Coping Questionnaire (Folkman & Lazarus, 1988; Lazarus & Folkman, 1984). The definitions of stress and coping on which the WORCS was based parallel the concepts of cognitive appraisal and coping underlying the Ways of Coping Questionnaire (Folkman & Lazarus, 1988). In this model, stress refers to the subjective appraisal of situations as difficult or troubling because of the distress associated with the situation or the effort required to deal with it. Coping refers to the thoughts and actions used to handle with stressful situations. The coping behaviors specifically tapped by the WORCS are the subject's use of religious cognitions and behaviors used to manage stressful situations, hence the title "Ways of Religious Coping Scale."

Different types of coping strategies (e.g., active vs. passive) have been theorized to vary in terms of adaptive utility. The WORCS internal/external subscale design was based on the distinction often made in the general coping literature between passive versus active or emotion-focused versus problem-focused coping strategies (Cohen, 1991). Therefore, the WORCS can be utilized to further explore the utility of these coping styles in regard to religious coping behaviors.

Summary of Research

Scale Development

A description of the item selection and scale construction of the WORCS is provided elsewhere (Boudreaux et al.,

1995). The preliminary version of the WORCS consisted of 68 items constructed from a review of the available religious coping literature. The 68-item version was administered to a pilot sample of 18 interdenominational subjects, including university religion department faculty and members of college religious organizations. The initial item pool was refined to avoid confusion and denominational bias prior to field testing.

A field trial of the modified 68-item WORCS was conducted with a sample of 341 college students from various religious affiliations. An exploratory principal components analysis was performed, and items were selected based on a simple-structure criterion of single-factor loadings of 0.40 or greater. With the removal of redundant items, the item pool was reduced to 40 items. Initial reliability and validity data for the 40-item WORCS was collected using a sample of 163 college students (Boudreaux et al. 1995).

An exploratory principal components analysis with varimax rotation was performed on the 40-item version of the WORCS. Factors were retained on the basis of a Scree plot, eigenvalues greater than one, and the presence of two or more items with loadings of 0.40 or greater. The factors were reduced to two main factors labeled Internal/Private and External/Social.

Reliability

Cronbach alphas were computed on the WORCS and its two main factor scales. The analysis yielded a high estimate of internal consistency for the total WORCS, $r = .95$, the Internal WORCS subscale ($r = .97$), and the External WORCS subscale ($r = .93$).

Validity

Construct validity was assessed by correlating the working version of the WORCS with a number of other measures. The WORCS was moderately correlated with self-reported religious service attendance ($r = .57$) and self-ratings of the life importance of religion ($r = .78$). Correlations between WORCS scores and the six Religious Coping Activities scales ranged from low to high and demonstrated adequate levels of convergent and divergent validity. For example, the religious discontent scale correlated negatively with the WORCS ($r = -.29$), while the spirituality scale and the good deeds scales (which are theoretically consistent with WORCS internal/external domains) were strongly and positively correlated with the WORCS ($r = .86$ and $r = .75$, respectively). Divergent validity was also demonstrated by weak correlations between the WORCS and measures of social desirability and locus of control.

As a further assessment of construct validity, the WORCS has been used to assess the impact of religious coping on psychological symptomatology in a variety of medical populations. The following investigations represent the preliminary data from a series of validity studies using the WORCS with general medical and chronically ill populations.

First, an investigation of 104 family practice outpatients found that higher use of religious behaviors to cope with stress was associated with fewer psychological symptoms (Catz, Davis, Boudreaux, Brantley, & Howe, 1996). As hypothesized, religious coping added significantly to major and minor life stressors as a predictor of global psychological distress and depression on the Symptom Checklist 90 (SCL-90) (Degrogatis, 1983). Convergent validity was supported by the positive relation between the WORCS and religiosity measures (i.e., religious services attendance) and correlations with general coping strategies.

Next, a study assessing coping behavior in 159 outpatient hemodialysis patients found an inverse relation between depression and external religious coping (Davis, Catz, Springer, McKnight, & Brantley, 1997). The finding that external (i.e., church attendance) rather than internal (i.e., prayer) religious coping was associated with fewer symptoms of depression suggests that the social support, distraction or increased activity associated with external behaviors may act as a stress buffer.

Additionally, an investigation of 127 outpatients at a hospital-based HIV clinic found that religious coping was inversely related to distress when potential confounds such as disease status, major life stressors, health locus of control, and social support were statistically controlled (Catz et al., 1997). Construct validity was demonstrated by the inverse association between religious coping and hopelessness and anxiety.

Finally, the WORCS was used in a normative sample including 451 primary care medical patients who were participating in a project supported by the National Institutes of Health investigating stress, psychopathology, and medical utilization (Brantley, Jones, Scarinci, Howe, & Springer, 1995). Results indicated that people with a psychiatric treatment history had lower WORCS total and Internal scores, but no differences were noted for WORCS External scores. This may indicate that lower use of cognitive religious coping strategies may be associated with the utilization of psychiatric services.

In summary, the preliminary results suggest that there is a consistent inverse relation between religious coping behaviors and psychological distress in various medical populations (Catz et al., 1996, 1997; Davis et al., 1997). These studies lend further support for the construct validity of the WORCS and indicate that the WORCS is valid for use with medical patients.

Conditions for Use

The WORCS was developed for use as a research instrument to measure religious behaviors used to cope with stressful situations. It was not designed as a measure of general coping styles. Research and normative studies support the use of the WORCS with college and medical adult populations from varied religious backgrounds. A fourth-grade reading level is required for valid completion of the WORCS.

Detailed instructions for administration and scoring, and psychometric properties of the WORCS are presented elsewhere (Boudreaux et al., 1995). Norms are currently being developed for a variety of medical populations. Preliminary data from 827 subjects representing a wide variety of medical populations are presented in Table 1. Additional normative data are currently being compiled.

Applications

The WORCS can be employed for any research question that requires the assessment of religious coping behaviors. It is particularly appropriate for subjects with limited educational experience and varied religious affiliations. As previously discussed, this instrument is for assessing the utility of internal versus external religious coping styles. Preliminary evidence also suggests that the WORCS is applicable for exploring the association between psychological symptoms and religious coping behaviors.

Future studies with the WORCS could build on existing studies exploring the relation between religious coping and psychological distress in medical populations or other related areas. Investigations using the WORCS in several medical populations suggest that further research is needed to explore the possible role of social support and activity management in

Table 1: Preliminary Norms for General Adult Medical Populations

Variable	Mean	Standard Deviation
Public subscale	14.78	11.30
Private subscale	44.04	14.42
Total WORCS score	96.94	33.97

the beneficial effect of public religious coping behaviors, the interrelations between religious coping and adjustment to life-threatening illnesses and the role of religious coping in physical symptomatology and health outcomes (Catz et al., 1996, 1997 and Davis et al., 1997).

Although the WORCS was originally developed for use with low-income medical samples and has been primarily used to explore the stress-pathology relation, its utility is not limited to these areas. Future applications of the WORCS may include assessing differences in patterns of religious coping between various populations or religious affiliations. For example, preliminary data suggest that Baptists score higher on the WORCS than Catholics and other Protestants (Boudreaux et al., 1997). Further investigations can be made to determine what factors play a role in this differentiation. Since the WORCS has been used primarily with Christian samples, studies investigating religious coping patterns of other religious affiliations should be conducted. Finally, preliminary data suggest that future use in mental health and psychiatric populations may be warranted.

To date, the WORCS has been used to explore the relation between religious coping and psychological distress in general medical and chronic illness populations. The first series of studies suggest that there is a consistent association between religious coping behaviors and psychological distress in general medical, hemodialysis, and HIV clinic attenders (Catz et al., 1966, 1997; Davis et al., 1997). In summary, these studies support the hypothesis that greater use of religious coping strategies as measured by the WORCS is associated with better psychosocial adjustment.

Benefits and Limitations

The WORCS addresses many of the problems found in other religious coping scales already in use. The readability level and item syntax is appropriate for populations with limited educational experience, requiring only a fourth-grade reading level. Also, it assesses the domain comprehensively and is worded in terms of specific behaviors. The WORCS demonstrates acceptable internal consistency for the subscales as well as the full scale, and a clear definition for "stressful" is provided in the instructions to reduce ambiguity. The WORCS also contributes to the literature by providing a means of measuring internal versus external religious coping strategies, which may differentially impact the psychological and physical consequences of stress.

Despite the strengths of the WORCS, it has some potential weaknesses. The initial normative population was college students and skewed in the white, female, Catholic direction. Therefore, generalizability across race, gender, and religious affiliation is somewhat limited. Local norms should be developed to reflect the proportions of religious affiliations among different research samples; we are currently developing norms for medical populations. Despite improvements over other scales, there remains a Western/Christian slant to several of the items. These items were retained to capture the religious behaviors of Christian populations with whom the scale is likely to be used in the future. Given the higher than average scores on the WORCS obtained by Buddhist and Muslim subjects, the inclusion of some Christian-specific items does not appear to make the scale inappropriate for use with non-Christian populations. There also may be some limitations associated with the stability of the factor structure across different samples. It would be beneficial to replicate the two-factor structure of the WORCS with a variety of community and medical populations.

The importance of religion in psychology is a rapidly expanding area of interest (American Psychological Association, 1994; Larson & Larson, 1992; Rowan, 1996). The initial results indicate the WORCS is a psychometrically sound measure that may be a valuable research tool for future investigations. Additional studies investigating religious coping among chronically ill patients, as well as further norming research with over 800 patients from various populations, are currently being completed. The exploration of religious coping and its impact on psychological distress and physical health clearly warrants further study.

Chapter References

Acklin, M. W., Brown, E. C., & Mauger, P. A. (1983). The role of religious values in coping with cancer. *Journal of Religion and Health, 22,* 322–333.

American Psychological Association. (1994). Spiritual problems included in DSM-IV. *American Psychological Association Monitor, 25(6),* 8.

Anson, O., Carmel, S., & Bonneh, D. Y. (1990). Recent life events, religiosity, and health: An individual or collective effect. *Human Relations, 43,* 1051–1066.

Boudreaux, E., Catz, S., Ryan, L., Amaral-Melendez, M., & Brantley, P. J. (1995). The Ways of Religious Coping Scale: Reliability, validity and scale development. *Assessment, 2,* 233—244.

Boudreaux, E., Catz, S. L., Martin, P. D., Scarinci, I., Springer, A., & Brantley, P. J. (1997). *The Ways of Religious Coping Scale (Part II): Extension to several medical samples.* Unpublished manuscript.

Brantley, P. J., Jones, G. N., Scarinci, I., Howe, J., & Springer, A. (1995). *Stress and psychopathology in medical utilization.* Unpublished manuscript, Louisiana State University.

Cannon, W. B. (1929). *Bodily changes in pain, hunger, fear, and rage.* New York: Appleton.

Catz, S. L., Davis, P. G., Boudreaux, E., Brantley, P. J., & Howe, J. (1996). Validation of the WORCS with primary care medical patients. *Annals of Behavioral Medicine (Suppl.),* 145.

Catz, S. L., McClure, J. B., Smith, C. F., Jeffries, S. K., Brantley, P. J., & Jones, G. N. (1997). Coping, distress and life-threatening illness: WORCS validation with an HIV sample. *Annals of Behavioral Medicine, 19 (Suppl.),* 182.

Cohen, F. (1991). Measurement of coping. In A. Monat & R. S. Lazarus (Eds.), *Stress and coping: An anthology* (pp. 228–244).

Davis, P. G., Catz, S. L., Springer, A., McKnight, G. T., & Brantley, P. J. (1997). Internal versus External coping as predictors of depression in hemodialysis patients. *Annals of Behavioral Medicine, 19(Suppl.)*, 120.

Derogatis, L. R. (1983). *SCL-90-R Administration, scoring, and procedures manual—II*. Baltimore, MD: Clinical Psychometric Research.

Everly, G. S., Jr., & Rosenfeld, R. (1981). *The nature and treatment of the stress response: A practical guide for clinicians*. New York: Plenum.

Folkman, S., & Lazarus, R. S. (1988). *Manual for the Ways of Coping Questionnaire*. Palo Alto, CA: Consulting Psychologists Press.

Gallup, G. (1985). *Religion in America—50 years, 1935–1985, the Gallup report*. Princeton, NJ: Princeton Religious Research Center.

Gibbs, H. W., & Achterberg-Lawlis, J. (1978). Spiritual values and death anxiety: Implications for counseling with terminal cancer patients. *Journal of Counseling Psychology, 25*, 563–569.

Hathaway, W. L., & Pargament, K. I. (1990). Intrinsic religious coping and psychosocial competence: A covariance structure analysis. *Journal for the Scientific Study of Religion, 29*, 423–441.

Jenkins, R., & Pargament, K. (1988). Cognitive appraisals in cancer patients. *Social Science and Medicine, 26*, 625–633.

Kaczorowski, J. M. (1989). Spiritual well-being and anxiety in adults diagnosed with cancer. *Hospice Journal, 5*, 105–116.

Larson, D. B., & Larson, S. S. (1992). *The forgotten factor in physical and mental health: What does the research show?* Arlington, VA: Authors.

Lazarus, R. S., & Folkman, S. (1984). *Stress appraisal and coping*. New York: Springer.

Levin, J. S., & Vanderpool, H. Y. (1991). Religious factors in physical health and the prevention of illness. *Prevention in Human Services, 9*, 41–64.

McCrae, R. R. (1984). Situational determinants of coping responses: Loss, threat and challenge. *Journal of Personality and Social Psychology, 46*, 919–928.

Pargament, K. I., Ensing, D. S., Falgout, K., Olsen, H., Reilly, B., Van Haitsma, K., & Warren, R. (1990). God help me: I.) Religious coping efforts as predictors of the outcomes to significant negative life events. *American Journal of Community Psychology, 18*, 793–823.

Rabkin, J. G., & Struening, E. L. (1976). Life events, stress, and illness. *Science, 194*, 1013–1020.

Rowan, A. B. (1996). The relevance of religious issues in behavioral assessment. *The Behavior Therapist, 19*, 55–57.

Schafer, W. E., & King, M. (1990). Religiousness and stress among college students: A survey report. *Journal of College Student Development, 31*, 336–341.

Selye, H. (1956). *The stress of life*. New York: McGraw-Hill.

Yates, J., Chalmer, B., St. James, P., Follansbee, M., & McKegney, F. (1981). Religion in patients with advanced cancer. *Medical and Pediatric Oncology, 9*, 121–128.

Names Index

Subject Index

This index includes keywords, topics, and subjects mentioned in the chapters on the stress instruments, as well as the introduction of this book. It does not contain journal or book titles and their authors. Please refer to the Names Index for names of authors, editors, or instrument developers cited in this book.

About the Authors

Carlos P. Zalaquett is the assistant director of the Counseling Center at Sam Houston State University (SHSU). He obtained his M.A. from SHSU and his Ph.D. from the University of Texas at Austin. He currently directs SHSU's Stress Management and Biofeedback Laboratory and is the effectiveness evaluation coordinator at the university Counseling Center. He also teaches psychology of adjustment and supervises students in their practicum training in the Psychology and Philosophy Department at the university.

Zalaquett has published several articles in scientific journals and is the author of *Un Acercamiento a la Perspectiva Ericksonians* (An Approach to the Ericksonian Perspective; Cuadernos EPUC, Universidad Catolica de Chile, 1986), and the "Succeeding in the Twenty-First Century" World Wide Web home page. He frequently lectures on counseling and stress management at university and state organizations, as well as internationally. His area of research is stress and anxiety. He is particularly interested in the evaluation of stress; the behavioral, physiological, and neuroimmuniological effects of stress; and the development of strategies to reverse or ameliorate those effects. Part of his research has focused on counseling, psychotherapy, and techniques to reduce stress, anxiety, and psychosomatic disorders.

Zalaquett is a member of the American Psychological Association, the Southwestern Psychological Association, and the Biofeedback Society of Texas. His dedication and commitment to his work have resulted in several awards and honors, such as citation in the *Who's Who among America's Teachers* (1996), the Counseling Center's Outstanding Employee of

377

the Year award (1995), the Honor Diploma for Outstanding Contributions to the International Hispanic Association of Sam Houston State University (1988), and the Honor Diploma for his Contribution to Psychology, given by the Chilean Society of Clinical Psychologists (1979).

Richard J. Wood has served as the director of Library Services, Sam Houston State University, in Huntsville, Texas, since August 1990. From 1986 to then Wood was director of library services at The Citadel, the Military College of South Carolina, in Charleston. He was head of circulation (1971–1986) and coordinator of user services (1979–1986) at Slippery Rock State College of Slippery Rock, Pennsylvania. Previously, he was the Millcreek Branch librarian of the Erie County Public Library in Erie, Pennsylvania. He has authored numerous articles and, with Frank Hoffmann, recently coedited *Library Collection Development Policies: A Reference and Writer's Handbook* (Scarecrow, 1996) and the fourth and fifth editions of *Guide to Popular U.S. Government Publications* (Libraries Unlimited, 1997, 1998). With Katina Strauch, he coedited *Collection Assessment: A Look at the RLG Conspectus* (Haworth, 1992). He is currently a contributing editor to Sage Periodical Press's *Library Software Review* and has published many articles in this serial publication. Since 1986, Wood has evaluated stress among librarians in both South Carolina and Texas and has published research papers in this area. He was awarded a master's in library science (1969) and Ph.D. (1979) from the University of Pittsburgh.